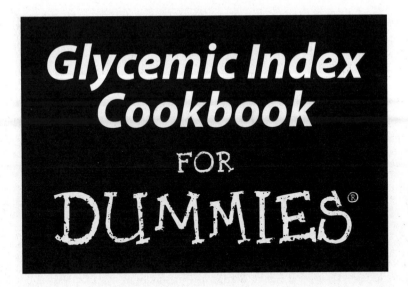

Glycemic Index Cookbook

FOR

DUMMIES®

by Meri Raffetto, RD, and
Rosanne Rust, MS, RD, LDN

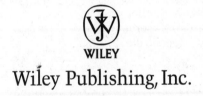

WILEY

Wiley Publishing, Inc.

Glycemic Index Cookbook For Dummies®

Published by
Wiley Publishing, Inc.
111 River St.
Hoboken, NJ 07030-5774
www.wiley.com

WILEY

About the Authors

Meri Raffetto is a registered dietitian and recognized professional in the area of nutrition and wellness. She has extensive experience in nutrition counseling, education, and medical nutrition therapy working in many areas, including eating disorders, weight management, and heart health. She's the founder of Real Living Nutrition Services (www.reallivingnutrition.com), providing one of the only interactive online weight-loss programs where people can work one-on-one with a dietitian to get advice, support, and coaching to create sustainable lifestyle changes. Meri also develops custom online corporate wellness programs for small to large companies. She is the author of *The Glycemic Index Diet For Dummies* and the coauthor of *The Calorie Counter For Dummies* (both published by Wiley).

She is a wife and mother of triplets; loves great food; and enjoys camping, swimming, and hiking with her family.

Rosanne Rust is a registered, licensed dietitian with nearly 25 years of experience in the dietetics field. She has a master's degree in clinical dietetics and nutrition from the University of Pittsburgh. Rosanne is an author, teacher, and spokesperson. She currently provides virtual weight-loss coaching as a licensed provider for Real Living Nutrition Services (www.realliving nutrition.com) and is an online nutrition instructor for Penn State World Campus. Her private practice includes freelance writing, online nutrition coaching, media and spokesperson work, and corporate wellness consulting. Rosanne is the coauthor of *The Calorie Counter For Dummies* (Wiley) and a regular health columnist for *The Meadville Tribune*.

She is a wife and mother of three boys. She practices what she preaches and enjoys running, weightlifting, yoga, cycling, tennis, hiking, boating, skiing, snowboarding . . . and, of course, eating!

Dedication

We both come from large Italian families, so it only makes sense to dedicate this book to our parents, Joe and Iolanda and Frank and Toni, who instilled in us from an early age a love of food and cooking and the importance of enjoying every moment of life — especially those spent with family and friends.

Authors' Acknowledgments

To start, we want to thank Matt Wagner from Fresh Books and our acquisitions editor, Erin Calligan Mooney, for all their work spearheading this project. Our project editor, Georgette Beatty, was such a pleasure to work with, and we greatly appreciate her time and cheerful support in making this cookbook organized and fun to read — not to mention her complete understanding of our crazy lives during the writing of this book.

A major thank you to our copy editor, Amanda Langferman, for her dedication to helping us find the perfect wording, especially for the recipes, and our technical editor, Rachel Nix, for ensuring that the information in the book is accurate.

Writing a cookbook and developing recipes was truly a fun experience with a whole lot of recipe testing. We'd like to send a special thanks to Miriam and Jonathon, Joe and Iolanda, and Marla and Jillian for helping us test recipes. You guys are the greatest! And, of course, to our final recipe reviewer, Emily Nolan, and our nutritional analyst, Patty Santelli — thank you!

Publisher's Acknowledgments

We're proud of this book; please send us your comments at http://dummies.custhelp.com. For other comments, please contact our Customer Care Department within the U.S. at 877-762-2974, outside the U.S. at 317-572-3993, or fax 317-572-4002.

Some of the people who helped bring this book to market include the following:

Acquisitions, Editorial, and Media Development

Senior Project Editor: Georgette Beatty

Acquisitions Editor: Erin Calligan Mooney

Copy Editor: Amanda M. Langferman

Assistant Editor: David Lutton

Technical Editor: Rachel C. Nix, RD, CD, CLC

Recipe Tester: Emily Nolan

Nutritional Analyst: Patty Santelli

Editorial Manager: Michelle Hacker

Editorial Assistant: Jennette ElNaggar

Art Coordinator: Alicia B. South

Cover Photo: T.J. Hine Photography

Cartoons: Rich Tennant (www.the5thwave.com)

Composition Services

Project Coordinator: Sheree Montgomery

Layout and Graphics: Claudia Bell, Carl Byers, Brent Savage

Proofreaders: Laura Bowman, Melissa Cossell

Indexer: Estalita Slivoskey

Illustrator: Elizabeth Kurtzman

Photographer: T.J. Hine Photography

Food Stylist: Lisa Bishop

Publishing and Editorial for Consumer Dummies

 Diane Graves Steele, Vice President and Publisher, Consumer Dummies

 Kristin Ferguson-Wagstaffe, Product Development Director, Consumer Dummies

 Ensley Eikenburg, Associate Publisher, Travel

 Kelly Regan, Editorial Director, Travel

Publishing for Technology Dummies

 Andy Cummings, Vice President and Publisher, Dummies Technology/General User

Composition Services

 Debbie Stailey, Director of Composition Services

Contents at a Glance

Recipes at a Glance

Soups, Stews, and Chilies

Salads

Vegetable Side Dishes

Beef and Pork Entrees

Seafood Entrees

Vegetarian Entrees

Desserts

Table of Contents

Introduction

●●●

*T*he glycemic index is a scientific method for calculating the way carbohydrates in food act in the body. The glycemic index is a great tool you can
use to help manage many health issues, including diabetes, heart disease,
and polycystic ovary syndrome. You can also use it to help you achieve or
maintain general good health and wellness. It isn't a "diet" in a gimmicky way.
Instead, it's a new way to look at your carbohydrate-containing foods to help
you make the best choices for your particular situation.

No matter what inspired you to pick up this book, we know that incorporating any kind of dietary change into your life can bring with it a whole new set
of challenges. Our goal in this book is to show you that implementing a low-
glycemic diet can be simple and delicious. You don't have to feel deprived
because this concept works well with moderation. So stop worrying that
you'll never be able to eat another potato or pasta dish again. This book is
here to help make your transition to a low-glycemic lifestyle a little easier by
giving you ideas for how to cook low-glycemic meals for yourself, your family,
and even guests.

About This Book

If you're implementing a low-glycemic diet into your lifestyle (or just thinking
about doing so), *Glycemic Index Cookbook For Dummies* is the perfect book
for you. In the following pages, you find delicious recipes that you can begin
to make and that we hope will become some of your favorites. This book also
covers the basics of the glycemic index and glycemic load as well as practical, necessary information about grocery shopping, meal planning, getting
your kitchen prepared, and much more.

You can use this book as a resource and, like any cookbook, you don't have
to read it from cover to cover. Instead, you can find that perfect recipe
you've been looking for or go straight to the chapter on stocking your pantry.
Everything you need to know about cooking the low-glycemic way is here.

Conventions Used in This Book

In this book, we use data from individual foods that have been tested for
their glycemic index and then calculate an estimated glycemic load for each

recipe based on the sum of the ingredients used in that recipe. Take note that the recipes themselves haven't been tested in clinical human studies. Without human studies, no recipes can state with complete accuracy what their glycemic index or load will be. But rest easy that the estimates we provide are close enough to help you live a low-glycemic lifestyle.

When we use the terms *low, medium,* and *high glycemic* in conjunction with a particular food or recipe in this book, we're referring to its glycemic load, not its glycemic index measurement (see Chapter 4 for the difference between the two).

Like with all cookbooks, we recommend that you read through each recipe in its entirety before you start making it. That way, you can add the necessary refrigerating time, standing time, or freezing time to your overall cooking schedule. Reading through the recipe's directions beforehand also clues you in to any special tools, like immersion blenders, grill pans, or presoaked skewers, you may need to complete that particular recipe.

Here are a few other guidelines to keep in mind about the recipes in this book:

✔ All butter is unsalted. Margarine is not a suitable substitute for butter unless we state you can use either one.

✔ All eggs are large.

✔ All milk is lowfat unless otherwise specified.

✔ All onions are yellow unless otherwise specified.

✔ All pepper is freshly ground black pepper unless otherwise specified.

✔ All salt is kosher.

✔ All dry ingredient measurements are level.

To make sure your measurements are also level, use a dry ingredient measuring cup, fill it to the top, and scrape it even with a straight object, such as the flat side of a knife.

✔ All temperatures are Fahrenheit (see Appendix B to convert Fahrenheit temperatures to Celsius).

✔ All lemon and lime juice is freshly squeezed.

✔ All sugar is white granulated unless otherwise noted.

✔ All flour is all-purpose unless otherwise noted.

✔ When the recipe says to beat until frothy or foamy, take a fork and beat the liquid rapidly until small bubbles start to form and it thickens slightly.

✔ When a recipe says to steam a vegetable, the amount of water you need to use in your pot or steamer depends on your steaming method, so we don't include the water in the ingredients list. As a general rule of thumb, if you're using a basket in a pot, the water level should be just under the basket.

And finally, we include the following basic conventions throughout the rest of the book:

✔ We use **boldface** to highlight keywords and the specific action steps in numbered lists.

✔ We use *italics* to define or emphasize a word or phrase.

☉ We use this little tomato icon to highlight the vegetarian recipes in this book.

✔ Web sites appear in `monofont`; we haven't added any extra spaces or punctuation in them, so type exactly what you see in the text.

What You're Not to Read

Like all *For Dummies* books, this one has gray-shaded boxes called *sidebars* that contain interesting but nonessential information. If you aren't interested in the nitty-gritty, you can skip these sidebars. We promise not to include that information on the test (just kidding — there's no test, of course!). You can also safely skip any information marked with the Technical Stuff icon (see the section "Icons Used in This Book" for more details).

Foolish Assumptions

We assume that you're looking for meal-planning tips and recipes that will help you succeed with your weight-loss goals and healthier living by using the glycemic index diet. We also assume that you've done some cooking. In other words, you're familiar with the right knife to use to slice a tomato without cutting your finger, and you can tell one pot from another.

If you need to brush up on your cooking skills, check out *Cooking Basics For Dummies,* 3rd Edition, by Bryan Miller and Marie Rama (Wiley) before you get rolling.

How This Book Is Organized

This book is divided into six parts to help you incorporate the benefits of a low-glycemic diet into your life with recipes, helpful pointers, and more.

Part 1: The Science behind the Glycemic Index Diet

The glycemic index shows how different foods that contain carbohydrates — fruits, vegetables, grains, legumes, and dairy products — affect blood sugar levels. Keeping blood sugar levels stable is important for managing weight loss, diabetes, heart disease, and other health issues. It's also good practice for general wellness.

This part discusses how the glycemic index plays a role in general wellness, disease prevention, and weight loss. Here, we offer you the clinical side of a low-glycemic diet as well as practical tools on how you can use a low-glycemic diet to help you achieve your personal health goals.

Part 11: Creating a Healthy Lifestyle with Low-Glycemic Cooking

Figuring out how the glycemic index works is the first step, but how do you put it to work in your everyday life? In this part, we show you how to make moderate changes so you can easily make a low-glycemic diet fit your life-style. This part is full of meal-planning strategies, sample meal plans, low-glycemic cooking skills, tips for stocking your kitchen, and our very own grocery shopping tour. After reading the chapters here, you'll have no problem creating the recipes we include in this book.

Part 111: Serving Up Starters, Snacks, and Sides

You definitely don't have to give up taste to use low-glycemic foods in your cooking. The chapters in this part show you how to make some tasty breakfast dishes, wholesome baked goods, appealing appetizers, and hearty vegetable and grain sides that prove you can have plenty of flavor even when you're following a low-glycemic diet. And don't forget the soups, stews, chilies, and salads! These recipes are perfect to share with your family at home or guests at a party.

Part IV: Making Memorable Main Dishes and Desserts

Making delicious, low-glycemic main entrees is pretty easy to do. After all, the main protein sources like poultry, beef, pork, and seafood are naturally low glycemic because they don't contain carbohydrates. So as long as you stick to lowfat, lean protein sources, you're good to go! In this part, you find new and tasty ways to prepare entrees with these protein sources that you can eat every day as well as serve to guests. We also include a vegetarian chapter to show you how to use low-glycemic meatless protein sources like beans and nuts to make delicious, hearty entrees.

What about dessert? Can you have dessert in a low-glycemic lifestyle? We say yes! At the end of this part, you find a whole chapter dedicated to showing you how to make some sweet treats that are low to medium glycemic and also lower in fat and calories. See? You can satisfy your sweet tooth and still meet your overall health and wellness goals!

Part V: The Part of Tens

In this part, we provide ten healthy lifestyle steps to go along with your low-glycemic diet so you can create a complete health plan. Focusing on the whole picture will help you stay your healthiest. Here, you also find ten tips for maintaining your low-glycemic lifestyle during special occasions like parties, vacations, and holidays so you can continue to make progress toward your health goals even during those challenging times.

Part VI: Appendixes

The appendixes contain some great hands-on information to help you start implementing a low-glycemic diet in your life right away. Appendix A shows you some popular low-glycemic foods you can use whenever you like and explains which medium- to high-glycemic foods you need to use in moderation.

If you'd rather use the metric system, Appendix B provides simple conversion tables to make switching from ounces to grams (and other measurements) simple.

Icons Used in This Book

The icons in this book are like bookmarks, pointing out information that we think is especially important. Here are the icons we use and the kind of info they point out:

 Even if you forget everything else in this book, remember the paragraphs marked with this icon. They'll help you make good low-glycemic choices and stay on track with your health goals.

 The information marked with this icon is interesting to know, but it goes beyond what's essential for your basic understanding of the glycemic index. If you're the type of person who likes to know more about any particular topic, you'll enjoy these tidbits. If not, feel free to skip 'em.

 This helpful icon marks important information that can save you time and energy, so make sure you don't overlook it.

 Watch out for this icon; it warns you about potential problems and common pitfalls of implementing a low-glycemic diet into your lifestyle.

Where to Go from Here

Where you go from here depends on your immediate needs. Are you a newbie to the glycemic index and want to learn a little before you head to the kitchen? Then check out Part I for some basic information. If you're interested in meal planning, start with Chapters 4 and 5. If you're not sure where you want to begin, peruse the table of contents and pick out the topics that mean the most to you and start there. (We just want to remind you not to skip our personal favorite, Chapter 19, which covers desserts, of course! You definitely don't want to miss out on the yummy treats we offer you there!)

Part I

The Science behind the Glycemic Index Diet

The 5th Wave   By Rich Tennant

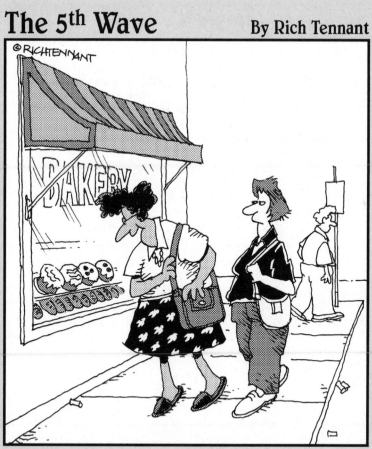

"This Glycemic Index Diet should work as long as my Looks So Good Gotta Have It Index doesn't kick in."

In this part . . .

The glycemic index was originally created as a way to scientifically determine how different foods that contain carbohydrates — fruits, vegetables, grains, legumes, and dairy products — affect blood sugar levels. Since that initial research took place more than 30 years ago, scientists have come to understand that the glycemic index can be an effective tool for improving and maintaining health and wellness.

In this part, we cover the science behind using low-glycemic foods to potentially prevent and manage conditions such as heart disease, diabetes, polycystic ovary syndrome, and metabolic syndrome. We also provide practical tools that can help you use a low-glycemic diet to work toward your individual weight-loss goals.

Chapter 1

What Is the Glycemic Index?

In This Chapter

▶ Defining the glycemic index by focusing on carbohydrates

▶ Getting a feel for how glycemic index measurements work

*W*hen the glycemic index was first introduced in the 1980s, its main focus was on helping people with diabetes gain better control of their blood sugar. The original glycemic index research included only 62 foods, but if you fast forward to today, you see that hundreds of foods are now included. Although the glycemic index is a fairly new science, you can find all sorts of mainstream diet programs that incorporate it into their daily guidelines. To keep up with the glycemic index trend, many food companies are focusing on developing lower-glycemic food options, and glycemic testing institutions are creating special food labeling to make it easier for you to find the low-glycemic foods you're looking for.

So if you're thinking about starting a gimmick-free lifestyle change that's based on science (yes, we mean the glycemic index diet), get ready to dive right in! In this chapter, we give you a quick rundown of what the glycemic index is and how the glycemic index is measured.

Introducing the Main Event behind the Glycemic Index: The Effect of Carbs

The *glycemic index* isn't a diet in the sense that you have to follow specific meal plans or eliminate certain foods from your daily meals and snacks. Instead, it's a scientific way of looking at how different carbohydrates in foods affect *blood glucose,* or blood sugar, levels. Although all carbohydrates raise blood sugar to some degree, the glycemic index takes this notion a step further by figuring out how much a specific food raises blood sugar. This information is especially important to know if you want to lose weight or if you have diabetes, heart disease, or certain other health issues. (See Chapter 2 for details on how the glycemic index diet can help you manage different health conditions.)

The glycemic index applies only to foods that contain carbohydrates, which include vegetables, fruits, grains, lentils, legumes, sugars, and the dairy portions of your meals. It shows you how these foods impact your blood sugar, which then affects everything from your energy levels to food cravings.

The following sections give you the scoop on how different types of carbohydrates impact your blood sugar and insulin levels.

Understanding the differences between carbohydrates

Most foods are made up of the following three calorie-containing macronutrients:

- ✔ **Carbohydrates:** As the body's primary fuel source, carbohydrates provide energy for the brain, muscles, and organs.

- ✔ **Protein:** The body rarely uses protein for energy because protein has other, more valuable uses — like being the building blocks of body tissues.

- ✔ **Fat:** The body uses fat for energy, but only when it has used up all the available carbohydrates.

Although health experts recommend that people get 40 to 60 percent of their total calorie intake from carbohydrates, active people need more carbohydrates to fuel their muscles, and children and adolescents need more carbohydrates to fuel growth. On the other hand, people who are sedentary or who have health issues related to *insulin resistance* (which occurs when your body produces insulin but doesn't use it properly) need smaller amounts of carbohydrates. (See Chapter 2 for details on how a low-glycemic diet can benefit folks with certain health issues.)

Because carbohydrates are the body's primary source of energy, it makes sense that just about every food group contains them. For instance, fruits, vegetables, grains, beans, lentils, and dairy products all contain different amounts of carbohydrates.

In general, carbohydrates come in these two varieties:

- ✔ **Simple carbohydrates:** Contain one or two sugar units
- ✔ **Complex carbohydrates:** Contain multiple sugar units

In the past, scientists thought simple carbohydrates raised blood sugar levels faster than complex carbohydrates because their sugar units are shorter and, thus, would break down more quickly. However, the glycemic index has shown that all carbohydrates, both simple and complex, vary greatly in regard to their blood sugar responses. For example, past reasoning dictated that a baked russet potato, which is a complex carbohydrate, would make a person's blood sugar rise more slowly than a teaspoon of sugar, which is a simple carbohydrate. But when these two foods were tested in clinical human studies, the opposite was true. The potato increased blood sugar more quickly than the sugar.

You can't tell how different foods will impact blood sugar or whether those foods are high or low glycemic just by looking at their food categories. Instead, researchers have to test specific foods to determine how the human body will respond to them. The same is true for recipes. The recipes we include in Parts III and IV are made up of low-glycemic ingredients that have been tested, but the recipes themselves haven't undergone any human clinical tests. For this reason, we can make an educated guess that the recipes will stay low glycemic when you make them, but we can't know for sure without the clinical testing. (Check out Appendix A to find the tested glycemic levels of many common foods.)

Knowing how blood sugar can work for you and against you

All carbohydrates, whether they're low glycemic or high glycemic, break down into blood sugar, which plays a crucial role in the body's ability to function properly. The body uses blood sugar as fuel for energy — much like a car uses gasoline — which is why athletes depend on carbohydrates to fuel their bodies so they can participate at peak performance.

The problem with blood sugar (and carbohydrates) arises when your blood sugar levels spike high throughout the day on a regular basis. These spikes occur when you eat mostly high-glycemic foods or large portion sizes of carbohydrate-containing foods. For many people, these spikes don't have a noticeable impact on their lives, but for others, these spikes can lead to food cravings, mood swings, energy crashes, and more serious issues like high clinical blood sugar (for diabetics or those with prediabetes), high cholesterol, or high *triglycerides* (fats found in the bloodstream that can increase your risk of heart disease when their levels are high). In addition, regular blood sugar spikes can impact how your body stores fat. How blood sugar spikes affect you personally depends on your body and genetics.

Choosing low-glycemic foods most of the time is one way to help keep blood sugar under control. We explain how to use a low-glycemic diet to battle cravings, suppress your appetite, and keep calories under control in Chapter 3.

Considering the role insulin plays in storing blood sugar

As we note in the previous section, when you eat carbohydrates, your body breaks them down into blood sugar. As soon as your blood sugar levels start to rise, your pancreas releases a hormone called *insulin*. Insulin acts like a key that unlocks the door to your cells so the blood sugar can enter them and be used as energy (see Figure 1-1).

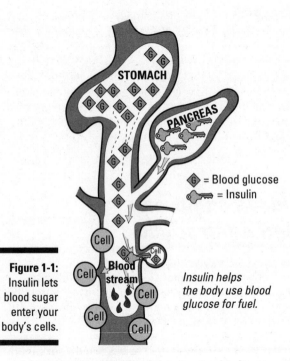

STOMACH

PANCREAS

G = Blood glucose

= Insulin

Cell

Cell

Cell

Blood stream

Cell

Cell

Cell

Insulin helps the body use blood glucose for fuel.

Figure 1-1:
Insulin lets blood sugar enter your body's cells.

Even though insulin transports blood sugar directly to your cells, your body doesn't turn all that blood sugar into energy right away. When blood sugar levels rise above normal (in part because you're eating high-glycemic foods), insulin signals your liver, muscles, and other cells to store the extra sugar. Your body stores some of this excess blood in your muscles and liver as *glycogen* (long-term stored energy) and converts some to body fat. Eating low-glycemic foods helps you regulate insulin and blood sugar levels that could become unstable because of a health condition or because you eat excess amounts of carbohydrates or calories.

Keep in mind that your body is extremely efficient. You won't become overweight just because you have one high-glycemic meal or because you eat one too many servings of stuffing at Thanksgiving. Your body stores fat over time when you continually take in more calories than you need. (See Chapter 3 for details on how to use a low-glycemic diet to control calories.)

Measuring a Food's Glycemic Index

The *glycemic level* of a food measures how fast that food is likely to raise your blood sugar. A food that is rapidly digested and absorbed with a high increase in blood sugar is considered *high glycemic,* and a food that is slowly digested and absorbed with a gradual rise in blood sugar is considered *low glycemic.* Foods that fall in the middle are considered *medium glycemic.* The following sections describe the index measurement process; define low-, medium-, and high-glycemic foods; explain the importance of nutrition when looking at categories of foods; and spell out some of the limitations of the glycemic index.

Only carbohydrate-containing foods can be considered low, medium, or high glycemic. Other food groups, like meats and fats (think oil and butter), don't contain carbohydrates, so you have to use your nutrition know-how to determine the best choices for you.

Be sure that you don't confuse the glycemic index with the *glycemic load,* which is a measurement based on the glycemic index and which you can use to start planning meals that fit the glycemic index diet. Flip to Part II for the scoop on glycemic load and meal planning.

Graphing responses to different foods

Measuring a food's glycemic index is actually a very expensive and involved process that requires human test subjects. Researchers feed 50 grams of *available carbohydrates* (that's total carbohydrates minus fiber) from a particular food item to ten or more volunteers to test how the food raises their blood sugar levels at different intervals over a two-hour period after it's consumed. The researchers plot the changes in blood sugar levels on a graph and then follow the same procedure with 50 grams of available carbohydrates from pure sugar or white bread. To determine the glycemic index of the tested food item, they compare the average blood sugar response of all ten volunteers to the tested food item and the average response to the sugar or white bread.

Researchers use pure sugar for comparison purposes because it's the simplest form of energy used by the human body. However, because most people don't typically eat sugar by itself, researchers sometimes use white bread instead to test comparisons of staple foods.

Here are a few examples that show you how this testing process may look on a graph:

- ✔ Figure 1-2 shows the sharp rise in blood sugar response when test subjects consume pure sugar. You can see the quick rise and ensuing drop over a short amount of time. Notice that the maximum blood sugar spike occurs around 45 minutes after consumption. After this peak, the blood sugar levels drop quickly.

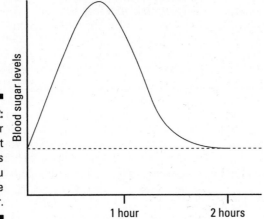

Glucose (Reference Food)

Figure 1-2:
Blood sugar spikes about 45 minutes after you consume sugar.

Blood sugar levels

1 hour   2 hours

- ✔ Figure 1-3 shows what happens when test subjects consume a high-glycemic food. Notice how the rise is similar to what you see in Figure 1-2.

- ✔ Figure 1-4 shows how the curve changes when test subjects consume a low-glycemic food. Notice that the maximum spike is much lower and occurs much later than the spike that occurs after subjects eat pure sugar or high-glycemic foods; it happens about an hour after consumption with a slow drop back to the baseline.

Because this type of blood sugar response requires lower levels of insulin, it results in better control of food cravings, hunger, and mood. For diabetics or anyone with insulin resistance, this means that your body won't require as much insulin and what insulin is needed will be required at a slower rate.

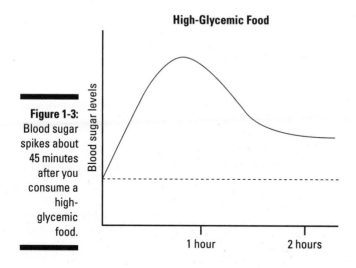

High-Glycemic Food

Figure 1-3:
Blood sugar
spikes about
45 minutes
after you
consume a
high-
glycemic
food.

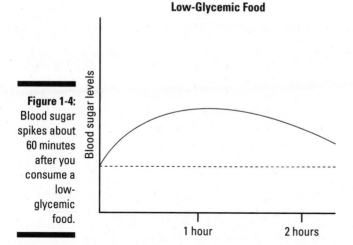

Low-Glycemic Food

Figure 1-4:
Blood sugar
spikes about
60 minutes
after you
consume a
low-
glycemic
food.

Keeping nutrition in mind when defining low- to high-glycemic foods

After a food undergoes glycemic index testing, determining whether it's low, medium, or high glycemic is pretty straightforward. High-glycemic foods have the fastest blood sugar responses, and low-glycemic foods have the slowest.

Here are the glycemic index measurements on a scale of 0 to 100:

- ✔ **Low glycemic index:** 55 or lower
- ✔ **Medium glycemic index:** 56 to 69
- ✔ **High glycemic index:** 70 or higher

High-glycemic foods aren't necessarily unhealthy foods. Similarly, low-glycemic foods aren't always healthy. The glycemic index measurement simply lets you know how quickly your blood sugar will rise from eating a particular food.

Basing your food choices solely on the glycemic index can get you into trouble because it means you're looking at only one aspect of the food and ignoring other important aspects, such as calories, fiber, vitamins, and minerals. (Chapter 3 explains why considering calories and fiber is important, especially when you're trying to lose weight.)

Many people think that whole grains, fruits, and vegetables naturally fall into the low-glycemic category. Although this estimation is true most of the time, it isn't always the case. On the same note, many non-nutritious foods are considered low glycemic. Table 1-1 shows you the glycemic index measurements of some popular healthy and unhealthy foods. As you can see, some foods fall right where you thought they'd be. For example, brown rice is a low-glycemic food. In contrast, other foods may surprise you. Notice that peanut M&M's and Snickers bars have low-glycemic indexes. Does that mean they're healthy and nutritious? No. Although they aren't a bad snack to choose once in a while, they're still a low-nutrient, high-fat, and high-calorie food.

The point at which specific types of products vary is where the glycemic index gets tricky. For example, notice that jasmine rice has a significantly higher glycemic index than basmati rice even though both types of rice are white. To help you figure out which common foods, including different rice and pasta varieties, fall into the different glycemic categories, turn to Appendix A.

Table 1-1   The Glycemic Lowdown on Some Popular Foods

Food	Glycemic Index Number	Measurement
Peanut M&M's	33	Low
Snickers bar	43	Low
Brown rice	48	Low
Whole-wheat bread	52	Low
Basmati white rice	57	Medium

Food	Glycemic Index Number	Measurement
Spaghetti	58	Medium
Plain bagel	69	Medium
Watermelon	72	High
Jasmine rice	89	High
Baked potato without skin	98	High

Beware of labeling all low-glycemic foods as "healthy." That's what happened during the lowfat craze of the 80s and 90s. People started eating lowfat everything, even if it meant higher sugar and calorie contents. To help you make the best food choices, use the glycemic index in combination with everything you already know about healthy eating, and incorporate high-nutrient, low-calorie foods into your everyday diet.

Watching out for a few limitations

The glycemic index is a great tool, but it does have a few limitations you need to know about:

- ✔ **The lists are limited.** Glycemic index testing has only been around for about 20 years, and it isn't required by federal guidelines in the United States. The testing process is quite expensive and time-consuming because each variation of every food must be tested before researchers can finalize their results. Also, only a small number of researchers actually conduct the glycemic index testing, and they can't possibly keep up with the thousands of new food products that manufacturers develop each year.

  The recipes in Parts III and IV use low-glycemic ingredients with estimated glycemic loads (described in Chapter 4), but the recipes themselves haven't been officially tested.

- ✔ **The findings vary.** Researchers have to observe humans to determine glycemic index measurements, and no two humans are alike. That means the rate at which people digest carbohydrates, their insulin responses, and even the time of day when they're tested can cause variation in testing results. To account for these variations, researchers have to test each food on many people and then take the average.

  Furthermore, the food world is full of variety. For example, you may find one long-grain rice variety with a glycemic index of 62 and another with an index of 68. The differences can result from where the grains were grown, how long they were cooked, how they were cooked, and so on.

The measurement process isn't a perfect science, but, for the most part, the same types of foods turn out to be around the same glycemic index. For example, even if one long-grain rice variety has a glycemic index of 62 and the other 68, both still fall into the medium-glycemic category. The important message to take home is focusing on whether a food generally ends up low, medium, or high glycemic and then trying to select lower-glycemic foods.

✔ **Combining foods in meals complicates things.** Putting foods with different glycemic index measurements together in one meal means creating a different glycemic index for that whole meal. With an infinite number of meal combinations out there, you can understand why you won't find a complete list of high-, low-, and medium-glycemic meals anytime soon. Even so, some packaged frozen meals like lasagna or macaroni and cheese have been tested. (Go to www.nutritiondata.com to find out if researchers have determined the glycemic level of the particular food or meal you want to eat.)

Despite these limitations, the glycemic index can be a very useful tool in helping you achieve your goals in health and fitness. Turn to Chapter 2 to find out how following a low-glycemic diet can help you work toward disease prevention and Chapter 3 to see how you can use a low-glycemic diet for weight loss.

Chapter 2

Surveying the Many Health Benefits of a Low-Glycemic Diet

*O*ne great thing about following a low-glycemic diet and eating more fruits, vegetables, whole grains, beans, and lentils is that doing so can benefit you in many different ways. You may just want to eat healthy and perhaps lose some weight (flip to Chapter 3 for more details), or you may be managing a disease like diabetes or polycystic ovary syndrome (PCOS). Either way, the strategies and recipes in this book can help you accomplish your health goals. In this chapter, we discuss how a low-glycemic eating plan can help you fight diseases as well as manage existing health conditions.

A low-glycemic diet isn't just another quick-fix gimmick; it's a way to make the best choices when deciding which and how many carbohydrates to eat. Following the guidelines in this book can help you not only if you're dealing with a health issue but also if you're working toward overall wellness and disease prevention.

Working toward Disease Prevention

Did you know you can prevent quite a few diseases with some basic lifestyle changes that include diet? Well, it's true, and it's especially important for those of you who have a family history of chronic disease. As dietitians, we know the importance of working toward disease prevention all too well, but we also know it from a personal standpoint (heart disease runs in both our families). As you find out in the following sections, a low-glycemic lifestyle can significantly lower your risk factors for certain diseases, increase your levels of antioxidants, and help you get important phytonutrients.

Although eating a low-glycemic, plant-based diet contributes a great deal to good health, it can't work alone. Other lifestyle components, such as exercising regularly, reducing stress, getting enough sleep, and making time for fun and relaxation, play an important role, too. The goal is to take a holistic approach to your health; see the nearby sidebar "Setting lifestyle goals to improve your health" for more information.

Setting lifestyle goals to improve your health

Working on all aspects of your lifestyle (including diet, exercise, stress management, sleep, and relaxation) is important when your main goals are to prevent disease and feel your best. After all, you have a lot of control in your life to set the clock back on aging and make sure you stay healthy for the long haul. Don't get us wrong, though; some things, like genetics and age, are out of your control, but to get the most benefits from your efforts, focus on the changes you can make. Use this worksheet to help you set goals for better health in each area of your life.

For each category, list one to three goals you'd like to work on.

Diet:

Example: I am going to include fruit with my breakfast each morning.

_____

_____

_____

Exercise:

Example: I am going to go on a strenuous walk four days a week.

_____

_____

_____

Stress Management:

Example: I am going to attend a yoga class two days a week.

_____

_____

_____

Sleep:

Example: I am going to go to bed by 10 p.m. each night.

_____

_____

_____

Fun and Relaxation:

Example: I am going to give myself a half-hour of "me time" each night to read a good book.

_____

_____

_____

Reducing risk factors for chronic diseases

When we talk about *risk factors* for chronic diseases, we mean both genetic factors (like having a family history of high cholesterol or high blood pressure) and lifestyle factors (like smoking and making unhealthy food choices) that can lead you down the path to chronic disease. For example, simply eating a diet high in saturated fat can be a risk factor for heart disease.

When it comes to reducing risk factors for chronic diseases, a low-glycemic diet works well for most people for two reasons. First, it's a moderate approach rather than a drastic and restrictive one. Second, it focuses on high-nutrient, plant-based foods, which offer you loads of vitamins, minerals, and antioxidants that work together to protect your body from diseases like heart disease, cancer, and diabetes.

The following research statistics show how making simple dietary changes can help protect you from developing chronic diseases:

- If you're overweight, losing 5 to 7 percent of your body weight reduces the risk of chronic illnesses such as diabetes and heart disease. (You can easily lose weight with the help of a low-glycemic diet.)

- Estimates from a multi-study report show that if the only lifestyle change people made was to include five servings of fruits and vegetables daily (an important part of a low-glycemic diet), their overall cancer risk could decline by 20 percent.

✔ According to an article in *The Journal of the American Medical Association*, men and women with the highest consumption of fruits and vegetables — a median of 5.8 servings per day among women and 5.1 servings per day among men — were found to have a 31-percent lower risk of suffering from a stroke.

✔ The Linus Pauling Institute at Oregon State University looked at a meta-analysis of 11 studies in 2005 and found that people consuming four or more servings of fruits and vegetables a day had a decreased risk of coronary artery disease. Those with an intake of at least eight servings a day produced an even greater decrease. Green leafy vegetables and fruits and vegetables rich in vitamin C appeared to contribute the most to the apparent protective effect of total fruit and vegetable intake.

✔ The Nurses' Health Study found that women who ate the most high-glycemic foods had a 50-percent greater risk of developing diabetes than those who primarily ate a diet of low-glycemic foods.

✔ In a study of almost 48,000 adults (published in the journal *Archives of Internal Medicine* in 2010), researchers found that eating high-glycemic foods was strongly linked to a greater risk of coronary heart disease, whereas eating low-glycemic foods was not.

Raising your antioxidant levels

Antioxidants are substances that help slow down the process of *oxidation* (when your body's cells burn oxygen), thus decreasing the number of *free radicals,* or unstable molecules, that rip through your body, causing damage to your cells, tissues, and DNA. Antioxidants are found in many of the foods you eat and are one of your body's best defenses against these harmful free radicals. Think about your day and the many things you're exposed to, such as car exhaust, sunlight, unhealthy foods, and air pollution. These types of exposures can cause free radicals to spin out of control in your body, damaging everything in their path and maybe even leaving you at an increased risk of chronic diseases like heart disease and cancer.

Consider this simplified example: Have you ever sliced an apple and left it for a while only to come back to a brown apple? This browning occurs because of oxidation. When you add orange juice or lemon juice to the apple right after you cut it, it stays white longer because it's protected by the antioxidant vitamin C.

Avoiding free radicals entirely is next to impossible, so instead, you need to combat them with a diet high in antioxidants like vitamin C, vitamin E, and beta carotene, which are found in the fruits and vegetables that are important in a low-glycemic diet. Try to incorporate five to nine different fruits and veggies into your diet each day; a good variety of fruits and vegetables assures you'll get ample amounts of all the antioxidants. Table 2-1 lists some low-glycemic foods that are rich in certain antioxidant vitamins.

Table 2-1	Antioxidant-Rich, Low-Glycemic Foods
Antioxidant	*Low-Glycemic Foods That Contain It*
Vitamin C	Asparagus
	Broccoli
	Cantaloupe
	Cauliflower
	Dark leafy greens, such as spinach, kale, and collard greens
	Grapefruit
	Green and red bell peppers
	Guava
	Oranges
	Pineapple
	Strawberries
	Tangerines
	Tomatoes
Vitamin E	Dark leafy greens, such as mustard greens, Swiss chard, spinach, and turnip and collard greens
	Dry roasted almonds
	Peanut butter
	Raw sunflower seeds
Beta carotene	Broccoli
	Cantaloupe
	Carrots
	Cilantro
	Dark leafy greens, such as kale, spinach, and turnip and collard greens
	Romaine lettuce

Scientists suggest that there may be some sort of synergy between the different vitamins and the other chemicals in the food you eat that gives your body the antioxidant benefits it needs. Therefore, taking a vitamin C supplement may not provide the same benefit as eating an orange.

Filling up on phytonutrients

Did you know the colorful fruits and vegetables in a low-glycemic diet offer more than just vitamins and minerals? Well, it's true; plant-based foods also contain *phytonutrients,* which are naturally occurring compounds that offer your body potential health benefits. Research in this area is new and exciting; to date, certain phytonutrients have been shown to work as antioxidants (see the previous section), contain anti-inflammatory properties (which help prevent inflammation that occurs in the body with many diseases like heart disease), and promote heart health.

Phytonutrients provide the pigment to your fruits and vegetables, so you can literally know which class of phytonutrients you're consuming simply by the color of the food you're eating. Table 2-2 shows the specific health benefits and phytonutrients of certain colors of foods. Pretty cool, right?

Table 2-2	Health Benefits of Low-Glycemic Foods by Color	
Color	**Health Benefits**	**Low-Glycemic Foods of That Color**
Blue/purple	A lower risk of some cancers, improved memory function, and healthy aging	Blueberries, eggplants, grapes, and plums
Green	A lower risk of some cancers, healthy vision, and strong bones and teeth	Broccoli, green peppers, honeydew melon, kiwi, salad greens, and spinach
Red	A healthy heart, improved memory function, and a lower risk of some cancers	Pink watermelon, red bell peppers, and strawberries
White	A healthy heart and a lower risk of some cancers	Bananas, garlic, and onions
Yellow/orange	A healthy heart, healthy vision, a stronger immune system, and a lower risk of some cancers	Carrots, oranges, yellow and orange bell peppers, and yellow watermelon

Managing Current Health Problems

For many of you, using a low-glycemic diet goes beyond wanting to lose weight or prevent disease; instead, it may be more about managing a particular health condition. Most health issues that you can manage using a low-glycemic diet have one thing in common: *insulin resistance,* a condition in which the body doesn't utilize the sugar in the blood properly, making the body resistant to the insulin it's producing and leading to high blood sugars and high insulin levels. (In case you're wondering, *insulin* is a hormone that transports blood sugar into the cells, where it is used as energy.) Some health issues associated with insulin resistance include metabolic syndrome, polycystic ovary syndrome, and various forms of diabetes.

Other than insulin resistance, new research now shows that a low-glycemic diet may also help with other health conditions like heart disease.

In this section, we touch on some of the research and potential benefits of using low-glycemic foods and recipes if you have one of these health issues or if you're at an increased risk of developing one of them based on your family history.

Metabolic syndrome

Metabolic syndrome (also known as *syndrome X* or *insulin resistance syndrome*) is a cluster of symptoms that include high cholesterol, high inflammation markers (inflammation inside the body is associated with greater risk of heart disease), high blood sugar, high blood pressure, high *triglycerides* (fats in the body that can lead to heart disease if their levels get too high), increased abdominal weight, and elevated insulin levels. Not surprisingly, this condition can be very difficult to manage. You can't focus only on cholesterol or blood sugar; you have to manage all the symptoms simultaneously. Sound overwhelming? It can be, but the good news is that a low-glycemic diet can help you tackle many of the issues at the same time.

A low-glycemic diet can help you manage metabolic syndrome in the following ways:

- ✔ **It helps reduce inflammation in the body.** One study, published in the *American Journal of Clinical Nutrition* in 2002, showed that women who ate higher amounts of whole grains, bran, and cereal fiber — most of which are low glycemic — had lower inflammation markers. Women who specifically followed a low-glycemic diet also had lower inflammation markers.

- ✔ **It can decrease triglycerides by lowering the number of excess calories that your body can convert to triglycerides.** A low-glycemic diet can also decrease insulin levels, which are also associated with high triglycerides.

- ✔ **It helps lower bad cholesterol and increase good cholesterol.** Research shows that a low-glycemic diet offers consistent benefits for heart health by increasing HDL (good cholesterol). Researchers aren't certain whether it's simply the higher fiber content or something else to do with low-glycemic foods that lowers the bad cholesterol; more research is needed to confirm the specific cause.

✔ **It helps lower insulin levels and stabilize blood sugar levels.** Eating lower-glycemic foods helps you avoid blood sugar and insulin spikes.

✔ **It can help with weight management by helping you control insulin levels, stave off food cravings, and feel more satisfied.** Research shows that a 6.5-percent reduction in weight can significantly reduce blood pressure, cholesterol, blood sugar, and triglycerides.

A low-glycemic diet is a great tool for those of you with metabolic syndrome to use because it can help you manage each symptom. Here are some tips to get you started:

✔ Choose low-glycemic carbohydrates, such as brown rice, quinoa, fruits, and veggies (see Appendix A for a list of other low-glycemic foods), for your meals and snacks, and use appropriate portion sizes (see Chapter 4 for more about portions).

✔ Avoid eating carbohydrates by themselves; instead, pair them with a protein or fat source like meats or nuts.

✔ Decrease the amount of saturated and trans fats in your diet to 10 percent of your daily calories. (You can completely eliminate trans fats because your body doesn't need them at all.)

✔ Start eating fatty fish, walnuts, and/or flaxseeds for their omega-3 fatty acids, which help people with metabolic syndrome by decreasing inflammation and lowering triglycerides.

✔ Incorporate at least five servings of fruits and vegetables into your diet each day.

Polycystic ovary syndrome

Polycystic ovary syndrome (PCOS) is a condition that affects women and causes a hormonal imbalance that leads to several problems, including ovarian cysts, irregular menstrual cycles, fertility issues, weight gain, acne, skin tags, excess body and facial hair, and thinning hair on the scalp. If left untreated, PCOS can lead to diabetes and heart disease (both of which we discuss in this chapter). The exact reason why PCOS occurs is unknown, but there does seem to be a link between insulin resistance and PCOS, which is where a low-glycemic diet comes into play.

Insulin resistance reduces your body's insulin sensitivity, which means that less blood sugar from the foods you eat actually enters into your cells. As a result, the cells become resistant to insulin, and the pancreas responds by releasing more and more insulin to regulate metabolism. In return, these high insulin levels stimulate the ovaries to produce large amounts of the male hormone testosterone, causing symptoms like infertility, ovarian cysts, and loss of menstrual cycles. Meanwhile, the extra buildup of blood sugar is sent to the liver and muscles. The liver converts it into fat, which is then stored throughout the body, leading to weight gain and obesity. Note that you can still manage your weight if you have PCOS; doing so just takes more focus on food choices and exercise.

Managing blood sugar is a key factor in treating people with PCOS, and following a low-glycemic diet can help reduce blood sugar spikes and keep insulin levels down. Although more research needs to be done to confirm the clinical effects of using a low-glycemic diet with PCOS, this diet plan offers a good strategy for most people who are trying to manage blood sugar and insulin levels.

If you have PCOS, follow these tips to start using a low-glycemic diet to manage it:

✔ Choose low-glycemic carbohydrates, such as brown rice, quinoa, fruits, and veggies (see Appendix A for a list of other low-glycemic foods), and use appropriate portion sizes for meals and snacks (see Chapter 4 for details on portions).

✔ Eat a diet that gets 40 to 50 percent of your calories from carbohydrates (compared to the normal 55 percent). Although research is needed in this area, many professionals agree that women with PCOS do better with a slightly lower carbohydrate diet.

✔ Space out your carbohydrates during the day to avoid blood sugar spikes at one meal.

✔ Choose high-nutrient carbohydrates, like fruits and vegetables, and limit your intake of low-nutrient foods, like cookies and chips. For instance, instead of going for a bag of chips from the vending machine, have an apple and an ounce of nuts.

If you're having a hard time maintaining your diet and lifestyle changes, visit www.incyst.com for sound advice and information from a network of dietitians who specialize in PCOS. Also, check out *Managing PCOS For Dummies* by Gaynor Bussell (Wiley).

Prediabetes and type 2 diabetes

As we discuss earlier in this section, your body uses insulin to convert sugars from the carbohydrates you eat into energy needed for daily life. Think of insulin like a key that unlocks the door to your body's cells to let the sugar into your bloodstream. People with *diabetes* either don't produce enough insulin or don't use the insulin they do produce properly, resulting in excess blood sugar and insulin levels. The two main types of diabetes that you may be able to impact, at least in part, by using a low-glycemic diet are

- ✔ **Type 2 diabetes:** When the body produces insulin but doesn't use it properly, leading to excess blood sugar and insulin levels
- ✔ **Prediabetes:** When your blood sugar is higher than normal but not high enough to be diagnosed as type 2 diabetes

Type 1 diabetes, or *juvenile onset diabetes,* mostly begins in childhood and is a condition in which the body doesn't make insulin. Managing type 1 diabetes requires insulin injections; while diet changes are essential, you need more detailed information on how to manage type 1 diabetes than simply following a low-glycemic diet. See your doctor for details on how to deal with this type of diabetes.

If you don't control your diabetes, it can put almost every organ in your body at risk, including

- ✔ Heart and blood vessels
- ✔ Eyes
- ✔ Kidneys
- ✔ Nerves
- ✔ Gums and teeth

The scientific community continues to debate whether or not a low-glycemic diet has a major impact on diabetes because so many variables, including portion sizes and the way individuals metabolize sugars, come into play. Although more research is needed, current studies show that following a low-glycemic diet has a small but positive effect on a person's blood sugar levels.

A recent review of current research conducted by the Human Nutrition Unit of the School of Molecular and Microbial Biosciences at the University of Sydney, Australia looked at whether a low-glycemic diet helps people with type 2 diabetes manage their blood sugar levels. The end results showed that a low-glycemic diet does indeed help. Specifically, a low-glycemic diet decreased Hgb A1C levels by 0.5 percent. (*Hgb A1C* is a blood test that gives the big picture of how a person is managing his or her blood sugar over a particular period of time, such as two weeks or several months.) Another review resulted in similar findings with a decreased Hgb A1C of 0.43 percent. The conclusion from these reviews is that following a low-glycemic diet has a small but clinically useful effect on blood sugar control.

As far as prediabetes is concerned, all people with type 2 diabetes had prediabetes at one time. The goal is to control prediabetes before it turns into type 2 diabetes. Data collected from the Nurses' Health Study in 1997 showed that women with the highest dietary glycemic load were 37 percent more likely to develop type 2 diabetes over a six-year period than women with a low gly-cemic load intake (see Chapter 4 for details on glycemic load). Data from the Black Women's Health Study in 2007 found that women who followed a high-glycemic diet were 23 percent more likely to develop type 2 diabetes within eight years than those who followed a low-glycemic diet.

Here are some simple dietary guidelines for using a low-glycemic diet to help manage your diabetes:

✔ **Eat appropriate portion sizes.** Overeating any carbohydrates, including low-glycemic ones, increases your blood sugar. Portion sizes are key to successful blood sugar management.

✔ **Incorporate protein and fat into your meals to balance the carbohy-drates.** Eating protein and fat with your carbohydrates can help slow down digestion and lower the rise in blood sugar as well as help you feel more satisfied.

✔ **Eat a low-glycemic snack or meal every four to five hours.** Make sure not to let your blood sugar get too low, especially if you're taking insulin or oral medications.

✔ **Always test your blood sugar so you can monitor how your dietary choices are stacking up.** Your body is different from all other diabetic patients, which means you may metabolize certain foods differently. Watching your daily blood sugar can help you discover which foods and how much of those foods affect your blood sugar in different ways.

If you have diabetes, you're probably familiar with tools like carbohydrate counting and the exchange system. Don't throw these tools out the window! They can work well with low-glycemic foods. If you haven't seen a registered dietitian, now is a great time to get some guidance, especially if your blood sugars are running high often (Hgb A1C more than 7).

If you want more information on diabetes and diet, check out *Diabetes For Dummies,* 3rd Edition, *Prediabetes For Dummies,* and *Diabetes Cookbook For Dummies,* 3rd Edition, by Alan Rubin (Wiley).

Heart disease

Heart disease is still the number-one cause of death in the United States. The only warning sign of heart disease you may have is high blood pressure, high cholesterol, or high triglycerides. In some cases, you may not have any risk fac-tors. For this reason and because the warning signs are almost commonplace these days, being proactive in preventing this disease is especially important.

In 2008, *The American Journal of Clinical Nutrition* published reviews from 37 studies showing on average that following a low-glycemic diet has a consis-tent benefit for heart health. Specifically, findings demonstrate that eating a low-glycemic diet increases HDL (good cholesterol) and lowers triglycerides. This result may have something to do with the fact that many low-glycemic foods aren't processed and/or are higher in fiber than high-glycemic foods — either way, it's a great benefit.

When it comes to managing heart disease, eating healthy fats and including high-fiber foods in your daily diet are a big part of the picture. Use what you know about healthy fats, high-fiber foods, and low-glycemic foods — like keeping your saturated-fat intake low and incorporating 25 to 35 grams of fiber a day (see Chapter 3 for details) — to help keep your heart healthy, especially if you already have known risk factors like high cholesterol or high blood pressure or if you have a family history of heart disease.

Here are a few tips to help you get started toward heart health:

- ✔ Choose low-glycemic carbohydrates, such as brown rice, quinoa, fruits, and veggies, rather than high-glycemic carbohydrates, like white bread or russet potatoes.

- ✔ Use appropriate portion sizes for all your food groups (see Chapter 4 for guidance).

- ✔ Incorporate five to nine fruits and vegetables into your daily diet.

- ✔ Avoid trans fats, and limit your intake of saturated fats (think high-fat cuts of meat and dairy).

- ✔ Increase your fiber intake with a goal of eating 25 to 35 grams per day.

- ✔ Eat plenty of omega-3 fatty acids, which are found in fish, walnuts, and flaxseeds. *Note:* Fatty fish, such as salmon, tuna, and halibut, are better sources of omega-3 fatty acids than plant-based sources.

For more information on heart disease, check out *Heart Disease For Dummies* by James Rippe (Wiley).

Chapter 3

Losing Weight with a Low-Glycemic Diet

*I*f you search for low-glycemic diets on the Internet, you'll find gimmicks promising weight-loss miracles along with some evidence-based science. Looking over all this information, you're sure to run into inconsistencies because the glycemic index isn't black and white as many gimmicks claim. Even so, researchers are finding more and more benefits associated with eating low-glycemic foods, and some of those benefits can indeed help you lose weight.

This chapter discusses the legitimate science behind the glycemic index and shows you how incorporating low-glycemic foods into your daily diet is an important piece of the weight-loss puzzle because those foods help minimize cravings and suppress your appetite. We also describe how a low-glycemic diet fits into other weight-loss strategies, like controlling your caloric intake, incorporating the right balance of foods, and making the most of your metabolism.

Using a low-glycemic diet for weight loss is a successful strategy, but it isn't a stand-alone fix.

Regulating Blood Sugar and Curbing Cravings with Low-Glycemic Foods

When you eat carbohydrate-containing foods, your body breaks down those carbohydrates into *glucose,* or blood sugar. Your pancreas releases *insulin,* a hormone that acts like a key to unlock the door to your cells so the blood sugar can enter your cells and be used as energy. Your body doesn't turn all of that glucose into energy at once, however. When glucose levels rise above normal, insulin signals your liver, muscles, and other cells to store the extra glucose. Some gets stored in your muscles as *glycogen* (long-term stored energy), and some gets converted to body fat. Basically, your body becomes the storage unit for all the excess energy you aren't using, which is great for athletes who need to burn lots of calories for the next day's competition, but not so good for the average person who doesn't burn those extra calories. (We discuss the importance of calories during weight loss in the later section "Keeping Calories under Control.")

When you eat high-glycemic foods (like white processed breads or sugar-based foods), your blood sugar spikes high and fast, and your pancreas releases large amounts of insulin to deal with those spikes. That increased amount of insulin rushing to the scene of the crime takes care of the blood sugar as rapidly as the spikes occurred, so your blood sugar comes crashing down quickly — not low enough to see in a blood test, but low enough to make you feel hungry. That blood sugar crash can mean food cravings even if you just ate an ample number of calories.

As you may know, food cravings occur for many different reasons, including both psychological and physiological reasons. Erratic changes in your blood sugar levels, as we just explained, are one factor that has been linked to food cravings. Couple those blood sugar spikes with stress or even conditioned cues from childhood and you have a recipe for a significant craving.

For example, let's say you have a stressful meeting at work. You don't have time to eat a balanced breakfast, so you grab a bowl of high-glycemic cereal to eat as you rush through your morning routine. After the adrenaline of your meeting is over, you're starving! Have you ever experienced that intense mid-morning hunger even though you ate breakfast? Instead of eating a healthy snack like yogurt or some fruit and nuts, you go straight for a sleeve of cookies. You want a treat for a job well done!

Consider the combination of events at work here:

- ✔ You ate a low-calorie, high-glycemic breakfast that made your blood sugar spike and then drop, leading to extreme hunger and cravings for some sort of carbohydrate.
- ✔ The stress from the meeting triggered cravings for sugar.

✔ You felt like you deserved the box of cookies because you grew up receiving treats after you did something well.

✔ You eat the whole sleeve of cookies rather than just two or three cookies because you're hungry, the food is there, you deserve a reward, and your body wants carbohydrates.

If you would've decided to have a more balanced breakfast of oatmeal with nuts and fruit (or one of our breakfast recipes in Chapter 8 that balance low-glycemic carbs with protein and fat), you may not have been as hungry after the meeting. As a result, you could've decided not to eat the cookies in the first place or enjoyed a few cookies slowly instead of eating the whole sleeve ravenously. Tweaking just one link in this chain of events could've given you a little more control.

To help keep your food cravings under control (and therefore help keep your weight down), follow these three guidelines:

✔ Choose low-glycemic foods for your meals and snacks. Low-glycemic foods play a crucial role in keeping your blood sugar levels stable because your body converts these foods into blood glucose more slowly and with smaller spikes. This stability means you'll feel more satisfied during the day and won't have excess insulin tugging at your hunger levels.

✔ Match these low-glycemic foods with protein and fat sources to help you feel full for a longer period of time.

✔ Eat consistently (at least every 4 to 5 hours).

Many of our recipes in this book follow these general guidelines. Those that don't are meant to be side dishes as part of a meal, not a whole meal on their own. To help you get a handle on how to achieve the right balance in every meal, we often suggest what foods to pair with certain recipes so you don't have to do any guesswork.

Keeping your blood sugar stable can result in some wonderful benefits when it comes to weight loss, but don't get us wrong: Calories are still king when it comes to weight loss, and we discuss this topic in detail later in this chapter.

Suppressing Your Appetite the Low-Glycemic Way

Low-glycemic foods can serve as a natural appetite suppressant. In fact, just eating certain foods can suppress your appetite as much as or even more than the pills you see advertised all over. You know what we're talking about — the ads for new, revolutionary appetite suppressants that really work!

The great news is you don't have to spend money or pop any pills to get the weight-loss results you're looking for. Instead, you can simply enjoy food! The following sections highlight how a low-glycemic diet can help you control your appetite.

Including fiber in your daily menu

Imagine that there's a part of food that isn't digested, has few to no calories, and helps you feel full longer. Okay, stop imagining and start eating! This amazing food item actually exists, and it's called fiber! Fiber is literally nature's appetite suppressant because it adds more bulk to your meals and isn't digested like other food parts. Eating a diet high in fiber (about 25 to 35 grams a day) is truly one of your best weight-loss strategies.

So what does fiber have to do with low-glycemic foods? Well, many, albeit not all, low-glycemic foods are high in fiber. And you may naturally increase your fiber intake by increasing the amount of low-glycemic foods you use in your cooking, depending on what your diet looked like before. Because a large majority of low-glycemic foods are good sources of fiber, you may just find you've upped your daily fiber intake by increasing your low-glycemic-food intake.

Releasing your fullness hormones

Several different hormones control your appetite by triggering hunger and fullness. Together these hormones make up your body's internal appetite-control mechanism that tells you when to eat and when to stop eating. Think about the times when you wait too long to eat and, as a result, you're starving; you can thank your hunger hormones for those intense hunger pains.

On the flip side, think about times when you overeat, like on Thanksgiving when you're so stuffed after dinner that all you want to do is curl up on the couch in sweats and take a nap. These stuffed feelings are the effects of your fullness hormones.

So what do these hormones have to do with a low-glycemic diet? Preliminary studies show that one of your body's fullness hormones, called *GLP-1,* may have a direct connection to a low-glycemic diet. GLP-1 is one of two hormones that work by telling your brain you've had enough to eat. Basically, it tells your stomach to stop moving anything along in your intestines until what's already there has been broken down. For example, you know your

GLP-1's at work when you go beyond full to eat that one last bite of dessert after a big dinner. Your GLP-1-inspired expression may be something like, "I can't eat another bite, or I'll explode!"

For a more scientific example, consider this study: In 2009, researchers from King's College in London took a close look at GLP-1 in relation to a low-glycemic diet. Volunteers who ate a low-glycemic breakfast ended up with 20-percent-higher levels of GLP-1 in their blood after breakfast compared to those who ate a high-glycemic breakfast. Although it's just one study, it shows a direct correlation between low-glycemic foods and GLP-1.

Although more research is needed, the good news is that you can try out your own personal study on the subject simply by adding more low-glycemic foods to your diet. Pay attention to your true-hunger levels (the sensations in your stomach, not your mind), and see whether eating low-glycemic foods helps you feel full longer.

Keeping Calories under Control

The glycemic index is certainly a part of the weight-loss puzzle — primarily how you choose to eat carbohydrates — but you have to look at your daily calorie levels, too. This section explains why you need to control the number of calories you consume and how calories relate to a low-glycemic diet.

Knowing that calories still count when you want to lose weight

Calories are simply a measurement of energy. If you don't use the calories you consume as energy, your body stores them as body fat. When you begin to use up that stored energy, you lose weight. To get your body to lose body fat, you need to reduce your calorie intake through dietary changes and increase your calorie output through exercise. For example, if your body requires 2,200 calories a day to maintain your current weight, to lose weight, you need to make a calorie deficit, perhaps decreasing your calorie intake by 200 calories a day by skipping your large morning latte and then starting up a spin-cycle class to burn even more calories through exercise.

Table 3-1 gives you an idea of the different calorie deficits needed to lose specific amounts of weight (one pound equals 3,500 calories).

Table 3-1	Calorie Deficits and Weight Loss
Rate of Weight Loss (Pounds per Week)	Calorie Deficit Per Day (from Diet and Exercise)
0.5	250
1	500
1.5	750
2	1,000

To lose weight, you don't have to eat an extremely low-calorie diet. In fact, for better success, we recommend decreasing your calorie intake only by 250 to 500 calories a day so you can live with the changes you're making and don't feel deprived. So, for example, if you currently eat 2,200 calories a day, try eating just 1,950 calories a day. (Note that if you aim to eat 1,950 calories, you'll more likely eat between 1,700 and 1,900 calories because no one eats an exact calorie level each day.) Of course, every person is different and you may have to tweak your calorie level and exercise to fit your body's needs. The point is not to go too low (below 1,200 calories).

Yes, going this route may result in slower weight loss, but would you rather lose 25 pounds in four weeks only to gain it back by the end of the year or lose 25 pounds over the course of the year and keep it off for a lifetime? If you're in favor of the latter scenario, you can use a low-glycemic diet, with its focus on fruits, vegetables, and whole grains, to help you start trimming your daily intake of calories.

You don't need to literally count your calories every day. We can't imagine counting our calories day in and day out, so we can't ask you to do it! The only time we suggest counting calories is when you want to get a baseline of what your current intake is. Otherwise, you can easily lower your calories just by making simple dietary and lifestyle changes. So instead of worrying about numbers, focus on the steps you can take to reduce your calories.

Here are a few examples of how making simple dietary and lifestyle changes can help you decrease your daily calorie intake:

- Choosing a 4-ounce steak rather than an 8-ounce steak can save you about 200 calories.
- Skipping the loaded baked potato at dinner and replacing it with a low-glycemic side salad can save you about 300 calories.
- Choosing half a sandwich with a cup of soup at the deli in place of a whole sandwich can save you about 250 calories.
- Grabbing a low-glycemic apple as a side with your deli sandwich in place of chips can save you 50 to 100 calories.
- Going for a brisk 30-minute walk can burn about 150 calories.

✔ Going for a light 30-minute swim can burn about 300 calories.

✔ Playing a game of tennis with your family can burn about 210 calories.

The point of these examples is to show you that just focusing on small changes, related to both food choices and exercise, can lead to a daily calorie deficit that can help you lose weight in a healthy way without being too rigid. The small changes really do add up quickly! Just think: Simply by eating a smaller steak and going for a short walk, you can make a calorie deficit of 350 calories for one day. If you made this calorie deficit daily, you could lose 0.5 to 1 pound each week without drastically changing your lifestyle.

Understanding that low glycemic doesn't always mean low calorie

Although you may find that you eat fewer calories with a low-glycemic diet, low-glycemic foods aren't always low calorie. For example, brown rice is lower glycemic than jasmine rice, yet they both have equal calorie levels.

The calorie decrease you get from a low-glycemic diet really depends on the diet you maintained before your switch. If you were eating a lot of processed, high-calorie foods before you switched to low-glycemic foods, you'll likely see a noticeable calorie deficit. However, if you were eating fairly healthy, whole foods and are just doing some minor tweaking, you won't see much difference in your overall calorie level.

You may be surprised to find out that many treats like peanut M&M's and other types of candy have low-glycemic indexes. Beware that just because a food is low glycemic doesn't mean you can eat it in unlimited quantities. One package of peanut M&M's may be low glycemic, but it also contains 243 calories. So if you're looking for a once-in-a-while treat, feel free to purchase a package of peanut M&M's from the vending machine; just don't make it an everyday snack!

Here are some examples of low-glycemic foods with high calorie levels:

✔ **½ cup of ice cream:** About 250 calories per serving

✔ **Two peanut butter cookies:** 270 calories

✔ **One 60-gram slice of pound cake:** 200 calories

Don't forget the non-carbohydrate-containing foods — namely meat — that are always low glycemic but high in calories like the following:

✔ **8-ounce fillet mignon steak:** 590 calories

✔ **4 fried chicken wings:** 408 calories

Watch out for gimmicks that try to simplify the glycemic index by making you think you can eat anything you want as long as it's low glycemic. Without also managing your overall calorie level, you can end up gaining weight by eating low-glycemic foods, depending on the particular foods you eat. Looking at the whole picture of weight loss (the foods you eat, the amounts of those foods, and the amount of exercise you get) will help you achieve the results you're looking for and reap the rewards low-glycemic foods can provide.

Taking a closer look at portion sizes (They aren't what they used to be)

Research shows that about 80 percent of people underestimate their food intake. Underestimating how much you're eating is easy to do because portion sizes have gotten so large in restaurants and other places that serve food that your estimate of 1 cup of rice or 3 ounces of meat is much larger than reality. One study done at St. Luke-Roosevelt Hospital Obesity Research Center in 1992 found that participants estimated that they were eating about 1,000 calories each day when, in fact, they were eating 2,000 calories.

Another study, this one conducted by the Department of Nutritional Sciences at Pennsylvania State University in 2002, showed that the larger the portion size on your plate, the more you'll eat. It found that most people don't stop eating when they feel their fullness hormones at work in their stomach (see the earlier section "Releasing your fullness hormones" for details). Instead, they eat more food simply because it's in front of them.

The main problem is that portion sizes are growing at an alarming rate. As they continue to grow, people become immune to the increasing sizes and begin to see them as "normal," resulting in the consumption of more and more calories. For example, in the 1970s, the typical size beverage you'd get as a fountain drink from a restaurant or from a cooler at a quick stop was 12 ounces; today the typical size is 20 ounces and goes all the way up to 100 ounces! Bagels used to weigh 2 to 3 ounces; today they weigh 4 to 7 ounces. And the regular size serving of French fries from McDonald's (you remember . . . the one that came in the little white paper bag) weighed one-third of the weight of the largest size today.

Unfortunately, these extra-large portions have become so normal that when people today see the "smaller" servings, they think they're getting a tiny amount of food that surely can't fill them up. This problem is even bigger for today's youth because all they know are the current portion sizes, and when they see what a portion size is supposed to look like, it appears very small.

Even today's plates are a lot larger than they were in the 1950s and 1960s. Heck, most dinner plates today don't fit in traditional-sized cupboards or dishwashers. Doesn't it seem a little crazy that people today have to re-engineer cupboards and dishwashers to fit their enormous plates? Using large plates can lead you to overeat because your eyes are used to seeing a certain amount of food on the plate; as a result, you fill up the plate to that capacity regardless of how big the plate actually is.

Watching portion sizes

Even if you switch high-glycemic foods for healthier low-glycemic options, you won't see the weight-loss results you want if you don't use appropriate portion sizes. Eating large portion sizes can hurt you in two ways:

- ✔ **Low-glycemic foods can become high-glycemic foods if you eat too much in one serving.** A food's low-glycemic measurement is based on a specific amount of food eaten, which is why the glycemic load is so important. The *glycemic load* shows how high the glycemic index is when you eat a very specific portion size. So, if you eat two servings of medium-glycemic pasta, that pasta can turn into a high-glycemic food. (See more about the glycemic load in Chapter 4.)

- ✔ **Larger portion sizes equal higher calories.** If you don't burn the calories you consume, your body will store them as fat. It doesn't matter if the foods are low glycemic, high glycemic, or somewhere in between — they still add up to calories. (Check out the section "Knowing that calories still count when you want to lose weight" for more details.)

Flip to Chapter 4 for more information about using correct portion sizes as you plan low-glycemic meals.

Sticking to the right number of servings each day

Your ideal daily calorie level depends on your metabolism, height, weight, gender, and a whole slew of other factors. However, simply knowing how much of each food group you should be eating each day can help you control your overall calorie intake. For instance, if you know a serving of rice is about ½ cup, you also know that eating 2 cups raises your calorie level and counts as four servings of grains rather than just one. This information alone can be very helpful when you're deciding how much to eat.

The United States Department of Agriculture (USDA) provides the MyPyramid guide to demonstrate how much you should be eating of each food group per day. You can get details at www.mypyramid.gov/index.html. Here's a quick guide of what you should aim for:

- ✔ 1½ to 2 cups of fruits and 2½ to 3 cups of vegetables
- ✔ 6 to 8 servings of grains (mostly low glycemic), like ½ cup of rice or pasta, 1 slice of bread, or 1 cup of cereal

✔ 3 servings of lowfat dairy, like 1 cup of milk or yogurt, ¼ cup of cottage cheese, or 1½ ounces of cheese

✔ 5 to 6½ servings of protein (equivalent to 1 ounce per serving), like poultry, fish, or tofu

✔ 5 to 7 teaspoons of healthy oils and fats, like avocadoes, olive oil, or canola oil

✔ 100 to 300 "extra" calories from snacks and treats

Keep in mind that these guidelines aren't exact; they simply offer you some general recommendations on portion sizes. If you're a small woman who isn't very active, you want to stay toward the lower side of the recommendations. If you're an active male, you want to lean toward the higher side of the recommendations. If you aren't sure which recommendations are right for you, make an appointment with a registered dietitian to create a more specific meal plan.

Although the USDA MyPyramid guide doesn't specify the types of foods, try to stick to low-glycemic fruits, vegetables, and grains to get the most out of your diet plan.

Picking the Right Foods to Help You Lose More Weight

You may get the impression from the dieting world that you have to eat twigs and berries or tiny amounts of food to lose weight. We're here to tell you that just isn't true. If you want to lose weight and keep it off, the key is in how you balance your food choices. When you find the right balance, you can

✔ Enjoy all the foods you love without feeling restricted because no foods are off limits.

✔ Feel more satisfied throughout the day.

✔ Eat a good volume of food without going overboard in calories.

This section helps you pick the right foods to achieve this perfect balance.

A perfect meal includes a moderate amount of a low-glycemic grain (see Chapter 4 for more about such grains), a fruit or vegetable, a lean protein, and a small amount of unsaturated fats, whether you add them or they're found in your protein source.

Eating your fruits and vegetables (Just like your mother told you!)

Fruits and especially vegetables are low in calories, high in fiber, and high in nutrients. They're mostly low glycemic, too. As a matter of fact, most vegetables aren't even tested for glycemic index or load because the amounts of carbohydrates in them are so low.

When you want to lose weight, you can either eat tiny portions of high-calorie/ high-glycemic foods, or you can pump up the volume with fruits and vegetables and still maintain a lower calorie level. After all, a serving of vegetables has only 25 calories, and a serving of fruit contains only about 60 calories. What this little tidbit means for you is that you can up your vegetables during the day to get more volume and more fiber to help you feel full longer for far fewer calories than many other foods, including those that are low glycemic. (We discuss the benefits of fiber in the earlier section "Including fiber in your daily menu.")

To see what we mean, consider the following:

- 1 cup of steamed carrots = 50 calories
- 1 cup of fruit = 60 calories
- 1 cup of pasta = 160 calories
- 1 cup of 2% milk = 140 calories

The biggest issue with weight loss in the United States is that the plates are all messed up! People tend to eat more meats and starches and then add just small amounts of fruits and vegetables. Switch that trend around and you have a very successful weight-loss strategy. After all, fruits and vegetables are not only low in calories but are also crucial for providing important vitamins, minerals, and antioxidants that protect you from chronic diseases like heart disease, cancer, and type 2 diabetes (see Chapter 2 for details).

To take this idea one step further, we want to demonstrate how simply switching around your plate can save you calories and help keep your blood sugar from spiking too high. The following examples illustrate some quick swaps you can make to your meals that will set you on the path for success-ful weight loss (see Chapter 4 for more on glycemic load):

Breakfast

Before the switch: Large plain bagel with cream cheese = 464 calories (high glycemic load)

After the switch: 2 poached eggs with one slice of whole-wheat toast with 1 teaspoon of butter and a banana = 397 calories (medium glycemic load)

Total savings: 67 calories and a lower glycemic load

Lunch

Before the switch: Deli roast beef sandwich with mayonnaise on a white bun with a small bag of potato chips = 628 calories (high glycemic load)

After the switch: Half of a roast beef sandwich with mayonnaise on a white bun with a side salad and 1 tablespoon of vinaigrette salad dressing = 472 calories (medium glycemic load)

Total savings: 156 calories and a lower glycemic load

Dinner

Before the switch: 4 ounces of grilled garlic chicken served over 1½ cups of pasta = 345 calories (high glycemic load)

After the switch: 4 ounces of grilled lemon chicken over ½ cup of quinoa with 2 cups of steamed broccoli and red bell peppers = 260 calories (low glycemic load)

Total savings: 85 calories and a lower glycemic load

Dessert

Before the switch: 1 cup of ice cream with chocolate sauce = 440 calories (low glycemic load)

After the switch: ½ cup of ice cream with ½ cup of fresh sliced strawberries = 230 calories (low glycemic load)

Total savings: 210 calories

As you look at the preceding examples, notice that you can eat a lot more food for fewer calories when you incorporate more fruits and vegetables into your meals. Now you may be thinking, "There isn't a huge saving in calories for each meal," but by making these simple changes, you save 518 calories, which is enough to help you lose a pound a week. Think of it this way: By making a few simple shifts toward eating more fruits and vegetables in place of your meat and grain servings, you can easily lose those extra pounds without starving yourself or making drastic changes in your diet or life.

If you aren't used to eating a lot of fruits and veggies, you can explore new fruits and vegetables (or new ways of preparing them) with the recipes in Chapters 12 and 13. For full-on vegetarian meals, check out Chapter 18. Even if you like only a handful of vegetables, try to find different ways to prepare them so you eat more of them. You'll be amazed not only by how good you feel but also by how much easier it is to lose weight.

Including protein

Choosing lean protein sources to include in your meals is essential for good health as well as weight loss. Examples of lean protein include lean cuts of beef and pork, white meat of poultry, fish, eggs, soy, and beans. At the same time, you need to limit your intake of higher-fat cuts of meat, like chicken wings or rib-eye steak; they can easily add up in calories as well as saturated fat. (See Chapter 7 for more on the best cuts of meat for a low-glycemic diet.) Balancing each meal with protein-rich foods can help you feel more satisfied and help your body repair tissue, which is one of protein's main functions.

Meats and animal protein, like beef, poultry, eggs, and fish, don't have a glycemic level because they don't contain any carbohydrates (if they do, it's less than 1 gram). On the other hand, some plant-based proteins, like beans and nuts, do contain carbohydrates and have glycemic levels. You need to consider the glycemic levels of these proteins when calculating the glycemic levels of your meals. For example, if you're having rice with beans for dinner, although the beans offer protein, you need to consider both the rice and the beans in that meal's glycemic level because they both contain carbohydrates. (The good news is that a serving of beans — about ½ cup — is typically low glycemic.)

Aim to incorporate 2 to 4 ounces of protein-rich foods into each meal. Don't worry if one meal is a little lower, like if you decide to have only one ounce of nuts on top of your oatmeal for breakfast. You can just add a little more protein to your lunch and dinner meals for that day. Remember that these are general guidelines; depending on your needs, you may want to schedule some time with a registered dietitian to get a more personalized plan.

Sticking to a "good" fat diet rather than a lowfat diet

Lowfat diets were once a popular trend in the weight-loss world, and although fat is still an important nutrient to consider, you don't have to buy everything lowfat to lose weight. Fat does provide more calories per gram than protein and carbohydrates (9 versus 4), but the food industry and diet world may have gone a bit overboard in their lowfat recommendations.

Believe it or not, fat can actually help you lose weight by helping you feel fuller after your meals. Important fatty acids like omega-3s can also improve your overall mood and anxiety, which is definitely a plus for all the emotional eaters out there. Using both monounsaturated fats and omega-3 fatty acids in the appropriate serving sizes (typically 5 to 7 teaspoons each day) can also help you prevent heart disease and strokes, which is especially important for those of you who have a family history of these diseases.

In general, nutrition professionals recommend that you get 30 percent of your daily total calories from fat. Keep in mind, though, if you have a health condition like heart disease, your doctor may recommend less. The trick is to use primarily "good" fats in your diet and stay away from less healthy fats like saturated and trans fats.

Good fats include unsaturated fats you find in foods like

- ✔ Avocados
- ✔ Canola oil
- ✔ Nuts and seeds
- ✔ Olive oil and olives
- ✔ Peanut oil

Omega-3 fatty acids are found in

- ✔ Black walnuts
- ✔ Canola oil
- ✔ Fatty fish like salmon
- ✔ Flaxseeds
- ✔ Sardines

The saturated fats and trans fats you need to limit in your diet are found in

- ✔ High-fat meats like rib-eye steak, pork sausage, or chicken wings
- ✔ Whole-fat dairy products like whole-fat milk or whole-fat yogurt
- ✔ Packaged foods made with saturated fats or hydrogenated oils like certain frozen meals or cookies
- ✔ Margarines made with hydrogenated oils

Beware of commercial lowfat products. Your main goal should be to find the right balance of fats, calories, and overall sugar. Many lowfat products, especially cookies and pastries, simply increase the sugar content to decrease the fat content. For example, compare two blueberry muffins from Starbucks:

- ✔ **Regular blueberry muffin:** 380 calories, 19 grams of fat, and 28 grams of sugar
- ✔ **Lowfat blueberry muffin:** 430 calories, 2.5 grams of fat, and 57 grams of sugar

Yes, the lowfat muffin has much less fat than the regular muffin, but it's also higher in calories and contains double the amount of sugar. Eating the lowfat muffin won't really help you with your weight-loss efforts; in fact, it could actually make things worse because of its higher calorie level and higher glycemic load (see Chapter 4 for more on glycemic load).

Note: The recipes in this book primarily use lean meats and healthy fats. The saturated fats used are always in small quantities to keep the recipes true to our recommendations.

Making the Most of Your Metabolic Makeup

Have you ever been following the same exact diet as your spouse or some of your friends only to watch them lose more weight than you? Well, don't fret. They didn't lose more weight because they followed the diet better than you. They just have a speedier metabolism than you do.

Your *basal metabolic rate* (often simply called *metabolic rate*) is how many calories your body burns at rest. Each time you breathe, eat, or even sleep, your body uses energy by burning calories. In the following sections, we describe factors that influence metabolic rate, explain how to use your rate in your weight-loss plan, give you pointers on boosting your metabolic rate, and note the connection between metabolism and resistant starches.

Recognizing factors that affect your metabolic rate

The following factors influence your metabolic rate:

- ✔ **Age:** By the time you reach adulthood, around 25 years of age, your metabolic rate begins to decrease by about 2 to 5 percent every decade. You may not feel these effects in your 30s, but by the time you reach your 40s and 50s, you'll likely find yourself wondering why you gain weight so much more easily than you did when you were young.

- ✔ **Environment:** For those of you who live in an area that's very cold or very hot, you may have an edge over people who live in moderate climates. Why? Because your body naturally requires more calories to normalize body temperature when you're cold or hot. So if you endure the long winters of the Midwest or the hot summers of the Southwest, you can at least get some benefits!

- ✔ **Gender:** Ever wonder why men always seem to lose weight easier than women do? Well, genetically they have more muscle mass than women, and the more muscle you have, the higher your metabolic rate. Women also tend to store more fat than muscle as a natural reserve for pregnancy and breast-feeding.

- ✔ **Genetics:** Your genetic makeup and the shape of your body can affect your metabolic rate. For example, someone with a tall, thin frame may experience more heat loss than someone with a short, petite build, resulting in a higher metabolic rate to maintain normal temperature.

- ✔ **Health:** Many health conditions, such as hypothyroidism and other diseases that can lead to hypothyroidism, like polycystic ovarian disease, can affect your metabolic rate.

Putting your metabolic rate to use for weight loss

Knowing your metabolic rate, or how many calories you burn at rest each day, can be a helpful tool for weight loss because it gives you an idea of how many calories you need to eat per day to lose weight. For example, if you burn 1,400 calories at rest each day and you burn 500 calories during other activities, you burn a total of 1,900 calories each day. To lose half a pound to one full pound each week, you would need to make a 250- to 500-calorie deficit each day, bringing you to a range of 1,400 to 1,650 calories a day. (See the earlier section "Keeping Calories under Control" for more details.)

You can do several calculations to determine your average metabolic rate, but the only way to get a truly accurate reading is to do a test using *indirect calorimetry,* which measures respiratory gases to see just what you're burning. Some registered dietitians and gyms can do this test for you.

When you're trying to lose weight, we always recommend focusing on lifestyle goals, such as increasing exercise and making changes in your food choices and portion sizes, but just knowing the numbers can also be helpful. Not necessarily because we want you to count calories, but because you need to know if you have a very low metabolic rate for one reason or another. If your rate is super low, you may struggle a lot to lose weight. For example, imagine that your metabolic rate with activity is only 1,600 calories and you have to reduce your calorie level to 1,100 to 1,350 calories a day to lose half a pound to one full pound a week. That calorie range is pretty low and would be very restrictive, so we'd recommend that you put most of your focus on strategies to increase your metabolic rate instead of cutting calories (see the next section for details on how to do so).

Boosting your metabolic rate

The good news about your metabolic rate is that you can increase it at any time by following a few simple strategies. (Remember that holistic approach to weight loss we've mentioned before? These strategies are part of it.) Incorporating some of the following approaches will help you burn more calories so you can eat more and lose more:

> ✓ **Build lean muscle mass.** In the past, most weight-loss programs focused on burning calories with aerobic activity. Although aerobic exercise is important, you also need to build muscle at the same time. Muscle burns up to 90 percent more calories than fat. By adding 3 to 5 pounds of muscle, you can actually burn an estimated 100 to 250 additional calories a day. Weight lifting, resistance bands, walking, and strenuous yoga or Pilates are all activities that can help you build muscle.

✔ **Get your heart rate up.** Regular aerobic exercise that gets your heart rate pumping faster raises your metabolic rate during the activity and for several hours afterward. Participating in aerobic exercises, such as bike riding, jogging, brisk walking, swimming, and aerobic-style fitness classes, three or more times a week is a good strategy to follow.

✔ **Add up the small activities.** Any time you can increase your heart rate for even five minutes, you give your metabolic rate a small boost. Add up these five-minute chunks over the course of a day and you have yourself a successful strategy. Taking the stairs rather than the elevator, playing with your kids, walking, and dancing while you cook in your kitchen can all help you make the most of each day.

✔ **Avoid skipping meals.** These days, the increasingly popular on-the-run attitude makes it easy to skip meals; however, just because everyone else is doing it doesn't mean you should, too! The problem with regularly skipping meals is your body begins to compensate for the lack of incoming food by lowering your metabolic rate. Making time for your meals even if they're small goes a long way toward keeping your metabolic rate strong.

✔ **Eat enough calories.** Similar to skipping meals, if you regularly consume a very low number of calories, your body will go into starvation mode and lower your metabolic rate. Going too low in calories is often what makes people end up with rebound weight gain because their metabolic rates have decreased more than they realize. In most circumstances, maintaining a moderate calorie level is much more beneficial than trying to adhere to a very low calorie level. Avoid decreasing your calorie level below 1,200 a day.

Connecting metabolism to low-glycemic resistant starches

New research shows a connection between metabolism and the foods you eat, specifically food parts known as *resistant starches,* which are a type of fiber that "resists" being digested. Resistant starches ferment in the large intestine. We know it sounds gross, but it's actually a good thing! This fermentation process creates a beneficial fatty acid, called *butyrate,* which may block the body's ability to burn carbohydrates as its main source of fuel, causing it to burn stored fat instead. For this reason, resistant starches can be a great strategy in your weight-loss plan.

One particular study found that replacing just 5.4 percent of total carbohydrate intake with resistant starches created a 20- to 30-percent increase in fat burning after a meal.

The fatty acid butyrate has been shown to

- ✔ Increase your metabolic rate
- ✔ Decrease blood sugar and insulin responses
- ✔ Lower plasma cholesterol and triglycerides
- ✔ Increase feelings of fullness and reduce fat storage

The great news about resistant starches is that many of them are found in low-glycemic foods, making them a win-win food choice. The following list shares some common foods that contain these beneficial resistant starches and shows you some simple ways to enjoy them in your daily meal plan:

- ✔ **Beans:** Sprinkle kidney beans on a salad, snack on some hummus, or enjoy our Chunky Salsa with Black Beans and Tomatoes with a few tortilla chips (see Chapter 10 for the recipe).

- ✔ **Corn:** Add corn to a taco salad, or enjoy our Chunky Salsa with Black Beans and Tomatoes (see Chapter 10 for the recipe).

- ✔ **Pearl barley:** Prepare the Barley with Zucchini, Tomatoes, and Basil recipe found in Chapter 14, and serve it cold rather than hot.

- ✔ **Slightly green bananas:** Slice bananas in your cereal in the morning, or dip them in our Orange Cream Fruit Dip (see Chapter 10 for the recipe).

- ✔ **Yams:** Bake yams in 1-inch chunks, and refrigerate them for a quick snack.

One important note is that you have to eat resistant starches at room temperature or cold to get their full benefits; cooling a food with resistant starches after you cook it can increase its resistant starch content.

Part II

Creating a Healthy Lifestyle with Low-Glycemic Cooking

The 5th Wave   By Rich Tennant

MAKING HEALTHY SUBSTITUTIONS AT MEAL TIME.

In this part . . .

Knowing the glycemic load of certain foods is the first step you need to take to follow the glycemic index diet, but how do you fully incorporate it into your day-to-day life? This part dives into the practical tasks of meal planning, grocery shopping, and cooking. We know your life is busy, so we even show you how to incorporate low-glycemic convenience foods into your meal plans, as well as how to schedule time to cook recipes from this book.

Complete with meal-planning strategies, sample meal plans, low-glycemic cooking skills, tips on stocking your kitchen, and our personal grocery store tour, this part will help you start making — and eating — the recipes in this book with ease.

Chapter 4

Using the Glycemic Load to Create Meal-Planning Strategies

*T*he glycemic index is a great tool to use for choosing the best carbohydrates to eat on a daily basis. However, the glycemic index does have some limitations, specifically when it comes to how much of a food you can eat. In the past, many diet gurus recommended that people should simply avoid high-glycemic foods and eat only low-glycemic foods. This method seemed simple enough, but it wasn't as cut and dry as the gurus made it sound because they were judging the food on unrealistic portion sizes, giving many healthy fruits and vegetables a bad rap.

Portion size is where many of the early recommendations about the glycemic index fell short. The glycemic index requires human clinical tests with a very specific amount of food (the amount depends on the food being tested; see the section "Simplifying the Glycemic Index with the Glycemic Load" for details). So, even if a food ends up having a high glycemic index during its test, it may not maintain that label if you eat a smaller portion than what was tested. After all, a smaller portion means fewer carbohydrates. To give portion size the attention it deserves and to make the glycemic index more useful for dieters and lifestyle changers, researchers came up with the glycemic load.

While the glycemic index shows you the quality of a carbohydrate (in other words, how quickly your blood sugar will rise after you eat it), the *glycemic load* breaks that carbohydrate down into quantities you would typically eat, turning some previously taboo foods like carrots back into healthy choices. This chapter explores more details about the glycemic load and explains how to incorporate load information into your daily meal choices.

Simplifying the Glycemic Index with the Glycemic Load

The glycemic load is based on the fact that a smaller amount of a high-glycemic food will illicit the same blood sugar response as a low-glycemic food. Because the glycemic load represents the real portion sizes you would typically eat, it's a much better tool for you to use in your daily food choices than the glycemic index. Plus, it gives you more food choices — and no one wants to step in the way of more food choices! In the following sections, we explain how the glycemic load works, tell you how to calculate it, define different load categories, and show you the differences between the loads of various foods.

Defining the glycemic load

To measure the glycemic index of a given food, test subjects eat the amount of that food that supplies 50 grams of carbohydrates, which is the standard amount at which all foods are compared. Although the number of carbohydrate grams in each food tested is the same, the total amounts of food vary. For example, 50 grams of carbohydrates from bread is about three to four slices (depending on the bread), while 50 grams of carbohydrates from carrots is about a pound! Obviously, this 50-gram serving doesn't depict the amount of food people normally eat. This inconsistency is the reason why many nutrition experts have criticized the glycemic index over the years.

To address this issue, Harvard University's Dr. Walter Willet created the glycemic load in the late 1990s. The glycemic load adds the quantity of carbohydrates eaten at a meal to the calculation, which comes in handy because you're probably never going to sit down and eat an enormous amount of food, like a pound of carrots, at one time. (This is one of those don't-try-this-at-home moments. We're seriously afraid you might turn orange if you did!)

Check out Table 4-1 to get a better idea of the average amount of carbohydrates in each food group based on portion size.

Table 4-1	Average Carbohydrate Grams in Four Food Groups	
Food Group	*Carbohydrate Grams*	*Portion Size*
Starches	15	½ cup pasta; 1 slice bread; ⅓ cup rice
Fruits	15	1 small piece
Dairy products	12	1 cup lowfat milk; 1 cup lowfat yogurt
Non-starchy vegetables	5	½ cup cooked; 1 cup raw

Here's an example to help you sort out the info in Table 4-1: As you can see, the amount of carbohydrates found in ⅓ cup of rice (15 grams) is three times the amount you'd find in a serving of cooked vegetables (5 grams). So eating 50 grams of carbohydrates from cooked carrots would be about 5 cups, an amount you're not likely to eat, but eating 50 grams of carbohydrates from rice would be slightly more than 1½ cups, an amount you could easily eat. So you see, how a food affects your blood sugar depends on how much of it you eat. In the end, the glycemic load for the rice doesn't change too much from the glycemic index measurement. But the carrots are another story: Because you eat far less than the pound of carrots used in the glycemic index testing, carrots turn into a food with a low glycemic load when you actually eat them during a meal.

Calculating a food's glycemic load

Calculating the glycemic load for a particular food isn't too difficult as long as you have a few pieces of key information, namely the glycemic index of that food item and the grams of carbohydrates found in that food.

Here's the basic formula for calculating glycemic load:

Glycemic index × Grams of carbohydrates ÷ 100

Consider carrots as an example. They have about 8.6 grams of carbohydrates for a ½-cup serving and a glycemic index of 45 (feel free to round your numbers for simplicity). Plugging these numbers into the glycemic load formula gives you

$45 \times 8.6 \div 100 = 3.9$ glycemic load

Compare the carrots to instant white rice, which has more carbohydrate grams. A portion of about ⅔ cup of rice has about 36 grams of carbohydrates and a glycemic index of 72. Plugging these numbers into the glycemic load formula gives you

$72 \times 36 \div 100 = 26$ glycemic load

As you can see, the rice ends up with a much higher glycemic load than a serving of carrots.

Appendix A works out the glycemic load for many common foods for you. In case you're wondering, the recipes found in this book primarily use foods with a low to medium glycemic load.

Categorizing glycemic load measurements

Similar to the glycemic index, the glycemic load has its own measurements so you can easily tell whether a food has a low, medium, or high glycemic load. The measurements for glycemic load are

 ✔ **Low:** 10 or less

 ✔ **Medium:** 11 to 19

 ✔ **High:** 20 or more

Using the preceding calculations for carrots and instant white rice (the examples from the preceding section), you can see that carrots end up with a low glycemic load, meaning you just added another food to your good-to-go list! Instant white rice, on the other hand, ends up being a high glycemic load food, meaning you need to eat it in moderation.

Sometimes you won't be able to find glycemic loads for certain foods, so you won't know whether the foods are low, medium, or high. A good rule of thumb is to keep in mind the amount of carbohydrates in that food. Non-starchy vegetables, like broccoli, cauliflower, and asparagus, have very few carbohydrates and will always end up being low. In fact, most vegetables aren't even tested because of this fact. Dairy products also have fewer carbohydrates, especially for the serving size you typically consume. The foods that do contain more carbohydrates, and are therefore affected more by the glycemic index, are the starchy carbohydrates, like rice, bread, pasta, and potatoes.

Seeing how the glycemic load varies with different foods

Although you may think vegetables and higher-fiber foods always have lower glycemic loads than other types of food, they don't. For instance, you may think that a baked potato would have a medium to low glycemic load. After all, it's a vegetable and has a large amount of fiber. However, a russet potato has a very high glycemic load at 26. On the flip side, you may assume waffles would have a high glycemic load, with their flour content and low fiber, but they actually have a glycemic load of 10, which is considered low.

Foods like potatoes and waffles are what make glycemic loads so important. Years ago, people just assumed that all foods that contained complex carbohydrates (starchy foods like breads, rice, and pasta) would impact your blood sugar less than simple-carbohydrate-containing foods. However, thanks to the glycemic load, scientists and dieters alike can see that those rules aren't necessarily always correct. Sometimes complex carbohydrates impact your blood sugar more than simple carbohydrates like table sugar.

Table 4-2 shows some examples of common foods with their portion sizes and glycemic loads for comparison.

TIP

If you don't see the food you're looking for in the table, go to www.nutrition data.com and plug the food you're looking for into the search box at the top-right corner of the page. After you select the category that best fits your food and hit Search, you can alter the portion size. This Web site gives you all the nutrient information about that food and the estimated glycemic load.

Table 4-2	The Glycemic Load of Some Popular Foods		
Food	*Portion Size*	*Glycemic Load*	*Glycemic Measurement Level*
Apple	1 small (120 grams)	6	Low
Baked beans	Around ⅔ cup (150 grams)	7	Low
Baked russet potato	1 medium (150 grams)	26	High
Banana	1 medium (120 grams)	12	Medium
Carrots	About ⅓ cup (80 grams)	3	Low
Cherries	½ cup (120 grams)	3	Low
Chickpeas	About ⅔ cup (150 grams)	8	Low
Cooked white rice	About ⅔ cup (150 grams)	20	High
Cracked-wheat bread	1 piece (30 grams)	11	Medium
Fettuccine noodles	About ¾ cup (180 grams)	18	Medium
Full-fat ice cream	Less than ¼ cup (50 grams)	8	Low
Grapes	½ cup (120 grams)	8	Low
Green peas	About ⅓ cup (80 grams)	3	Low
Linguine	About ¾ cup (180 grams)	23	High
Macaroni	About ¾ cup (180 grams)	23	High
Oat-bran bread	1 piece (30 grams)	9	Low
Orange	1 small (120 grams)	5	Low
Reduced-fat yogurt	A little more than ¾ cup (200 grams)	7	Low
Spaghetti	About ¾ cup (180 grams)	18	Medium
Steamed brown rice	About ¾ cup (150 grams)	16	Medium
Waffle	1 small (35 grams)	10	Low
White bagel	1 small (70 grams)	25	High

Starting to Incorporate Low-Glycemic Foods into Your Meals

After you understand how the glycemic load works, you need to slowly incorporate foods with low glycemic loads (also known generally as *low-glycemic foods*) into your daily routine. The first step in the process of switching to a low-glycemic diet is simply familiarizing yourself with lists of glycemic information so you can begin to see which foods are low glycemic and which ones are high. After a while, you'll know how the foods you enjoy rank. Turn to Appendix A, and take a look at the foods you typically eat to get familiar with which ones are low glycemic and which ones are high.

After you're familiar with the foods you can eat, you can start shopping and cooking! We always suggest making gradual changes to your diet so you can get used to new foods and new ways of balancing your plate instead of jumping into too many changes all at once. Here are some tips to get you started (see Chapters 5 through 7 for more guidelines).

- ✔ Make one or two substitutions by choosing a low-glycemic food to replace one of your "staple" high-glycemic foods.

- ✔ Make a grocery shopping list of some staples to have on hand (milk, eggs, and fruits are good examples).

- ✔ Look over some of the recipes in this book, pick a few you'd like to try, and add those ingredients to your shopping list.

- ✔ Cook a few new recipes this week, and gradually increase your low-glycemic foods as you go along.

- ✔ Keep a food record as you start your switch to a low-glycemic diet so you can see how you're progressing. Include the time you ate, the type and amount of food you ate, and descriptions of your hunger feelings and/or mood before, during, and after you ate.

Make sure you always use the glycemic load measurement (not the glycemic index) so you don't feel restricted from using foods that truly won't affect your blood sugar in a negative way as long as you use the right portion sizes. If you've used only the glycemic index in the past, you're sure to find the glycemic load very freeing. Although no foods are completely taboo when you're following a low-glycemic diet, it's nice to know that some old favorites won't give you quite the blood sugar and insulin spikes you may have imagined — as long as you eat smaller portions, of course. Here are a few high glycemic index foods that have low glycemic loads:

- ✔ Carrots
- ✔ Honey
- ✔ Kiwi

✔ Papaya

✔ Plain popcorn

✔ Plain scone (Watch out for calories, though; see Chapter 3 for more information about the importance of calories.)

✔ Pumpkin

✔ Waffles

✔ Watermelon

✔ White-flour bread

The great thing about using the glycemic index diet is that it's all about moderation. The research that's been done so far is mostly based on subjects who incorporate a percentage of low-glycemic foods into their diets, so you don't have to use an all-or-nothing approach here. In fact, we recommend that you don't! (See the next section for more details on incorporating the right balance into your diet.)

Finding the Perfect Balance at Meal Time

Throughout this book, we talk a lot about balance, which is one of the most important factors you need to think about when it comes to nutrition. By *balance,* we mean how to incorporate the right amount of each food group and nutrients into your meals. With the right balance of foods, you can

✔ Eat a good amount of food and not feel like you're depriving yourself.

✔ Eat fewer calories and manage your weight more effectively.

✔ Decrease hunger and food cravings.

✔ Increase the amount of vitamins, minerals, and antioxidants you eat for better health.

✔ Improve your energy and mood.

On the flip side, consuming unbalanced amounts of protein, fat, and carbohydrates can lead to

✔ An unstable blood sugar that can stimulate your appetite and lead you to eat more

✔ A cycle of food cravings

✔ Hunger

✔ Lack of concentration

- An increase in total calories
- Cycles of emotional eating due to hunger and moodiness

We aren't talking about a specific science here, just simply the way you put your plate together. You can literally eat the same foods; you just have to change the amounts and types of food groups you include in your meals. This section takes a closer look at how to balance your meals effectively.

Combining carbohydrates, protein, and fat

When you start planning meals, do you ever think about what types of food you're putting together, or do you simply put together the same meals you had growing up? For instance, do you automatically pair a large plate of spaghetti with tomato sauce and bread? Most people lean toward preparing foods the way their parents did. The same is often true with cultural ways of eating foods, too. For example, when you think of a Fourth of July barbeque, you likely think of burgers, hot dogs, potato salad, and watermelon. Well, it's time to spice things up a little bit, and, no, we don't mean adding pepper to your watermelon! What we're talking about here is achieving balance in your meals by combining the right foods.

For each meal, make sure you have a good source of low-glycemic carbohydrate, protein, and fat. Achieving this balance on a daily basis helps you get all the nutrients you need, stabilize your blood sugar, and feel satisfied and energized without stimulating your appetite.

Finding the right balance of carbohydrates, protein, and fat isn't difficult to do. In fact, you may already do it with many of your meals and just need to tweak your day-to-day routine a bit. Here are some quick guidelines to help you add more balance to your meals:

- Include a low- or medium-glycemic whole grain like quinoa or brown rice.
- Add a protein source through lean meats, nuts, dairy, eggs, or beans.
- If you don't already have fat in your meat or other food source, add some healthy fats through avocados, olives, and nuts.
- Have a fruit or vegetable with every meal.

Using appropriate portion sizes

Correctly combining carbohydrates, protein, and fat at every meal is an important step in achieving overall balance, but using the right portion sizes is also a key piece to your meal-planning puzzle. The glycemic load depends on a certain portion size; for example, if ½ cup of rice has a medium glycemic load, increasing it to 2 cups of rice will lead you into a high glycemic load. Also, if you eat too much of any food group, your calorie level will go up — not a good thing if you're trying to lose weight.

In general, you want larger portions of fruits and vegetables and smaller portions of grains, meats, fats, and dairy. Use Table 4-3 to help guide you during meal planning.

Table 4-3	**Portion Size Chart**
Food Category	*Recommended Portion Size for Various Items*
Grains	1 slice of bread
	½ of an English muffin, hamburger bun, or bagel (Hockey-puck size is what you're looking for here; watch out for those extra-large bagels!)
	½ cup of cooked cereal, pasta, or other cooked grain
	⅓ cup of rice
	¾ cup of cold cereal
	One 6-inch tortilla
Other starchy carbohydrates	½ cup of beans (which have a small amount of protein)
	½ cup of lentils (which also have a small amount of protein)
Fruits	1 medium piece of fruit
	½ cup of canned or sliced fruit
	6 ounces (¾ cup) of 100% fruit juice
Vegetables	1 cup of raw veggies
	½ cup of cooked veggies
	6 ounces (¾ cup) of 100% vegetable juice

(continued)

Table 4-3 *(continued)*

Food Category	Recommended Portion Size for Various Items
Dairy or soy products	8 ounces of milk or yogurt
	⅓ cup of cottage cheese
	1 ounce of cheese
Proteins	½ cup of beans (which are also high in carbohydrates)
	3 to 4 ounces (the size of a deck of cards) of beef, poultry, pork, or fish
	1 ounce of cheese
	1 egg
	1 ounce of nuts
	1 tablespoon of nut spread (such as peanut or almond butter)
Fats	⅛ (2 tablespoons) of avocado
	1 teaspoon of oil, butter, margarine, or mayonnaise
	2 teaspoons of whipped butter
	8 olives
	1 tablespoon of regular salad dressing
	2 tablespoons of lowfat salad dressing

Portions can make a really big difference in how your meal affects your body. Consider this high-glycemic sample meal:

Protein: 12-ounce rib-eye steak

Grain: 2 cups of brown rice

Vegetable/fat: 1 cup of mixed greens salad with 1 tablespoon of salad dressing

Total calories/glycemic load: 1,335 calories; the higher portion of brown rice gives this meal a high glycemic load

All you have to do to make this meal lower glycemic and lower calorie is change the portion sizes as we do here (notice that we keep the same exact food items):

> **Protein:** 5-ounce rib-eye steak
>
> **Grain:** ⅔ cup of brown rice
>
> **Vegetable/fat:** 2 cups of mixed greens salad with 1 tablespoon of salad dressing
>
> **Total calories/glycemic load:** 655 calories; the smaller portion of brown rice gives this meal a medium glycemic load

You can see what a drastic difference portion sizes can make to the outcome of your meal. Simply by changing the portion sizes of the exact same foods, you save about 680 calories and make this meal medium glycemic so you don't experience such a large blood sugar spike after eating it. Plus, you get an extra load of vitamins, minerals, and antioxidants from the increased salad portion.

Making the balancing act easy with the plate method

One thing we're almost certain about is that you don't want to sit around and measure your food all day to make sure you're eating the right portion sizes. Lucky for you (and us), you don't have to be exact with your portions to achieve the right balance in your meals; you just have to be close.

To help you eat the right balance of foods and the right portion sizes at each meal, we recommend using the *plate method*. The idea behind the plate method is to fill your plate with the good-for-you, lower-calorie foods and limit the higher-calorie foods. According to the plate method, you should fill half of your plate with fruits and/or veggies, one-quarter with a protein source (such as meat, fish, or poultry), and one-quarter with a low-glycemic grain (such as barley or whole-grain bread). Figure 4-1 provides a template of the plate method for you to follow.

When people overeat, they tend to do so with starchy carbohydrates (like pasta, potatoes, and rice) and meats (like beef, poultry, and fish). These foods also contain more calories than low-glycemic fruits and veggies and can increase your blood sugar and saturated fat intake. Using the plate method gives you better control over these higher-calorie food groups and increases your intake of plant-based foods like fruits, vegetables, and beans, which you need to keep you healthy and reduce your risk of disease.

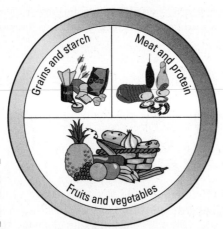

Figure 4-1:
The plate method.

The plate method is most effective when you use plates that are about the size of a standard paper plate — not the gigantic plates you find in today's markets. If you have a dish set that contains large dinner plates, medium salad plates, and small dessert plates, use the middle plate rather than the large one for your meals.

Aiming for a glycemic load of less than 25 for your meals

The good thing about a low-glycemic diet is that you don't have to track glycemic loads and other food-related numbers to be successful. But for those of you who like to track numbers and can't get enough of your calculator, feel free to keep track of the glycemic loads of all your meals. A good guideline is to consume a maximum glycemic load of 25 per meal. This load provides you good variety and also keeps your portion sizes in check. Here's an example of what a less-than-25-load meal might look like with recipes found in this book:

 2 cups of Fresh Garden Salad with Avocado and Lemon Vinaigrette (found in Chapter 12; estimated glycemic load = 1)

 5-ounce Marinated Sirloin Steak (found in Chapter 16; estimated glycemic load = 0)

 ⅔ cup of Quinoa with Veggies and Toasted Pine Nuts (found in Chapter 14; estimated glycemic load = 9)

You can have this entire meal, which features a grain (the quinoa), a protein (the steak), plenty of veggies, and some fat from the salad's avocado, for an estimated glycemic load of 10. Not too shabby! See what happens when you load up on veggies, which really don't affect your blood sugar too much, and hold back on the fat and grains?

For all you egg lovers out there, here's a less-than-25-load breakfast example:

Asiago Cheese and Tomato Omelet (found in Chapter 8; estimated glycemic load = 4)

1 slice of whole-wheat toast with 1 teaspoon of butter (estimated glycemic load = 6)

The fact that you can get an entire meal for a glycemic load of only 10 — far less than a glycemic load of 25 — proves you won't feel cheated from eating low-glycemic meals.

Keeping moderation in mind

You don't have to be perfect to follow a low-glycemic lifestyle. In fact, moderation often works better than rigidity. Incorporating all types of foods, including medium- and high-glycemic foods, into your new healthy lifestyle is easy to do.

Although moderation is an important concept to grasp when you're working toward a low-glycemic lifestyle, its definition can be a little unclear. For example, you may consider eating a small amount of a high-glycemic food with each meal to be moderation, but doing so may, in fact, be enough to cause blood sugar spikes, especially if you're diabetic or insulin resistant (see Chapter 2 for more about these conditions).

Here are a few quick guidelines to help you understand what we mean by *moderation:*

✔ Eat medium-glycemic foods once or twice a day or less.

✔ Eat high-glycemic foods two to three times a week or less.

By following these guidelines, you can eat all foods without restrictions and still keep up with your healthy, low-glycemic lifestyle. Keep in mind, though, that you won't ruin all your efforts if you occasionally end up eating three medium-glycemic foods in one day.

To help you balance all types of food in your diet, follow these tips:

✔ **Avoid eating multiple high-glycemic foods in one meal.** Indulge in one item at a time rather than several. For example, if you're at a barbeque, go for the hamburger bun in place of the potato salad, or skip the bun, get grilled chicken, and have the potato salad.

✔ **Consume smaller portions of high-glycemic foods.** Portion size matters when it comes to glycemic load (see the section "Using appropriate portion sizes" for details). Eating less of a typically high-glycemic food lowers the glycemic load for that particular meal. So eating ½ cup of rice instead of a full cup can make a big difference.

✔ **Split the portion size of two high-glycemic foods.** Imagine being at a party and seeing several of your favorite dishes on the food table; unfortunately, they're all high glycemic. To help you stick to your low-glycemic diet without depriving yourself, you can simply choose smaller portions of your two favorites and decrease your overall glycemic load for that meal.

Don't let your dietary guidelines become strict rules that you force yourself to follow every day. If you do, the rigidity will sabotage your efforts in the end. Instead, focus on making sure your meal plan follows the guidelines most of the time. Believe it or not, this task is actually easier than you may think because so many foods (like fruits, veggies, meats, and some fats) are low glycemic. All you really have to do is make some new choices with your grains and a few starchy vegetables and, of course, watch your portion sizes. Even then, you can still enjoy some of the higher-glycemic foods in moderation by following some of the guidelines we offer earlier in this section.

Use the recipes in this book to help you find some new favorites to add to your weekly meals. You may even discover ways to change some of your old recipes to make them lower glycemic (we provide some pointers in Chapter 5). Don't stress out by trying to follow a strict diet because you can reap all the same benefits with a moderate and much more enjoyable approach.

Chapter 5

Getting the Hang of Low-Glycemic Meal Planning

In This Chapter

▶ Alternating cooking with creating quick meals

▶ Giving your old high-glycemic recipes a new low-glycemic look

▶ Easing into low-glycemic meal planning with sample menus

A s we mention throughout this book, moderation and balance are key to finding success with a low-glycemic diet. You don't have to be perfect, and you certainly don't have to do heavy cooking all day every day. In this chapter, we explain the benefits of both cooking from scratch and pulling together fast meals, provide pointers on turning high-glycemic favorites into low-glycemic options, and show you a sample weeklong menu that fits into a low-glycemic plan.

Cooking versus Pulling Together Quick Meals: You Can Do Both!

Don't you just love diet and health books with meal plans that require you to cook full meals for breakfast, lunch, and dinner every day? Back in the real world, most people have busy schedules and simply don't have the time or energy to cook all day long.

If you look at your current habits, you probably do a mix of quick pull-together meals along with some actual cooking. You may overlook the division between cooking and pulling together quick meals, but we see it as a huge saboteur in the dieting and nutrition world. You see, if a diet of any kind doesn't work in their lifestyles, most people will just give up altogether. After all, people are creatures of habit. So, for example, if you're used to eating cereal for breakfast, following a meal plan that includes large cooked breakfasts every day probably isn't going to work for you. It's just not practical.

Luckily, in our version of a low-glycemic diet, it's perfectly fine for you to cook from scratch (when you have the time) *and* pull items together for a fast meal (when your schedule is jam-packed). This section goes into more detail about both options.

Scheduling time to cook full recipes

Let's face it: Cooking takes time, which we're sure can be a challenge to find in your busy world. It's easy to see why cooking so easily falls to the wayside when you have convenience foods, takeout, and fast food that are always there when you need them. And how many times have you bought fruits and vegetables with no real plan as to when or how you're going to cook them and, instead of eating them, wound up with a science experiment in your refrigerator? This scenario is more common than you may think.

If you want to incorporate more low-glycemic foods and recipes into your lifestyle (and we're guessing you do since you bought this book), we recommend that you do a little planning for your week so you can cook when time allows and don't end up wasting food. For example, before you buy that head of broccoli at the grocery store, decide that it's going in the stir-fry you're making on Tuesday or that you're having it as a steamed side dish with your burgers on Friday. This bit of planning not only saves you money on wasted food but also ensures that you're getting the health benefits of eating all the low-glycemic foods you buy.

To begin scheduling time to cook, follow these tips:

- ✔ **Sit down during the weekend and think about the events that are taking place during the week ahead.** If you have your kids' soccer match on Wednesday evening, don't plan to cook a big meal that night. Instead, plan a big meal the night before so you have leftovers ready to go after the match.

- ✔ **When you're looking at recipes for the coming week, consider the amount and type of prep and cooking time that's involved so you can make sure you have plenty of time in your schedule to make them.** For instance, you may see that a recipe like the Roasted Red-Skinned Potatoes with Shallots in Chapter 14 takes 10 minutes of prep time and about 45 minutes of cooking time. Although it seems like a lot of time, this recipe is one of our favorite sides to make when we're pretty short on time because all you have to do is cut up your potatoes and shallots, melt some butter in some oil, and throw them in the oven. Such recipes are great when you're going to be around the house but don't want to mess with a lot of time in the kitchen.

  On the other hand, you may have very little time for both prep and cook time during a particular week. In that case, you need to choose recipes that don't require much time to prepare, like the Grilled Salmon with Maple Glaze in Chapter 17. (Grilled recipes and salads are usually a safe bet in short-on-time situations.)

✔ **Cook more than you need for any recipe so you have leftovers for lunch or dinner the next day.** For soups, stews, and chilies (like the ones in Chapter 11), you can freeze them in individual freezer containers and have frozen meals when you're really in a hurry. You may even like to set aside a day to prepare quite a few meals to put in the freezer.

The important thing is to find the scheduling methods that work for you and your lifestyle so that cooking low-glycemic recipes becomes part of your normal routine and not a never-ending struggle.

Discovering some quick pull-together meals for those extra-busy days

Like just about everyone we've ever talked to, you probably have days and nights when you just don't have time to cook a full recipe. Believe it or not, those extra-busy days and nights don't mean you have to succumb to junk food, fast food, or takeout (although doing so once in a while isn't a big deal, even in a low-glycemic diet). Instead of relying on someone else to whip you up something fast, you can keep some basic food items on hand so you can pull together a quick low-glycemic meal whenever you're short on time or low on food supplies.

Here are some of our favorite low- to medium-glycemic pull-together meals for those super-busy days:

✔ **Poached eggs and toast:** For breakfast, poach an egg in the microwave for 1 minute (in other words, fill a small teacup halfway with water and crack an egg into the water). Add some toast and fruit, and you've got a great start to your day.

✔ **Cold cereal:** Let's face it, many of you are very used to eating cold cereal in the morning. This option works fine as long as you choose a low- to medium-glycemic cereal like bran flakes, Cheerios, or Special K. Add some fresh or frozen berries, a sprinkle of slivered almonds, and lowfat milk.

✔ **Grilled cheese sandwich and tomato soup:** Who doesn't love this old favorite — especially because it's in line with a low-glycemic diet just the way it is? (In case you're curious, the soup and cheese are low glycemic and the bread is medium.) This simple go-to meal works great when you need something quick, especially when you're in desperate need of a grocery run!

✔ **Grilled or roasted chicken over mixed greens:** All you need for this simple meal are mixed greens and some precooked chicken. You can either use leftover chicken from earlier in the week or pick up some already-grilled or roasted chicken from your local grocery store. Add some extra veggies or fruit, and top it off with a tablespoon of your favorite salad dressing.

- ✔ **Quick bean and cheese burrito:** Take a tortilla, throw in some black beans, cheese, and any leftover veggies you have in your fridge, and then warm everything in the microwave for about 30 seconds. This no-fuss version of a burrito is great when you're craving Mexican food but don't have a lot of time.

- ✔ **Rice and beans:** Black beans and brown rice make a quick and yummy dish, especially if you have some veggies, like tomatoes and bell peppers, lying around your kitchen. Add 1 tablespoon of shredded cheese, and prepare to be amazed by how good this basic meal tastes.

- ✔ **Salmon over mixed greens:** You may not have tried prepackaged salmon yet, but you can find it right next to the canned tuna fish in your local grocery store. It's often sold in a plastic pouch or canned. Keep a pack of salmon handy so you can throw it on a salad with extra veggies and avocado whenever you're in the mood for a quick and delicious meal for lunch or dinner.

- ✔ **Soup and salad:** Whether you have some leftover frozen soup or canned soup, you can make up a great low-glycemic meal in minutes. We recommend keeping a bag of fresh, prewashed greens in your fridge so you can make a simple salad to go along with your soup (or just about any other meal you decide to make).

If you want to be a little more adventurous than canned soup, take a look at what leftovers you have in your fridge . . . barley and a little chicken? Cut up the chicken, toss in the barley, add some frozen veggies and vegetable or chicken broth, and add a dash of your favorite herbs . . . voila! You have yourself a tasty soup!

Sprucing Up Your Favorite Recipes to Fit a Low-Glycemic Diet

Whether your favorite family recipes include your grandmother's lasagna or a simple dish of homemade macaroni and cheese, we're here to help you incorporate them into your low-glycemic diet. For those recipes that are high glycemic but too cherished to change, we encourage you to eat them as they are but to do so less frequently and with smaller portions. If you don't mind a little change in some of your favorites, though, you can make subtle modifications to your recipes to turn them into delicious low-glycemic meals.

One of the first steps you need to take when adopting a low-glycemic lifestyle is to take a look at the foods and recipes you typically eat. Many of them may already be low glycemic and don't need any changes, but others may require a little tweaking before you can add them to your regular menu.

Tips for dining out the low-glycemic way

Restaurant portion sizes are growing rapidly — so much so that you can't even recognize a normal-sized serving anymore. In fact, normal portion sizes look tiny compared to what you see when you're out to eat. For example, a normal portion of pasta is half a cup. Can you imagine getting a plate of pasta at a restaurant that small? The average restaurant portion size is big enough to feed three adults, which definitely gives you your money's worth but at what cost?

Science explains that the more you see, the more you eat, so, in the long run, you're likely to spend the money you saved by eating extra-large portions at restaurants on your health. After all, studies have found a direct correlation between eating out, higher caloric intakes, and higher body weights. Here are some tips to help you keep your restaurant portions in check and have better control over your calorie level and glycemic load:

✔ **Don't clean your plate.** Remember when your parents made you sit at the dinner table until you cleaned your plate? Well, now's the time to stop listening to them! Remember that you're likely getting enough food to feed three people, so eat only one-third or half of your meal. Take the rest home for leftovers. One good tip is to request your to-go box early. Before you start eating, portion out the food that you want to eat at that meal, and put the rest in your to-go box.

✔ **Split an entree with a friend.** You can save money and some extra inches on your waistline by splitting an entree with a friend. Don't worry; you'll certainly have enough food for two.

✔ **Opt for half a deli sandwich with a side soup or salad in place of a burger and fries.** If you eat out on a regular basis, save yourself a lot of calories, fat, and glycemic load by getting a deli sandwich at the grocery store rather than ordering a burger and fries from the local fast-food restaurant. Just eat half the sandwich because that's equivalent to a whole sandwich you'd make at home. Even the deli bread is gigantic!

✔ **Choose an appetizer and side salad as your main meal.** The size of an appetizer represents a better picture of what you should have for a meal. So combine an appetizer with a side salad to create a satisfyingly delicious main entree.

✔ **Get your salad dressings, sauces, mayonnaise, and gravies on the side.** If you leave it to the cooks, they may put more sauces on your meal than you like or really need. Having control of just how much you eat can save you a lot of calories.

✔ **Avoid specialty breads.** Choose whole-wheat or whole-grain bread rather than focaccia, rolls, or other specialty breads. Whole-wheat bread has a lower glycemic load than the others, and it's lower in calories, too.

Use these tips to help you turn your high-glycemic favorites into new low-glycemic meals:

  ✔ **Replace higher-glycemic foods with lower-glycemic alternatives.** For example, if your favorite stir-fry typically calls for jasmine rice, you can easily change it to brown rice without greatly affecting the overall recipe. Appendix A lists a wide variety of low-glycemic foods that you can use in place of higher-glycemic ones.

✔ **Use smaller portion sizes of high- or medium-glycemic foods.** If your favorite stew calls for russet potatoes, which are high glycemic, you can easily include them for effect and still maintain a low-glycemic meal. All you have to do is use fewer potatoes and more of the other vegetables in the dish.

✔ **Add healthy low-glycemic foods.** Instead of eating a dish entirely made up of pasta, add some low-glycemic veggies, like broccoli or bell peppers, and/or some protein, like chicken or salmon. That way, you decrease the amount of pasta you're eating, increase your nutrient intake, and lessen your glycemic load for that meal.

Surveying a Sample Weekly Menu Using Recipes from This Book

The goal of the following sections is to help demonstrate how to combine all the advice we provide earlier in this chapter (and in Chapter 4) in a practical way. Use it as a template to start your own menu planning for the week, and add as much or as little cooking as you want to make it work for your lifestyle.

We also added two snacks — one in the afternoon and one in the evening. You may be a one-snack-a-day person, or you may like an early snack. You can change around this schedule as much as you need.

Don't try to follow this sample menu like a diet. Instead, use it (and the guidelines we share with you throughout this chapter and Chapter 4) as a tool to help you make up your own meals for the week. Each meal in the following sections provides a good balance of protein, carbohydrates, and fat in the suggested portion size. Keep in mind, though, that appropriate portion sizes change depending on your gender and size. A 250-pound linebacker is certainly going to eat more than a 140-pound woman. For the following meals, we show you basic portion sizes with daily menus ranging from 1,600 to 1,900 calories. If you need more information about your particular size, we suggest contacting a registered dietitian to find out what's appropriate for you. Go to www.eatright.org to find a dietitian in your area, or get advice from a dietitian through one of the online programs at www.reallivingnutrition.com.

Sunday: Starting the week off right

For this day, we plan a cooked meal for breakfast followed by a light lunch of soup and a quick grilling and tortellini salad meal for dinner.

Sundays are a great time to make breakfast because you don't have to run off to work or school; you have a little extra time to cook.

Breakfast

3 ounces of Veggie Egg Bake (Chapter 8)

1 slice of whole-wheat bread with 1 teaspoon of butter or trans-fat-free margarine

½ cup of orange juice

1 cup of coffee or tea (optional)

Lunch

1½ cups of canned minestrone soup (regular or low sodium), or frozen soup if you have any left over

1 whole-wheat English muffin with 2 teaspoons of butter or trans-fat-free margarine

Snack

¼ cup of peanuts with 1 apple

Dinner

4 ounces of Garlic and Lime Grilled Chicken (Chapter 15) (***Note:*** Double this recipe to have leftovers for Monday's lunch.)

1 cup of Spicy Grilled Veggie Skewers (Chapter 13)

½ cup of Fresh Spinach and Tomato Tortellini Salad (Chapter 14)

Snack

½ cup of frozen yogurt

Monday: Keeping it simple

Mondays typically aren't the best days of the week to do a whole lot of cooking. You're trying to get back in the swing of things and are probably catching up on work or homework after a long weekend. So here we offer you some quick, ready-made ideas for breakfast and show you how to incorporate foods you made over the weekend into your lunch. We top it off with some of our easiest-to-prepare recipes for dinner.

Breakfast

¾ cup of quick-cook oatmeal (made with water)

½ cup of fresh blueberries

2 tablespoons of slivered almonds

1 cup of lowfat milk

1 cup of coffee or tea (optional)

Lunch

2 cups of mixed greens with sliced tomatoes and cucumbers (or any left-over veggies) and 3 ounces of chopped Garlic and Lime Grilled Chicken from Sunday night

1 tablespoon of lowfat vinaigrette salad dressing

3 whole-wheat Melba toast crackers

Snack

8 ounces of lowfat fruit yogurt or plain yogurt with ¼ cup of fresh berries

Dinner

4 ounces of Home-Baked Halibut Fish Sticks (Chapter 17)

1 cup of steamed broccoli

3 ounces (about the size of a deck of cards) of Roasted Sweet Potatoes (Chapter 14)

Snack

2 cups of lowfat, microwavable air-popped popcorn

Tuesday: Spending a little more time in the kitchen

If you have more time to cook on Tuesdays, try putting a little more umph into dinner those nights, as we do here. Also, by preparing the Oatmeal Raspberry Bars in the morning, you give yourself a quick breakfast and snack for the rest of the week.

Breakfast

1 Oatmeal Raspberry Bar (Chapter 8)

8 ounces of lowfat fruit yogurt or plain yogurt with ¼ cup of fresh berries

½ cup of fresh sliced melon (any assortment of watermelon, honeydew, and cantaloupe)

1 cup of coffee or tea (optional)

Lunch

Turkey sandwich on whole-wheat bread with provolone cheese, lettuce, tomato, and 1 teaspoon of mayonnaise or basil pesto

1 cup of canned vegetable soup (regular or low sodium), or frozen soup if you have any left over

Snack

¼ cup of trail mix made of assorted nuts and dried fruits

Dinner

4 ounces of Curry and Apple Pork Chops (Chapter 16)

½ cup of wild rice (box mix)

1 cup of Wilted Spinach Salad with Feta (Chapter 12)

Snack

½ cup of Easy Chocolate Mousse with ½ cup of fresh sliced strawberries (Chapter 19)

Wednesday: Spicing up dinner with steak

Halfway through the work week is a good day! You could easily have some leftover pork chops from Tuesday night or have steak and potatoes if you have time to cook something new.

Breakfast

1 poached or hard-boiled egg

1 slice of whole-grain toast with 1 teaspoon of whipped butter (lower in calories and fat than regular butter and easier to spread) or trans-fat-free margarine

1 small banana

1 cup of coffee or tea (optional)

Lunch

1 Chicken Caesar Wrap (Chapter 15) (**Note:** Make double the filling to have leftovers for Thursday's lunch.)

½ cup of fresh strawberries

Snack

1 Oatmeal Raspberry Bar (from Tuesday morning)

Dinner

5 ounces of Tenderloin Steaks with Mushroom Sauce (Chapter 16)

⅔ cup of Roasted Mixed Vegetables with Caramelized Shallots (Chapter 13)

Snack

2 cups of lowfat, microwavable air-popped popcorn

Thursday: Winding down the week with leftovers and turkey

The week is winding down, and the weekend is just one day away. Turkey cutlets are a great way to go for dinner, and you can easily have some leftovers from Wednesday for lunch. Making some quick muffins in the morning gives you a delightful breakfast and snacks for the rest of the week.

Breakfast

1 Carrot Cake Oat Muffin (Chapter 9)

½ cup of lowfat vanilla yogurt mixed with ¼ cup of assorted berries

1 cup of coffee or tea (optional)

Lunch

Leftover Chicken Caesar Wrap from Wednesday's lunch, or the Chicken Caesar Wrap filling over a bed of mixed greens

Snack

1 mozzarella cheese stick

1 apple

Dinner

1 Parmesan Turkey Cutlet (Chapter 15)

½ cup of Cheesy Quinoa with Spinach (Chapter 14)

1 cup of steamed broccoli

Snack

1 Baked Peach with Vanilla Frozen Yogurt (Chapter 19)

Friday: Using the grill to bring on the weekend

Friday is the start of the weekend, and there's nothing like grill night to get things started. We incorporate grilled salmon into the dinner for this menu to show an example of a week that incorporates two servings of fish, which we recommend to help you get your omega-3 fatty acids for the week. (Monday night featured Home-Baked Halibut Fish Sticks.)

Even if it's winter, you can still grill on an indoor grill pan.

Breakfast

¾ cup of quick-cook oatmeal (made with water)

2 tablespoons of slivered almonds

1 small banana

1 cup of coffee or tea (optional)

Lunch

Ham sandwich on whole-wheat bread with 1 slice of mozzarella cheese and 1 teaspoon of mayonnaise

2 cups of mixed greens with tomatoes, bell peppers, and cucumbers with 1 tablespoon of your favorite lowfat salad dressing

Snack

¼ cup of Chunky Salsa with Black Beans and Tomatoes (Chapter 10) with 12 baked tortilla chips

Dinner

4 ounces of Grilled Salmon with Mango Salsa (Chapter 17)

3 ounces of Baked Polenta with Tomatoes (Chapter 14)

Snack

½ cup of fresh strawberries

Saturday: Warming things up with soup and stir-fry

Saturdays are a great time to cook something to have for the week ahead. If it's winter, you can't go wrong with making a big pot of soup and using the leftovers during the next week. It's also a great day to have a hearty cooked breakfast. Notice that because we incorporate a big breakfast into this day's menu, we go light on lunch and dinner.

If you aren't a fan of tempeh, substitute it for the Ginger Chicken and Broccoli Stir-Fry in Chapter 15.

Breakfast

2 Banana Strawberry Oatmeal Pancakes (Chapter 8) with 2 teaspoons of whipped butter or trans-fat-free margarine and 1 tablespoon of maple syrup

2 slices of pan-fried Canadian bacon (*Tip:* Use nonstick cooking spray, and brown each side of the bacon over medium-high heat.)

Lunch

1½ cups of Summer Minestrone Soup (Chapter 11) (*Tip:* Use the leftovers for the week, or freeze them in individual serving containers to whip out when you need a quick frozen meal.)

1 ounce of whole-wheat crackers

Snack

8 ounces of lowfat fruit yogurt or plain yogurt mixed with ¼ cup of fresh berries

Dinner

1 cup of Tempeh Stir-Fry over ½ cup of brown rice (Chapter 18)

Snack

⅔ cup of Chocolate Peanut Butter Ice Dream (Chapter 19)

Chapter 6

Stocking Your Kitchen and Practicing New Cooking Methods

. . . .

In This Chapter

▶ Organizing your pantry, refrigerator, and freezer

▶ Adding the right tools to your kitchen toolbox

▶ Cooking up new grains and beans

▶ Incorporating more fruits and vegetables into your everyday meals

. . . .

*T*o live a low-glycemic lifestyle, you need to plan ahead and make sure you have the right ingredients and tools on hand so that you can create the delicious low-glycemic recipes we include in Parts III and IV of this book any day of the week. You also need to know the cooking methods that'll bring out the most flavor in your food (while keeping everything low glycemic) so that you and your family can truly get excited about mealtime. This chapter offers all the tips and tricks you need to know.

As you take a good look at your kitchen, you may be surprised to find out that you already have lots of low-glycemic foods in it. Items like tortellini, barley, oats, brown rice, cornmeal, whole-wheat flour, fruits, vegetables, meats, cheeses, canned tuna, soups, and dairy products all fit the bill. Even though you may want to shop for some new items to add to your regular stock, you certainly don't have to revamp everything. And keep in mind that we want you to enjoy cooking and eating, so don't get rid of all the higher-glycemic ingredients you have in your home if you don't want to. After all, everyone deserves a break from the routine once in a while, and you may need some of those ingredients to cook up an occasional treat for you and your family.

Restocking Your Pantry: Out with the Old, In with the New!

The following sections provide you with the tools you need to organize a healthy, low-glycemic pantry filled with dry foods, grains, pastas, beans, lentils, and soups. As you begin your pantry reorganization, you may find some items in your pantry that you never use or that are outdated. You may also find some high-glycemic foods that you could probably live without.

You don't have to throw out everything in your pantry right away, but you do need to reevaluate your shopping habits and slowly stock up on low-glycemic ingredients. By making small, gradual changes instead of trying to change everything at once, you provide a better foundation for long-term success.

To get started, sort each shelf of your pantry, and set aside the items that may not fit into a low-glycemic lifestyle. Take a look at what you typically buy, and compare it to the lists in Appendix A. Then keep a running grocery list; when you run out of a high-glycemic pantry item, replace it with a low-glycemic one. For example, if you have a box of biscuit mix on the shelf, don't throw it away, but add a low-glycemic mix (made with whole-wheat flour rather than white flour) to your grocery list so you can add it to your pantry the next time you need more biscuit mix.

Looking at handy low-glycemic dry foods

Dry foods, such as flour, seasonings, and baking mixes, are essential to the well-prepared kitchen. Having the right items on hand will save you time and effort when you want to prepare a meal or snack, so be sure to consider these common items as you prepare your new grocery list for stocking your pantry:

- Baking powder, baking soda, and cornstarch
- Dry yeast
- Cornmeal
- Extracts, such as pure vanilla, anise, and almond
- Flours, including whole-wheat, wheat-bran, and oat flour
- Oat-bran baking mix and oatmeal pancake mix
- Sugars (granulated, light or dark brown)
- Oils, including olive oil, extra-virgin olive oil, canola oil, and vegetable nonstick cooking spray

> ✔ Seasonings, including salt, sea salt, black pepper, white pepper, cumin, paprika, garlic powder, red pepper, chili powder, curry powder, ginger, cinnamon, dill, parsley, tarragon, basil, oregano, thyme, rosemary, no-salt herb blends, and your choice of other dried herbs
>
> ✔ Unsweetened cocoa

Note: Although sugar is very high glycemic, you need to have some on hand because some recipes in this book (and other recipes you make) call for small amounts.

Spices and herbs have no effect on the glycemic index, but you may find many in your pantry that are outdated. They add wonderful flavor and punch to dishes, but only if they're fresh. (In general, herbs and spices can lose aroma and flavor after a year or so.) Check dates on jarred spices and herbs, and rub the herbs between your fingers. If they don't let off a strong aroma, toss them. When you purchase new ones, try to purchase smaller jars to maintain freshness, and store them out of the light and away from heat. Herbs and spices are also available in bulk at some stores so that you can purchase smaller quantities or only the amount you may need for a special recipe.

If a recipe calls for fresh herbs, you can use ⅓ the amount of dried.

Exploring new low-glycemic grains

Although many grains are fairly high glycemic, they're still an important part of your diet. The good news is that you can replace many of the traditional high-glycemic grains with lower-glycemic ones that are not only healthier but also tastier. So when you go to restock your breadbox and pantry shelf, be sure to include the following low-glycemic grains:

> ✔ Bran cereals
>
> ✔ Brown rice or converted rice
>
> ✔ Pearl barley, quinoa, or bulgur wheat
>
> ✔ Steel-cut oatmeal, old-fashioned oats, or quick oats
>
> ✔ Whole-grain breads, such as 8 grain, 100% whole wheat, oat bran, and 7 grain
>
> ✔ Whole-wheat crisp crackers, such as water crackers, stoned wheat, whole-wheat matzo, and rye

When buying breads and cereals, be sure to read the labels carefully. Look for 100% whole-grain or whole-wheat products. Check labels for fiber content; look for 3 or more grams of fiber per serving.

Finding low-glycemic pastas

Although pasta often comes with a higher glycemic index, you can still include a variety of pasta dishes in your low-glycemic diet (which is excellent news for all you pasta lovers out there!). All you have to do is watch your portion sizes and stick to the following low- to medium-glycemic pasta choices (see Chapter 4 for more on portion size):

- **Dreamfield Pasta:** This brand is higher in fiber and protein and has a lower glycemic index than traditional pasta brands. It contains *inulin,* a fruit and vegetable fiber.

- **Spaghetti or fettuccine:** These types of pasta offer a medium glycemic load per serving.

- **Vermicelli:** This thin pasta is similar to spaghetti and has a medium glycemic load.

- **Tortellini:** The cheese in this small pasta helps reduce its glycemic load, and, because you end up eating less pasta per serving, tortellini is a low-glycemic pasta choice.

- **Ravioli:** This cheese- or meat-stuffed pasta offers a medium glycemic load due to its larger size (more pasta to filling ratio than tortellini).

Cook pasta in a large stockpot of water, and cook *al dente,* or firm to the bite. Overcooked pasta has a higher glycemic load than properly cooked pasta.

Stocking up on beans, lentils, and soups

Beans and lentils are loaded with nutrients and fiber, making them a perfect addition to your low-glycemic pantry (find out some tips for preparing beans and lentils in the later section "Fixing Beans as Part of a Healthy Meal"). When considering which beans and lentils to buy, consider the following:

- Any canned or dried beans (navy beans, kidney beans, garbanzo beans, and black beans, just to name a few) are great to have on hand. Canned beans have a long shelf life and are easy to add to any salad or side dish recipe. They make great dips, too. Dried beans are inexpensive and can last on the shelf for up to a year, but they do take longer to prepare.

- Although brown, green, and red lentils are available in stores, we prefer green lentils because they hold up best in cooking (the other types often crack or break apart). They're all high in fiber, iron, and B vitamins.

Soups such as lentil, black bean, vegetable, minestrone, and beef barley are also great to keep on hand for quick lunches. (When you have time, try some of the soup recipes in Chapter 11; they're easy to make and delicious to eat!)

 To make sure you always have what you need to prepare a quick meal, include other canned goods, such as canned vegetables, tomato paste, low-sodium broths, canned fruit packed in water, and canned tuna or salmon, on your pantry shelf as well.

Reinventing Your Refrigerator and Freezer

Keeping staple ingredients on hand in the fridge allows you to throw recipes together in a hurry. Not to mention it saves you a trip to the store, and who doesn't love that? Here are some low-glycemic basics you want to make sure you have in your refrigerator at all times:

- ✔ Fresh fruit (apples, nectarines, peaches, bananas, pears, berries, melons, and so on)
- ✔ Fresh vegetables (lettuce for salads, celery, onions, carrots, tomatoes, and so on)
- ✔ Eggs
- ✔ Lean deli meats
- ✔ Condiments (mustards, low-glycemic salad dressings, lowfat mayonnaise, Worcestershire sauce, salsas, relishes, grilling sauces, and so on)

Be sure to keep a few dairy staples on hand, too:

- ✔ Lowfat yogurt
- ✔ Fat-free or lowfat milk
- ✔ Lowfat cheeses
- ✔ Light cream cheese
- ✔ Lowfat cottage cheese

Stock your freezer to its fullest potential, as well. Having frozen meats, fish, or poultry that you can defrost quickly in the microwave at your disposal makes planning meals easier. Also consider keeping some frozen vegetables and fruits on hand for quick dishes. Add them to recipes, or use them as low-glycemic side dishes. Just be sure to choose plain vegetables and fruits that contain no added sauces or sugars. The following frozen items come in handy when you're planning menus:

- Frozen spinach
- Frozen peas
- Frozen broccoli or cauliflower
- Frozen chopped bell peppers, sliced carrots, or sliced onions
- Frozen fruit, such as unsweetened blueberries, peaches, or strawberries
- Skinless chicken pieces or boneless chicken breasts
- Salmon fillets and burgers
- Frozen shrimp
- Extra-lean ground beef in 1-pound packages
- Pork tenderloin

Don't forget about your own cooked leftovers! We include many recipes in this book — especially the soups, chilies, and stews in Chapter 11 — that you can freeze for later.

Getting Your Tools in Order

When it comes to healthy eating and meal planning, having a well-stocked pantry, refrigerator, and freezer is step one. Step two is having the proper tools to work with when you set out to actually make your meals. You don't need a gourmet kitchen, but the right cooking tools have the power to make cooking easier, more efficient, and more enjoyable. In the following sections, we cover the kitchen mainstay items you absolutely must have as well as some wish-list items that are nice but not vital to your success in the kitchen.

Cutting boards

You need a cutting board for almost every recipe in this book. We recommend that you have at least two — one you'll use for meats and the other you'll use for produce. The verdict is still out on whether wood or plastic is better, so the choice is up to you. The important thing is to have one for meat and one for fruits and veggies.

We like using plastic cutting boards because they're easy on your knives and easier to clean, but be sure to replace them when they become too nicked (bacteria can harbor within the grooves). As an added bonus, you can put most plastic boards into the dishwasher for easy cleanup.

Table 6-1 shows you the different types of cutting boards available and some advantages and disadvantages of each one.

Table 6-1	Types of Cutting Boards	
Type	*Advantages*	*Disadvantages*
Bamboo	Easy on knives	Not dishwasher safe
	Renewable resource	Need to be periodically seasoned with oil
	Attractive and durable	
	Natural bacteria-fighting properties	Vary in quality
		Will splinter if low in quality
Composite	Dishwasher safe	May give off odor when wet
	Durable	Harder on knives
	Easy to clean	Not eco-friendly
	Attractive	
Glass	Sanitary	Damage knives
	Easy to clean	Prone to chips and breaks
	Durable	
	Attractive	
Plastic	Easy on knives	Wear out quickly
	Easy to clean	Gouges and scratches can harbor bacteria
	Inexpensive	
	Can be color coded so you can keep track of which board you use for which products (for example, orange for produce, red for meats)	Not as attractive as wood or bamboo
		Vary in quality
		Not eco-friendly
	Dishwasher safe	
Wood	Easy on knives	Prone to nicks and scratches
	Can be refinished	Need to be periodically seasoned with oil
	Attractive	
	Can be as sanitary as plastic	Not dishwasher safe
		Vary in quality

Electrical appliances

Doing things by hand works just fine, but some people prefer the convenience of electrical tools to make prep work easier and save time. If you want to make your kitchen a little more tech-savvy, consider adding these appliances:

- **Blender:** A standard blender is a handy tool to have when you want to whip up a healthy smoothie. Plus, you can often use it in place of a food processor when making sauces and dips. An immersion blender is also useful. This hand-held device is quick to clean, great for making soups, and often includes a few helpful attachments.

- **Electric can opener:** Although it's a good idea to keep a hand-crank can opener in your drawer (just in case the electricity goes out when you're in the middle of making dinner!), an electric model opens cans in a jiffy.

- **Food processor:** You can choose either a large food processor or a small one, depending on how much storage space you have and what you plan to make with it. Processors are great for making sauces (such as tomato or pesto) and whole-grain bread crumbs, mixing bean dips, and chopping veggies. Smaller varieties take up less space but have smaller capacities.

- **Hand mixer or standing mixer:** Either or both of these are useful for mixing quick breads.

- **Steamer:** Although most steamers are called *rice steamers,* they work great for cooking rice, vegetables, and even stews and meats. Be prepared to shop around if you decide to add a steamer to your kitchen because they're available in many varieties and at many price ranges.

Pots and pans

No kitchen is complete without a few good pieces of cookware. Trust us, the results you get by cooking with decent pots and pans are well worth the money they cost upfront. Purchase the best style and brand you can afford. It's better to have a couple of really good pans that cook well and last than to buy a whole set of pans that wear out fast and don't perform well.

You can prepare just about anything as long as you have these kitchen mainstays in your cabinet:

- 12-inch sauté pan with lid
- Large stockpot (6 to 8 quart)
- 4-quart saucepan with lid
- 8-inch nonstick skillet

- Large roasting pan with lid
- Slow cooker (4 to 6 quart)

If you have those basic items covered, you may want to add the following wish-list items to your kitchen cabinet:

- 6-inch sauté pan with lid
- 10-inch sauté pan with lid
- 2-quart saucepan
- Dutch oven (a squat, lidded roaster, usually oval shaped, with two side handles)
- Grill pan
- Steamer pot or steam basket
- Wok

Utility tools

We know it's tempting to want to buy every little gadget you see on display at the kitchen store in your mall, but many of them really aren't necessary. When you're starting out, stick with the following basic utility tools; they can help you get rolling in the kitchen and will definitely save on storage space:

- 8-inch French or chef's knife
- Paring knife
- Serrated bread knife
- 6-inch utility knife
- Measuring cups and spoons
- Two glass measuring cups (one 2-cup, one 4-cup)
- Wooden spoon
- Slotted spoon
- Soup ladle
- Silicon spatula and turner
- Two rubber spatulas (one large, one small)
- Metal turner
- Metal whisk

  ✔ Peeler

  ✔ Tongs

  ✔ Kitchen shears

  ✔ Steel or plastic colander

  ✔ Two mixing bowls (one small, one medium)

  ✔ 9-inch baking pan (glass or metal)

  ✔ 13-x-9-inch glass baking dish

  ✔ Two cookie sheets

  ✔ Small ceramic or glass custard cups or ramekins

Here are some less essential but still nice-to-have items for your wish list:

  ✔ Filet knife

  ✔ Steak knives

  ✔ Butcher knife

  ✔ Garlic press

  ✔ Larger set of mixing bowls

  ✔ Flour sifter

  ✔ 8-x-8-inch glass baking dish

  ✔ More than two cookie sheets

Cooking Low-Glycemic Grains

Incorporating low-glycemic grains into your menus not only provides extra nutrition but also adds flavor and texture to your meals. Plus, grains are very enjoyable foods, so they help with satiety. The trick to using them as part of your low-glycemic lifestyle is to choose the right ones in the proper portions and then to prepare them properly. This section offers general cooking tips to keep in mind whenever you're handling grains, as well as suggestions for getting the most from the grain food group.

Checking out a whole-grain cooking chart

Table 6-2 gives you examples of some whole grains, their glycemic loads, and the time they take to cook. *Note:* You can cook most whole grains either in a microwave oven or on the stovetop; their packages often include directions for both methods.

Table 6-2	Whole-Grain Cooking Chart			
Type of Grain, 1 Cup Dry	*Glycemic Load*	*Amount of Water or Broth*	*Simmering Time after Boiling*	*Amount after Cooking*
Brown rice	Low	2½ cups	45–55 minutes	3 cups
Buckwheat	Low	2 cups	20 minutes	2½ cups
Cornmeal (polenta)	Low	4 cups	25–30 minutes	2½ cups
Pearl barley	Low	3 cups	45–60 minutes	3½ cups
Quinoa	Low	2 cups	12–15 minutes	About 3 cups
Steel-cut oats	Low	4 cups	20 minutes	2 cups
Wild rice	Medium	3 cups	45–55 minutes	3 cups

Adding some spark to your grains

We know what you're thinking: All this talk about how good whole grains taste must be a joke. Maybe you've had a negative experience with grains in the past, or you aren't really sure what we mean by *whole grains*. Either way, we're here to tell you not to write them off just yet. By trying out the recipes we include in this book, particularly in Chapter 14, you'll soon see that low-glycemic grains really can be a delicious addition to any meal.

Whenever you want to add a little grain to your meals, whether you're trying out the tasty recipes in Chapter 14 or you're making a recipe from some other source, keep the following tips in mind and you're sure to love the results:

✔ Add 1 to 2 teaspoons of extra-virgin olive oil to provide heart-healthy fat, add flavor, and keep the grain light and fluffy. (You can also use 1 to 2 teaspoons of butter to add a unique flavor that's a great match for some meals.)

✔ Instead of cooking the grain in water, cook it in low-sodium chicken or vegetable broth.

✔ Add fresh herbs like chopped cilantro, basil, or parsley.

✔ Add some dry ingredients like cumin or cayenne pepper for a little spice.

✔ Sauté some garlic, onions, mushrooms, and/or shallots, and then stir them into your cooked grain.

✔ Add chopped walnuts or slivered almonds to grains for a punch of flavor and a nice crunch.

✔ Add 1 to 2 tablespoons of Parmesan, feta, or crumbled goat cheese to add flavor and a creamy texture.

Fixing Beans as Part of a Healthy Meal

Beans are just plain good for you. Not only are they naturally lowfat, but they're also packed with fiber, B vitamins, and protein. With so many health benefits, it's no wonder we encourage you to look for new ways to incorporate them into your regular diet. To help you do so, we've included a plethora of recipes made with beans throughout this book, and in the following sections, we describe the different types of beans available and provide tips on how to cook them properly.

Beans are part of the legume family, along with lentils and peas:

✔ Lentils are sold dried; they're used in soups or side dishes. You can cook them by using 1½ cups of boiling water for every 1 cup of dried lentils. Place the lentils in the boiling water, and simmer over medium heat for 15 to 20 minutes. You can add your favorite herbs and spices or finely chopped onion for a bit more flavor.

✔ Peas are available fresh, frozen, dried, or canned. Peas are great on their own and work well as an addition to pasta dishes, salads, and stir-fries. Just make sure you don't overcook them; fresh or frozen only take about 4 to 7 minutes to cook. They should still be bright green.

Sifting through types of beans

When you start looking for new bean recipes or exploring your grocery store's bean selection, you may be surprised by how many kinds of beans you have to choose from. Each type has a different look, texture, and taste.

✔ **Black beans:** These beans are small, round, and black. They have a wonderful flavor by themselves and also are a great accompaniment to soups, chilies, salsas, and rice.

✔ **Garbanzo beans:** These beans, which are also called *chickpeas,* are small, round, tan-colored beans that are a favorite ingredient in Italian recipes and many popular Middle Eastern dishes. Garbanzo beans are also the basis of *hummus,* a delicious bean spread made with lemon juice, olive oil, garlic, and spices.

✔ **Kidney beans:** These beans come in two colors: red and white. They're large — about ¾ inch long — and have a kidney shape, hence their name. The red ones are often used in chili because they're hearty and hold their shape. Both colors of kidney beans work well in salads.

✔ **Lima beans:** These beans are flat and light green in color. They're mostly used in soups or as side dishes.

✔ **Navy beans:** These medium-sized, cream-colored beans work well in soups and dips.

 ✔ **Pinto beans:** These small, pinkish-brown beans are often used in Mexican cooking and are great when cooked and mashed for dips or side dishes.

 ✔ **Soybeans and edamame:** Soybeans can be used in soups, salads, dips, or baked dishes. Edamame, which are green, immature soybeans, can be eaten as a snack or made into a bean spread (like hummus).

Cooking canned beans versus dried beans

Beans are available either dried or canned. You can buy dried beans in bags or in bulk, depending on how many you need. They take longer to prepare than canned beans, but they're also lower in sodium.

To cook dried beans, first rinse and sort the beans, discarding any blemished ones or any dirt. Cover the dried beans with three times their volume of water, let them soak in the refrigerator for 12 hours, or overnight, and then drain them. Cooking times vary depending on the size and type of bean, as well as the cooking method you use.

You can also try the *quick soak method* by placing dried beans in a saucepan, covering them with three times their volume in water (you want the beans to be completely submerged), and then bringing them to a boil. Boil the beans for 2 minutes, and then remove from heat. Let them sit for 1 hour, and then drain them.

To cook dried beans in a stockpot, fill the pot with water and add the beans (they should be covered by water). Bring to a boil, and cook for about 1 to 1½ hours. To cook dried beans in your pressure cooker, follow the manufacturer's directions. You generally fill the cooker only half full when cooking dried beans; we also suggest adding 2 to 3 teaspoons of oil to the cooker. Cooking time depends on how long you've soaked the beans (the longer you soak them, the shorter the cooking time) but in general, it should take only about 10 to 15 minutes.

Note: One pound of dry beans (about 2½ cups) yields about 7½ cups of cooked beans; 1 cup of dry beans yields 3 cups of cooked beans.

The bean connoisseur may prefer only dried beans for their texture and flavor, but canned beans offer a quick and easy option to adding more beans to your daily meals. Simply open the can, drain the beans, rinse them, and use them in recipes.

The sodium content in canned beans can reach as high as 500 to 600 milligrams per ½-cup serving, so you need to rinse canned beans well. Rinsing can reduce sodium by as much as 40 percent. You can also look for low-sodium varieties.

Preparing Low-Glycemic Fruits and Vegetables

Just about every fruit and vegetable, with the exception of raisins, ripe bananas, and potatoes, has a low glycemic load. Incorporating fruits and veggies into your regular menu helps add wonderful colors and tastes to your meals, not to mention nutritional balance. In the following sections, we explain how to wash produce, describe methods for cooking veggies, and give you fresh ideas for incorporating more fruits and veggies into your diet.

Washing your fruits and veggies well

Because of the recent media reports that "the dirty dozen" — peaches, apples, bell peppers, celery, nectarines, strawberries, cherries, pears, imported grapes, spinach, lettuce, and potatoes — may contain the highest pesticide residues, you may be wary about adding more fruits and vegetables to your diet. But as long as you wash your produce properly before you cook it, you can ensure that your meals and snacks are safe to eat. And you definitely don't want to miss out on all the benefits you get from including fruits and vegetables in your diet.

When preparing produce, or any food for that matter, always start with clean hands. Trim off any spots or bruises from your fruits and veggies, and then wash them under cool water. Depending on your recipe, you may need to peel vegetables such as cucumbers, eggplant, potatoes, or carrots, but you can eat the skin of most vegetables if you want to. If you're keeping the skins on your veggies, be sure to rub them really well when rinsing.

Roasting and steaming and grilling, oh my!

You can prepare vegetables in a variety of ways, but we recommend roasting, steaming, or grilling rather than boiling. Boiling vegetables in large pots of water causes them to release their vitamins. (Ever boil carrots and find the drained water to be orange? You've lost a lot of Vitamin A down the drain!). By roasting, steaming, or grilling, you preserve as many nutrients as possible.

Raw veggies do have a lower glycemic load than cooked vegetables, and certain cooking methods (namely roasting) do raise the glycemic load a bit. But overall, you're looking at turning a low-glycemic food into a low-moderate glycemic food, so it's all good.

Roasting

Roasting gives vegetables a completely different and robust flavor. Specifically, roasting concentrates the sugars in veggies, bringing out a new, bold flavor. It also preserves all the nutrients because you're containing the vegetables in their juices.

To roast vegetables, simply place the sliced veggies and some minced garlic in an oven-safe dish, drizzle with 2 tablespoons of oil, salt lightly, and roast at 425 degrees for about 45 to 60 minutes, depending on how many veggies you're making. Check for doneness after 35 minutes, stir, and continue cooking as needed; the veggies should be very tender.

You can roast almost any vegetable, but our favorite ones to use for this particular cooking method are eggplant, onions, shallots, mushrooms, zucchini, and bell peppers. Of course, adding a good dose of garlic and olive oil really brings out the flavors and provides a beautiful glisten to the dish.

Steaming

Steaming is an easy technique that doesn't require special pots or equipment. You can steam in a variety of ways. For example:

- ✔ If you have a pot with a steamer basket insert, simply add water to the pot until it's just below the basket, allow it to come to a boil, place the vegetables in the basket, insert it into the pot over the boiling water, and cover the pot.

- ✔ You can also steam veggies by bringing about a half inch of water to boil in a medium-sized saucepan or pot; then add the vegetables, cover the pot, and steam. Watch closely to check for doneness. The water provides enough steam to cook the vegetables with minimal nutrient loss.

With the preceding techniques, most vegetables steam in about 5 to 7 minutes. For an even faster steam, you can fill a microwave-safe dish with up to an inch of water, add the veggies, and cook them in a microwave on high for about 2 to 3 minutes.

Grilling

Your outdoor or indoor grill is a no-mess way to prepare vegetables fast. Just make sure you select vegetables that can stand up to the grill. Squash, bell peppers, eggplant, and beets are good choices to cook directly on the grill. Onions taste great grilled as well, but you need to use aluminum foil or a grill basket to prevent them from slipping through the grill rack.

You can even steam veggies on the grill by chopping, seasoning, and wrapping them in foil. The foil pouch acts like a steamer and cooks the vegetables in 15 minutes or less.

Creating new ways to enjoy fruits and vegetables

People often get into a rut with the veggies they prepare or eat. But adding just a little variety to the way you prepare them turns the same old veggies into delicious side dishes and awesome main dishes. Chapters 13 and 18 provide you with all kinds of ideas.

Fresh fruit is also chock-full of flavor and nutrition, so try to find more ways to incorporate fruits into your snacks and meals. See Chapters 8, 12, and 19 for new tasty ways to add fruit to your meals.

Try out these ideas for adding more veggies and fruits into your daily intake:

- ✔ **Think beyond side dish, and focus on main dish.** For example, squash or zucchini takes center stage when it's stuffed as a main entree. All you have to do is cut the squash or zucchini in half, scoop out the pulp to make a "bowl" (you can reserve the pulp and add it into the stuffing mixture), stuff the bowls with a spinach and feta cheese mixture or ground sausage mixed with chopped carrots and onions. Place the stuffed squash or zucchini in a baking dish filled with about 1 inch of water. Bake it for 30 minutes, and enjoy a dish that's full of nutritious veggies.

- ✔ **Mix vegetables with other foods to try out some veggies you may otherwise not like.** For instance, you can try adding veggies to eggs (thinly sliced zucchini, green onions, and mushrooms work well) or bell peppers to salads or stir-fries.

- ✔ **Dip veggies like carrots, bell pepper strips, and cucumber slices in salsa or hummus for a double-veggie treat.** Check out some of our yummy dips in Chapter 10 for inspiration.

- ✔ **Use green-leaf lettuce to make lettuce wraps instead of relying on bread-based wraps.** Fill a large leaf of lettuce with your favorite sandwich filling (baked ham or turkey, chicken salad, or tuna, just to name a few), roll it up, and enjoy!

- ✔ **Grill fruits to add to meats.** Grilled pineapple or peaches are a great addition to pork or chicken.

- ✔ **Add fresh sliced or chopped fruit to your salads.** Turn to Chapter 12 for some delicious fruit-inspired salad recipes like the Cranberry Walnut Salad or the Tangerines, Pistachios, and Feta over Mixed Greens.

- ✔ **Make fresh fruit part of your morning and afternoon snacks, or use fruit as a dessert ingredient.** Fruit adds natural sweetness and color to your favorite snacks and desserts. See Chapter 8 for a few delicious snacks and Chapter 19 for some great dessert ideas.

Chapter 7

Making Your Way around the Grocery Store

Walking into a grocery store can be quite confusing when you're trying to stick to a low-glycemic diet. After all, very few food companies use low-glycemic labels, so you're left with a collection of nutrition facts panels that focus on carbohydrates, sugars, calories, and fat (among other categories). And as you walk up and down the aisles, you start to notice that many foods, including those in the seafood department, butcher's window, and bakery, don't have any labels at all. So how do you know which breads to buy or which cuts of meat are the best for you? Don't fret! We're here to help you answer tricky questions like these. In this chapter, we show you how to interpret the nutrition facts panel, choose the best baked goods, produce, dairy products, and meat, and create and use a shopping list that will truly make your next trip to the grocery store a breeze.

Using the Nutrition Facts Panel

The nutrition facts panel on a package of food doesn't tell you directly whether the food is low glycemic or not, but it can give you some useful information to help you make an informed decision. Knowing what to look for on the label can make life easier so you don't have to waste time at the grocery store wondering which bread is the best choice or which crackers fit best in your low-glycemic diet.

If using the nutrition facts panel is new for you, keep reading. This section covers the basics on how to interpret the categories and the ingredients listed on the panel.

Deciphering the categories

Using a low-glycemic diet in conjunction with a meal plan low in fat, high in fiber and nutrients, and moderate in calories is the goal for good health. So how do you tackle that goal when you're faced with so many different food items in the store? Getting the hang of reading the nutrition facts label is one way to help you make the best choices. The following sections walk you through the basic categories you find on a standard nutrition facts label in the United States. (Check out Figure 7-1 to see these categories on a sample label.)

Nutrition Facts
Serving Size: About 20g
Servings Per Container: 16

	Amount Per Serving	% Daily Value*
Total Calories	60	
Calories From Fat	15	
Total Fat	2 g	3%
Saturated Fat	1 g	4%
Trans Fat	0 g	
Cholesterol	0 mg	0%
Sodium	45 mg	2%
Total Carbohydrates	15 g	5%
Dietary Fiber	4 g	17%
Sugars	4 g	
Sugar Alcohols (Polyols)	3 g	
Protein	2 g	
Vitamin A		0%
Vitamin C		0%
Calcium		2%
Iron		2%

*Percent Daily Values are based on a 2,000 calorie diet.

Ingredients: Wheat flour, unsweetened chocolate, erythritol, inulin, oat flour, cocoa powder, evaporated cane juice, whey protein concentrate, corn starch (low glycemic), natural flavors, salt, baking soda, wheat gluten, guar gum

Figure 7-1:
A sample nutrition facts label.

Serving size and servings per container

The serving size is the first thing you need to look at on a nutrition facts label because it's what the rest of the information on the panel is based on. For example, if the package says one serving size is ½ the package and the calorie level is 100, you'll end up with 200 calories if you eat the whole package. The serving size is important because if you eat more than one serving of a particular food item, you'll be eating more calories and possibly a higher glycemic load as well.

The servings per container number tells you how many serving sizes are in the entire package. So the nutrition facts label on a box of crackers may tell you that 10 crackers are a serving size and that the box contains four 10-piece servings.

Total calories and calories from fat

The next item on a label is the calorie level per serving. When choosing which packaged foods to buy, aim for lower-calorie foods and consider your daily calorie requirements. To find out your daily requirements, check out nutritiondata.self.com/tools/calories-burned (see Chapter 3 for an introduction to calories).

The calories from fat entry shows you how many calories the serving size gives you from fat. In Figure 7-1, 15 of the total 60 calories come from fat. In other words, 25 percent of this food comes from fat (see the next section for details on fat). Keeping your fat intake low is part of your overall goal for a healthy diet.

Total fat, saturated fat, and trans fat

Fat is one of the three sources of calories for your body. Consuming a moderate amount of fats is important for your overall health, but eating too many can be bad for both your waistline and your health. Try to get 30 percent of your daily calories from fat. So if your daily calorie needs are 1,800, you want 30 percent of those calories, or 540 calories, to come from fat. To find out how much fat you should eat per day, break the calories into grams by dividing the calories from fat (540) by 9; you should eat no more than 60 grams of total fat a day. To get those 60 grams (or less), focus on eating healthy fats like those found in avocados, olive oil, canola oil, nuts, seeds, and fish (find out more about healthy fats in Chapter 4).

Saturated fat is a subgroup of total fat that you don't want to eat too much of. Unfortunately, saturated fats are not only a big part of some people's diets, but they're also associated with heart disease and some cancers. Try to get no more than 10 percent of your daily fat intake from saturated fats.

A good rule of thumb is to consume only 1 gram of saturated fat per 100 calories. So if you're looking at a food label for a food that has 200 calories per serving, make sure the food contains 2 grams or less of saturated fat.

Trans fats are human-made fats that are linked to heart disease. They aren't necessary in your diet and are used primarily because they help foods have longer shelf lives. Do your best to purchase products without trans fats. Look for trans fats on the nutrition facts label and in the ingredients list (often represented by terms like *hydrogenated* or *partially hydrogenated oil*).

Some food labels say they contain *0 percent trans fat* but also include partially hydrogenated soybean oil in their ingredients lists. That apparent contradiction means the foods themselves contain 0.5 grams or less of trans fat. If you eat more than a listed single serving of those foods, the amount of trans fats you eat also increases.

Cholesterol

Total cholesterol tells you the amount of cholesterol that's found in the food item. This information is especially important if you have heart disease or diabetes. The American Heart Association recommends that you keep your cholesterol intake below 300 milligrams a day and below 200 milligrams a day if you have coronary artery disease.

Sodium

Sodium is a natural-occurring mineral in some foods and is added to others to enhance flavor and give them longer shelf lives. Unfortunately, sodium is used excessively in the American diet. It's also been associated with high blood pressure and as an appetite stimulant.

Go easy on the salt shaker, and aim for lower-sodium foods. In terms of the nutrition facts label, try to stick with foods that contain 240 milligrams or less of sodium per serving. Aim to eat fewer than 2,300 milligrams a day if you're a healthy adult or 1,500 milligrams a day if you have high blood pressure or diabetes.

Total carbohydrates, dietary fiber, sugars, and sugar alcohols (polyols)

The total carbohydrates tell you how many carbohydrates are in one serving size. This information is important for overall health but is especially important for diabetics who are using carbohydrate counting as a tool to help them manage their diabetes.

Is something that has a higher amount of carbohydrates automatically considered to be a high-glycemic food? Not necessarily. If you take ¼ cup of dry quinoa, for example, you find about 30 grams of carbohydrates, which is enough to make it high glycemic. But that same amount cooked is considered low glycemic because it expands after being cooked with water and makes more servings. Once broken down into a cooked serving, the glycemic load becomes lower.

Dietary fiber is the indigestible portion of a plant-based food item. As we explain in Chapter 3, fiber helps control your blood sugar and helps you feel full for a longer period of time. It provides denseness to foods, has no calories, and can be found in fruits, vegetables, beans, lentils, and foods made with whole grains, including cereal, pasta, bread, and rice. Shoot for getting 3 grams or more of fiber per serving.

Sugars include added sugars like table sugar as well as natural sugars found in dairy, fruit, and vegetables. Because the sugar entry on the nutrition facts label includes both types, it's difficult to gage how much added sugar an item contains. For example, if you look at a container of yogurt that says it contains 30 grams of sugar, you don't know how many of those 30 grams are added sugars and how many are sugars naturally found in yogurt. When using a low-glycemic diet, you don't have to focus too much on the amount of sugars listed in the nutrition facts; instead, focus on eating the foods that have been tested for low- to medium-glycemic loads (see `nutritiondata. self.com` for details).

Sugar alcohols (polyols) are used in many packaged goods as sweeteners. They're usually absorbed incompletely in the bloodstream, causing a smaller rise in blood sugar than regular sugar. This characteristic makes them popular in the dieting world. Beware, though, this incomplete absorption can also cause symptoms like bloating and diarrhea. We don't recommend loading up on sugar alcohols; you can find plenty of sweet treats that don't include sugar alcohols.

Protein

The protein entry tells you how much protein is in a serving size of the food item you're looking at. Most of your protein is found in meats, beans, nuts, and soy products. However, you need to check the protein entry on the nutrition facts labels of foods like cereal so you can find one that has more protein (5 or more grams). Having protein with each meal is important, and if you like eating cold cereal for breakfast, try eating one with more protein.

Vitamins, calcium, and iron

Vitamins, calcium, and iron are important for good health and disease prevention. These entries on the nutrition facts panel let you know whether you're choosing a high-nutrient food or a low-nutrient food. The example in Figure 7-1 isn't a very high-nutrient food with only 2 percent of your daily value for calcium and iron.

Taking a closer look at the ingredients

The ingredients list is your best bet for determining whether a food has a low or high glycemic load because it gives you a good idea of whether or not you're buying a product that's made up of low-glycemic ingredients. You can find the ingredients list at the bottom of the nutrition facts panel (refer to Figure 7-1). Ingredients are listed from highest content to lowest. So the first ingredient makes up most of that food and the last ingredient makes up the least.

Suppose you're faced with an entire row of brown breads and you don't know which ones are low, medium, or high glycemic. By using the ingredients list, you can find out which grains make up a particular bread and how much of those grains are actually used. For example, say you find a bread with packaging that says whole grain (which is promising!), but when you look at the ingredients list, you see that white flour (which is high glycemic) is the main ingredient, with wheat flour (which is low glycemic) being one of the least-used ingredients, making the bread itself a higher-glycemic food. Good thing you know to keep searching for a better kind of bread!

Looking at the ingredients list for simple foods like pasta or bread is one thing, but what in the world do you do when you buy a mixed food like frozen lasagna or chicken noodle soup? The first step is to check out www.nutrition data.com to see whether the food you want to buy (maybe in a different brand) has been tested for glycemic load. Simply go to the Web site, and plug the food item into the search box in the upper-right corner of the page. For instance, when we plug vegetable lasagna into the Web site, we get an estimated glycemic load of 15 for one serving, which means it's a medium-glycemic food. On the other hand, when we plug in one cup of Campbell's Chunky Chicken Noodle Soup, we get an estimated glycemic load of 9, making the soup low glycemic.

The limitation of the glycemic index is that you never really know the glycemic index or load of a specific brand unless that food has been tested. Even so, you can at least make an educated guess about what a particular food's glycemic load should be if it contains the same ingredients as products that have been tested.

Buying Baked Goods, Grains, and Pasta

Ahhh . . . the bakery. Don't you love how grocery stores set up this particular department so that you have to walk by a huge collection of yummy breads, cookies, and pastries before you can make it to the shelves that contain whatever grains you actually have on your shopping list? It's like getting stuck in a sea of tasty treats every time you shop!

For the most part, you won't know the glycemic level of bakery foods because the types and amounts of carbohydrates in them vary so widely, but here are a few tips on how to make good grain choices:

- ✔ When buying bread and rolls, check out the ingredients list (which we explain in the earlier section "Taking a closer look at the ingredients"), and try to pick out the breads that are made with lower-glycemic ingredients like oat or wheat flour.

  If you're craving something different than whole grains, try out medium-glycemic sourdough bread, which has an estimated glycemic load of 11.

✔ When choosing desserts, try to stick with the ones that are low to medium glycemic, including peanut butter cookies (glycemic load 5), oatmeal raisin cookies (glycemic load 7), angel food cake (glycemic load 10), sponge cake (glycemic load 15), and chocolate cake with icing (glycemic load 19).

✔ Don't forget fat and calories! Glycemic load is only part of the picture; you need to consider how much fat and calories you're eating, too. If you're eating a treat only once in a while, don't worry too much, but if indulging your sweet tooth is a weekly ritual, pick desserts like angel food cake that are both low glycemic and low in fat.

✔ Put moderation into play. Everyone likes to have some great treats once in a while, especially for birthdays and parties. In these special situations, go ahead and enjoy some desserts. You won't wreck all your progress with one piece of cake.

When it comes to shopping for carbohydrates, you can't forget about grains (like rice) and pasta. Here are some guidelines on shopping for the best of the bunch:

✔ Choose low-glycemic grains like quinoa, bulgur wheat, or brown rice, and cook up your own low-glycemic recipes with them (see Chapter 14 for ideas) instead of buying packaged meals.

✔ Try out some pasta brands like Dreamfield pastas that have already been tested for their glycemic load.

✔ Look for whole-grain pasta instead of white pasta because it often has a lower glycemic load. Keep in mind, though, that not all whole-wheat pasta is low glycemic. Stick to spaghetti, vermicelli, or tortellini for lower glycemic loads (see Chapter 6 for more details on which pastas are lower glycemic).

Picking Produce

The glycemic level and nutrient value of produce varies depending on how it's packaged. Although the differences aren't drastic (most vegetables, with the exception of potatoes, are low glycemic), it's a good idea to keep them in mind while shopping. Here's what you need to know about fresh, frozen, and canned produce:

✔ **Fresh produce is the best at retaining nutrient value; it also has a lower glycemic load.** The closer your food is to its harvest time, the more nutrients it retains. Locally grown produce is your best bet because it hasn't traveled from other cities or states.

Watch out for bruises and wilting on produce; they can be signs that the produce has been handled improperly or that the food is past its peak. Ripeness matters; the glycemic loads of many foods, especially fruit, increase as the foods continue to ripen. (Notice how a ripe banana is much sweeter than its not-so-ripe counterpart.) Ripeness doesn't change the glycemic load dramatically, but it certainly doesn't hurt to stick with foods that aren't overly ripe.

✔ **Frozen produce has a slightly lower amount of retained nutrients than fresh produce and a similar glycemic load.** When products are frozen immediately after being cleaned and processed, they retain more of their nutrients (even though some nutrients are lost with the processing). Frozen produce can be a great economical value during off-seasons. Just make sure you skip the frozen fruit that has sugar added; that way, you don't increase your carbohydrates by buying frozen instead of fresh.

Frozen fruits and vegetables are easy to stock up on, so they can be super handy when you need a fast meal.

✔ **Canned produce loses some of its nutrient value and often has a bit higher glycemic load than fresh or frozen produce.** For example, raw apricots have a low glycemic load of 5, whereas canned apricots have a medium glycemic load of 12. This difference is due to the heating process that takes place during canning and the fact that most fruits are canned in heavy syrup. Look for fruits that are canned in water or light syrup.

Diving into Dairy

If you're a fan of dairy, you'll be happy to hear that virtually all dairy products, including ice cream, are low glycemic. Why? They're made up of carbohydrates as well as protein and fat, so the amount of carbohydrates in them is naturally lower, making them low glycemic. So the next time you're craving dairy, don't worry so much about glycemic load; instead, focus on the fat and added sugars.

Dairy contains saturated fats, which are associated with heart disease and certain cancers. To get your fat intake under control, try eating lowfat dairy products rather than their full-fat counterparts. You don't have to go all the way to fat free to see the difference; middle of the road, like 1% milk or 1% cottage cheese, is fine. You also want to choose dairy products that have no added sugars or ones that have the least amount (look on the ingredients list for the specific sugars included).

Be aware that some yogurts are really loaded with sugar! A quick tip is to buy plain yogurt and mix in all-fruit spread to make your own fruit yogurt with much less sugar.

Making Sense of Meats and Seafood

Meat and seafood are automatically low glycemic because they don't contain any carbohydrates. However, they do vary in how many saturated fats they contain, so you need to watch which cuts of meat and seafood you eat. But because many meat and seafood products don't come with nutrition facts panels, deciding which ones to buy can be a little confusing. To simplify things, we spend the following sections telling you which cuts of meats and seafood are the leanest so you know what to buy the next time you're in the butcher's section of the grocery store.

The best cuts of poultry

For the most part, poultry like chicken and turkey is a lean protein source. There are a few exceptions, however; dark meat and meat that contains the skin can often be higher in fat. In fact, in some cases, dark poultry meat is even higher in fat than beef.

To help you make the best choices in the grocery store, stick with the following leanest cuts of poultry (flip to Chapter 15 for some great poultry recipes):

- ✔ 99-percent lean ground turkey or chicken
- ✔ Skinless turkey or chicken breasts

The best cuts of beef

Shopping for beef can become pretty confusing because of the many cuts you have to choose from. In general, though, try to look for lean cuts of beef to keep your saturated fat and calorie levels down.

We suggest sticking to 10 grams of total fat or less per 3.5-ounce serving size. We use lean cuts of beef in the delicious recipes we include in Chapter 16 to help get you started. Here are some of the leanest beef picks:

- ✔ Bottom round roast
- ✔ Chuck shoulder roast
- ✔ Eye of round roast
- ✔ 95- to 99-percent lean ground beef

- ✔ Round steak
- ✔ Shoulder steak
- ✔ Strip steak
- ✔ T-bone steak
- ✔ Tenderloin steak
- ✔ Top round steak
- ✔ Top sirloin steak

The best cuts of pork

Many people think they have to ditch pork because of fat, but the reality is that most pork products are low in saturated fats, making them excellent entree choices for low-glycemic meals. As you can see, we use many different cuts of pork throughout this cookbook (see Chapter 16 for great recipes to try). Here are your best choices for lean pork:

- ✔ Bone-in center loin chop
- ✔ Bone-in rib chop
- ✔ Bone-in sirloin roast
- ✔ Boneless top loin chop
- ✔ Boneless top loin roast
- ✔ Pork tenderloin

The best bets on seafood

Although you can find both lean and fatty cuts of seafood, we actually recommend eating the fatty cuts (think cold-water fish like salmon) because they're high in healthy omega-3 fatty acids.

The biggest issue you need to be aware of with seafood is that different fish have different mercury levels. Pregnant women and young children need to be especially careful when eating mercury-containing fish. Too much mercury can pass into the bloodstream of the fetus and can harm the developing nervous system, leading to learning disabilities, developmental delays, and other serious health problems. These same issues can occur in young children who consume too much mercury.

Here are your best seafood choices because they contain the least amount of mercury:

- ✔ Canned light tuna (albacore is higher in mercury)
- ✔ Catfish
- ✔ Crab (domestic)
- ✔ Freshwater trout
- ✔ Haddock
- ✔ Halibut
- ✔ Pollock
- ✔ Salmon
- ✔ Shrimp
- ✔ Tilapia

Note: Cod and red snapper, two fish we use in Chapter 17, sometimes have higher mercury levels, so don't eat these types any more than once a week.

 The Monterey Bay Aquarium Seafood Watch provides useful information on seafood specifically for different regions. For more information, go to www. montereybayaquarium.org/cr/seafoodwatch.aspx.

Simplifying Shopping with a Low-Glycemic List

Are you one of those people who goes to the store and buys miscellaneous fruits, vegetables, and meats with no plan on how to use them? If so, you probably end up throwing most of them out because they never really fit in with a meal, at least not before they start to rot! At this point, you're not only wasting food but also throwing away money. But don't worry. A simple shopping list can come to the rescue! It helps you buy what you need, use the food you buy, and save money in the long run.

In addition to using a shopping list whenever you go to the store, we also recommend stocking up on low-glycemic, lowfat staple foods to make your life a little simpler. Note that when we say *staple foods,* we mean items that will keep in your pantry or freezer or that you're sure you'll find use for during the week. For instance, cheese may not be something that lasts a long time in your refrigerator, but if you're like us, you'll easily find plenty of uses for it during the week like on sandwiches or in your eggs.

Stocking up on low-glycemic staples when they're on sale or when you have coupons can actually help you slash your food budget. Keep in mind, though, that your staples are only items you know you'll use regularly. For instance, you probably don't want to stock up on fresh broccoli when it's on sale because it'll probably go bad before you can use it all. But if you're a salad person and know you'll be eating at least a few salads during the week for quick meals, it makes more sense to buy salad ingredients when they go on sale.

In Chapter 6, we share some pantry, freezer, and refrigerator favorites to include on your grocery list so you know what to stock up on. You can edit this list to fit your own tastes and lifestyle.

When making your shopping list, plan what you're going to make for the week. That way, you won't just buy random produce and meats without knowing what to do with them. Instead, you'll know that you're having polenta lasagna on Monday, minestrone soup with salad on Tuesday, and so on. You can then buy the exact ingredients you need for the week all in one grocery trip. (Flip to Chapters 4 and 5 for full details on meal-planning strategies.)

Part III
Serving Up Starters, Snacks, and Sides

The 5th Wave

By Rich Tennant

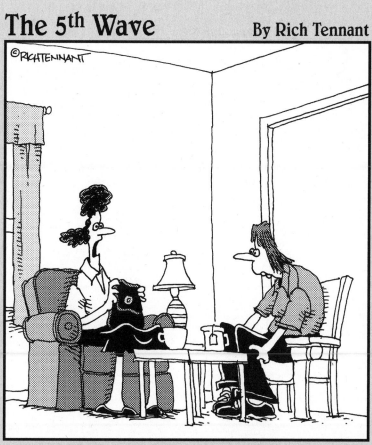

"Of course I'm concerned about the food you're serving your family. Let's face it, you named your first three children Twinkie, Ding Dong, and Fluffernutter."

In this part . . .

You definitely don't have to give up taste to use low-glycemic foods in your cooking; you can create delicious low-glycemic recipes that incorporate all your favorite foods.

This part includes tasty breakfast recipes that you can use whether you want a fast on-the-go breakfast or a big Sunday brunch. It also shows you a handful of baked goods and appetizers that are perfect for serving at a party or keeping around the house as snacks. Finally, the side dishes you find here (vegetables, grains, pasta, and potatoes) introduce you to a whole new world beyond boring old boiled vegetables and white rice so you can explore just how tasty a low-glycemic lifestyle can be.

Chapter 8

Beginning Your Day Right with a Healthy Breakfast

. . . .

In This Chapter

▶ Starting off the day with some quick breakfast recipes

▶ Sweetening your morning with pancakes and waffles

▶ Creating savory and healthy egg dishes

. . . .

Starting off your day with a healthy breakfast is one of the most important strategies for improving your health and well-being. We know . . . this statement conjures up memories of your mother or grandmother telling you that breakfast is the most important meal of the day as they whip up a batch of tasty pancakes and bacon. Somewhere along the way the idea of breakfast foods became taboo. Waffles and pancakes packed with refined high-glycemic starches, high-sugar cereals lacking in protein, and eggs rich in cholesterol started to scare people away from breakfast. However, research shows that eating a healthy breakfast is linked to

✔ Improved energy levels

✔ Weight control (thanks to decreased hunger during the day)

✔ Better endurance for physical activities

✔ Improved concentration at work or in the classroom

With all these benefits, breakfast is still the most commonly skipped meal of the day. We're sure you've been there before — you either don't know what to eat or you simply get too busy with work, school, kids, and whatever else fills your mornings, and before you know it, it's noon and you haven't eaten anything. Some of you may skip breakfast once in a while, but others of you may skip it every day. Well, it's time to listen to Grandma's advice — and bring back breakfast!

The idea is to transform the old refined-starch and high-fat breakfast into a healthier meal that's appropriate for a low-glycemic diet. We promise you can make this change without losing flavor. Whether you like a quick cereal or you enjoy more elaborate dishes, our goal in this chapter is to help you find some ideas that are low glycemic, low in fat, and high in nutrients so you can enjoy all the health and wellness benefits of a tasty breakfast meal.

Running-Out-the-Door Breakfast Ideas

Let's face it, part of the reason why many people skip breakfast is the fast-paced lifestyle that has become today's norm; people simply don't have time to eat a meal before running out the door to begin the day. The last thing you need is a list of elaborate breakfast recipes that'll work only on the weekends or during the holidays.

Reinventing a healthy breakfast to fit a low-glycemic diet starts with quick weekday ideas. This section includes healthy foods you can prepare in advance to have as quick grab-and-go breakfast meals all week long. These recipes are the perfect fit for a busy lifestyle.

Grab-and-go starters to begin your day

In general, we've seen the following two main reasons why people don't eat breakfast:

✔ Some days people just don't have enough time to sit down and make a breakfast meal.

✔ Many people feel sick or queasy if they eat first thing in the morning.

The good news for both sets of people is that you don't have to eat a big breakfast to get the health benefits an early meal has to offer. Eating a few grab-and-go starters to begin your day keeps your metabolism strong, provides energy for your day, and helps you concentrate and focus on your daily tasks. So it's perfectly fine to have a few snacks throughout the morning to equal one larger breakfast. For instance, you may grab a yogurt on your way out the door in the morning and an hour later eat a banana with peanut butter as you enjoy your coffee at your desk. Just make sure you have a plan so you don't end up grazing on whatever is around all morning. A couple of planned healthy snacks

can equal a breakfast. Too many small snacks can end up adding to your waistline.

If you just can't fit a full breakfast into your schedule or your life, try out these simple low-glycemic starters to begin your day the right way:

✔ Slice of whole-grain toast with peanut butter or other nut butter

✔ Banana or apple slices with peanut butter or other nut butter

✔ Slice of whole-grain toast with a slice of melted cheese

✔ Peanut butter and jelly on a toasted whole-wheat English muffin

✔ 8 ounces of lowfat yogurt

✔ Hard-boiled egg with a slice of toast

✔ Oatmeal Raspberry Bar (see the recipe in this chapter)

✔ Cottage cheese with fruit

Very Berry Dry Muesli

Prep time: 4 min • **Cook time:** 8–10 min • **Yield:** 8 servings

Ingredients	*Directions*
2 cups old-fashioned oats	**1** Preheat the oven to 350 degrees.
½ cup slivered almonds	
1 cup bran flakes	**2** Spread the oats and almonds on a small cookie sheet. Bake the oats and almonds for about 8 to 10 minutes, or until lightly toasted, stirring every 2 minutes.
½ teaspoon ground cinnamon	
2 cups sliced strawberries	**3** Let the mixture cool, and then pour it into a medium bowl. Add the bran flakes and cinnamon. Mix them thoroughly into the oat-almond mixture.
2 cups blueberries	
4 cups lowfat vanilla or fruit-flavored yogurt	**4** Mix the strawberries and blueberries together in a medium bowl. Serve ⅓ cup of muesli with ½ cup of mixed berries and ½ cup of lowfat yogurt for each serving.

Per serving: Calories 263 (From Fat 62); Glycemic Load 7 (Low); Fat 7g (Saturated 2g); Cholesterol 6mg; Sodium 94mg; Carbohydrate 43g (Dietary Fiber 5g); Protein 11g.

Vary It! Feel free to add other fresh or dried fruits (like fresh nectarines or dried apples) if you don't have berries on hand. For those of you who aren't yogurt fans, go ahead and drizzle each serving with ½ teaspoon of honey, and serve with 8 ounces of milk.

Tip: You can store the muesli in an airtight container for up to two weeks.

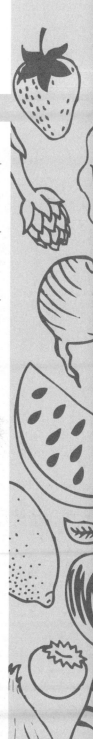

Pumpkin and Sunflower Seed Granola with Dried Blueberries

Prep time: 5 min • **Cook time:** 25–30 min • **Yield:** 8 servings

Ingredients	Directions
⅓ cup canola oil	**1** Preheat the oven to 375 degrees.
⅓ cup maple syrup	
1 tablespoon vanilla extract	**2** In a large bowl, stir together the oil, maple syrup, vanilla, and salt.
⅛ teaspoon salt	
½ teaspoon ground cinnamon	**3** In a separate bowl, mix together the cinnamon, oats, pumpkin seeds, and sunflower seeds.
3 cups old-fashioned oats	
½ cup unsalted pumpkin seeds	**4** Stir the maple syrup mixture into the oats and seeds until they're well coated.
½ cup unsalted sunflower seeds	
Nonstick cooking spray	**5** Spray a 9-x-13-inch baking pan or glass dish with nonstick cooking spray. Place the granola mixture into the pan.
1 cup dried, unsweetened blueberries	**6** Bake the coated oat-seed mixture for 10 minutes on the middle oven rack, and then stir it. Continue to bake the mixture for 15 to 20 more minutes, or until golden brown, checking and stirring every few minutes. For chunky granola, don't break up the chunks too much when stirring.
4 cups lowfat yogurt or lowfat milk	
	7 Top ⅓ cup of granola with 2 tablespoons of dried blueberries and ½ cup of lowfat yogurt or milk for each serving.

Per serving: *Calories 451 (From Fat 165); Glycemic Load 9 (Low); Fat 18g (Saturated 8g); Cholesterol 8mg; Sodium 134mg; Carbohydrate 60g (Dietary Fiber 6g); Protein 14g.*

Vary It! You can experiment by adding nuts to the recipe for a little variety. For example, you can replace the pumpkin and sunflower seeds with the same amount of almonds, cashews, walnuts, or even peanuts to change it up a bit. You can also change up the fruit by replacing the blueberries with 1 cup of dried apples, blackberries, strawberries, or whatever other dried fruits you have on hand.

Note: Don't mix the dried fruit into the whole batch because doing so will moisten the granola and make it less crisp after a few days.

Oatmeal Raspberry Bars

Prep time: 10 min • **Cook time:** 25–30 min • **Yield:** 12 servings

Ingredients	Directions
Nonstick cooking spray	**1** Preheat the oven to 350 degrees, and grease an 8-x-8-inch glass baking dish with nonstick cooking spray.
1½ cups rolled oats	
⅔ cup slivered almonds	**2** In a large bowl, stir together the rolled oats, almonds, cinnamon, and nutmeg. Set aside.
½ teaspoon ground cinnamon	
⅛ teaspoon ground nutmeg	**3** Melt the butter in a small saucepan over medium heat. Stir the brown sugar and honey into the melted butter; bring the mixture to a boil. Remove the pan from heat.
⅓ cup butter	
¼ cup packed brown sugar	
¼ cup honey	**4** Pour the butter mixture over the oats mixture. Stir until the oats mixture is well coated.
⅔ cup no-sugar-added raspberry preserves	
	5 Press half of the oats mixture into the baking dish. With a knife or spatula, spread a thin layer of raspberry preserves over the first layer of oats. Then press the second half of the oats mixture on top of the preserves.
	6 Bake for 25 to 30 minutes, or until slightly browned around the edges. While the oatmeal bar is warm, press the surface gently with the back of a spoon to flatten the mixture. Then use a knife to score it into 12 bars.

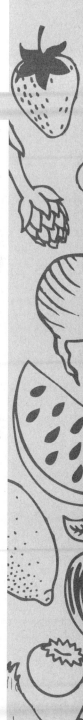

Per serving: Calories 192 (From Fat 9); Glycemic Load 7 (Low); Fat 9g (Saturated 4g); Cholesterol 14mg; Sodium 3mg; Carbohydrate 27g (Dietary Fiber 2g); Protein 3g.

Tip: These bars provide a great smaller option for those of you who don't like eating a big meal in the morning. For a larger meal, pair one of these bars with 8 ounces of lowfat yogurt and a slice of fresh fruit. (Check out these bars in the color section.)

Note: You can store the oatmeal bars in an airtight container for up to one week.

Giving Breakfast a Sweet Side

Following a low-glycemic diet means reducing many of the refined grains and sugars in your diet. That being said, you can still enjoy some sweet breakfast choices, like pancakes and waffles. Decreasing the amount of white flour and adding some bulk with fruits or nuts can turn a high-glycemic meal into a low to medium one. Using a few tricks like these, you can enjoy some old favorites while staying on the low-glycemic side.

Just make sure to keep your butter and syrup toppings to a minimum to avoid turning our lower-glycemic recipes into higher-glycemic ones, not to mention adding too many calories. Keep your butter to 1 teaspoon per serving size and your maple syrup to 1 to 2 tablespoons, or skip it altogether and add ¼ cup of fruit to sweeten things up.

Keep in mind that going low glycemic is really about moderation, so you can still enjoy your high-glycemic breakfasts once in a while. But for those of you who crave pancakes on a weekly basis, this section is for you!

Banana Strawberry Oatmeal Pancakes

Prep time: 12 min • **Cook time:** 18 min • **Yield:** 6 servings

Ingredients	Directions
1¼ cups reduced-fat (light) oat-bran pancake mix or reduced-fat oatmeal pancake mix	*1* In a large bowl, mix together the pancake mix, oats, cinnamon, and nutmeg. Add the milk, and let sit for 1 to 2 minutes.
½ cup quick-cooking oats	
1 teaspoon ground cinnamon	*2* Add the mashed bananas to the oat mixture. Stir in the beaten eggs and orange zest (batter will be thick).
¼ teaspoon ground nutmeg	
1 cup lowfat milk	*3* Spray a large nonstick skillet with nonstick cooking spray, and heat the skillet over medium heat. Using ¼ cup of batter for each pancake, drop 4 pancakes in the skillet, spacing them about 1½ inches apart. (Because the batter is thick, try to pat down the batter to make pancakes that are approximately 3 inches in diameter.)
1 cup mashed ripe bananas (about 2 medium bananas)	
2 eggs, beaten to blend	
½ teaspoon orange zest	
Nonstick cooking spray	*4* Cook the pancakes until they're brown on the bottom and some bubbles begin to break around the edges, about 3 minutes. Gently turn the pancakes over. Cook until they're brown on the bottom and firm to the touch in the center, about 3 minutes (pancakes will be thick).
6 tablespoons maple syrup (optional)	
1½ cups sliced strawberries	
1½ cups sliced bananas	
	5 Repeat Steps 3 and 4 for the remaining batter to cook 12 pancakes total. Coat the pan with cooking spray before each batch.
	6 For each serving, serve 2 pancakes with 1 tablespoon of syrup (if desired), ¼ cup of sliced strawberries, and ¼ cup of sliced bananas.

Per serving: Calories 240 (From Fat 37); Glycemic Load 10 (Low); Fat 4g (Saturated 1g); Cholesterol 73mg; Sodium 144mg; Carbohydrate 43g (Dietary Fiber 8g); Protein 10g.

Note: This recipe uses a thick batter for hearty pancakes; you can find oat-bran pancake mix in most major grocery stores.

Vary It! The banana-strawberry topping really makes this recipe wonderful, but feel free to experiment with other fruit toppings, as well!

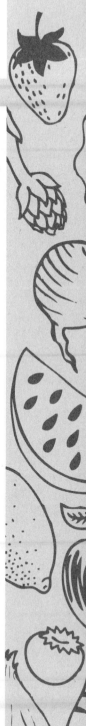

Peanut Butter Pancakes

Prep time: 7 min • **Cook time:** 6 min • **Yield:** 4 servings

Ingredients	*Directions*
½ cup all-purpose flour	*1* In a large bowl, mix together the all-purpose flour, oat flour, baking powder, and sugar.
⅔ cup oat flour	
2 teaspoons baking powder	*2* In a separate bowl, beat together the egg, peanut butter, vanilla, milk, and oil until everything is blended together and the egg is separated.
2 tablespoons sugar	
1 egg, beaten	
½ cup chunky peanut butter, no sugar added	*3* Add the liquid mixture to the flour mixture, and stir until just combined.
½ teaspoon vanilla	
1 cup skim milk	*4* Spray a large nonstick skillet with cooking spray, and heat the skillet over medium-low heat. Using ¼ cup of batter for each pancake, drop 4 pancakes in the skillet, spacing them about 1½ inches apart.
2 tablespoons peanut oil or canola oil	
Nonstick cooking spray	
2 cups sliced bananas or other fresh fruit	*5* Cook the pancakes until they're brown on the bottom and some bubbles begin to break around the edges, about 2 minutes. Gently turn the pancakes over. Cook them until they're brown on the bottom and firm to the touch in the center, about 1 minute.
	6 Repeat Steps 4 and 5 with the remaining batter so you cook 8 pancakes total. Recoat the pan with cooking spray before the second batch.
	7 For each serving, serve 2 pancakes with ½ cup of sliced bananas or other fresh fruit.

Per serving: *Calories 501 (From Fat 231); Glycemic Load 19 (Medium); Fat 26g (Saturated 5g); Cholesterol 54mg; Sodium 394mg; Carbohydrate 56g (Dietary Fiber 6g); Protein 16g.*

Note: When you try this recipe, notice that the peanut butter makes these a bit higher in calories. Trust us, the protein and healthy fat in these pancakes make for such a filling and hearty breakfast that you won't need to eat more than 2 per serving.

Tip: You definitely don't need to doctor these pancakes up with maple syrup and butter. We recommend serving them with a sliced banana or other favorite fruit — that way, you don't ruin the delicious peanut butter flavor.

Cornmeal Waffles

Prep time: 12 min • **Cook time:** 18 min • **Yield:** 9 servings

Ingredients	*Directions*
Nonstick cooking spray 1½ cups all-purpose flour 1½ cups cornmeal 1 tablespoon baking powder ¼ teaspoon salt 2 tablespoons sugar 2 eggs, lightly beaten 1 teaspoon vanilla 2 cups skim milk 3 tablespoons canola oil 4½ cups berries 9 tablespoons maple syrup or honey	*1* Spray the waffle iron with nonstick cooking spray, and heat it on the high setting. (If you don't have a high setting, simply turn it on.) *2* In a large bowl, mix together the flour, cornmeal, baking powder, salt, and sugar. *3* In a separate bowl, beat together the eggs, vanilla, milk, and oil. *4* Add the liquid mixture to the flour mixture, and stir until just combined. *5* Pour ¼ cup of the batter onto the waffle iron, or enough to evenly fill the grates on the waffle iron. Cook each waffle separately, and don't open the waffle iron until it's in finished/ready mode, about 2 minutes. *6* Repeat Step 5 with the remaining batter so you cook 9 waffles total. Recoat the iron with cooking spray before you cook each new waffle. *7* For each serving, serve 1 waffle with ½ cup of fresh berries and 1 tablespoon (or less) of maple syrup or honey.

Per serving: *Calories 342 (From Fat 61); Glycemic Load 16 (Medium); Fat 7g (Saturated 1g); Cholesterol 48mg; Sodium 241mg; Carbohydrate 63g (Dietary Fiber 4g); Protein 8g.*

Note: Make these waffles (shown in the color section) in a Belgian waffle maker, and serve them with your favorite fruit.

Tip: If you have leftovers, freeze the extra waffles, and throw them in the toaster oven for a quick meal later in the week.

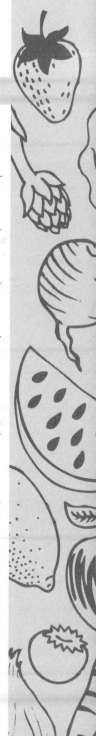

Making Eggs Part of a Healthy Breakfast

Eggs are one of your best bets for a healthy, low-glycemic breakfast; they're a great source of protein and important vitamins and minerals. Yes, the yolk is rich in cholesterol, but eating eggs in moderation hasn't shown adverse affects on heart health. In fact, a review of 224 studies carried out over the last 25 years has now determined that you can eat one to two eggs daily without raising your cholesterol levels.

If you have high cholesterol or a heart condition, be sure to follow your physician's specific recommendations in regards to diet and eggs. Every person's situation is different.

In this section, we show you how to dress up your eggs by adding other healthy ingredients to make a hearty, delicious breakfast that isn't loaded in fat or calories. Served with a slice of whole-wheat toast or eaten alone, the foods in this section will start your day off with a bang. You'll feel full for a longer period of time and may even experience an increase in energy.

We feature two types of egg dishes in this section:

- ✔ **A Tex-Mex twist:** Who says Tex-Mex is only for lunches and dinners? We love the idea of adding a little fun and a whole lot of flavor to breakfast with some favorite south-of-the-border ingredients like salsa and peppers. The best part about these recipes is that you can change them up to fit your own preference. If you love hot and spicy, replace medium or mild salsa with hot, or add a few jalapeños to get some more heat. Because these particular ingredients are low glycemic and low calorie, you can add as many as you'd like.

- ✔ **Cheesy does it:** We love that cheese is a low-glycemic food option because it's not only a great source of calcium but also a delicious addition to almost any meal. You don't want to get too carried away, though, because it is higher in fat and can add up in calories quickly. The best thing about adding cheese to egg dishes is that you need just a little to really bring out the flavor of your eggs.

Breakfast Burritos

Prep time: 10 min • **Cook time:** 12 min • **Yield:** 4 servings

Ingredients	*Directions*
1 tablespoon canola oil	*1* Heat the canola oil in a large nonstick skillet over medium-high heat. Cook the onions and peppers until they begin to soften, about 3 minutes.
½ small sweet onion, finely chopped	
1 red bell pepper, finely chopped	*2* Add the mushrooms, and cook them until soft, about 5 minutes.
1 small portobello mushroom, diced	
4 eggs	*3* Meanwhile, whisk together the eggs, egg substitute, milk, salt, and pepper. Reduce the heat to low, and add the egg mixture to the vegetable mixture, scrambling until cooked through, about 3 minutes.
1 cup egg substitute	
2 tablespoons lowfat milk	
Salt and pepper to taste	
⅓ cup shredded Mexican blend cheese	*4* Add the cheese, and stir it into the mixture until melted, about 1 minute.
Four 10-inch whole-wheat tortillas	*5* Spread each tortilla with ¼ of the scrambled eggs, salsa (to taste), and ¼ of the avocado. Roll up the tortillas burrito-style and serve.
Salsa to taste	
1 ripe avocado, peeled, pitted, and sliced	

Per serving: *Calories 399 (From Fat 462); Glycemic Load 9 (Low); Fat 18g (Saturated 4g); Cholesterol 213mg; Sodium 492mg; Carbohydrate 43g (Dietary Fiber 7g); Protein 23g.*

Vary It! We stick to a pretty standard recipe here, but if you like a little spice, go ahead and add some cayenne pepper or hot sauce.

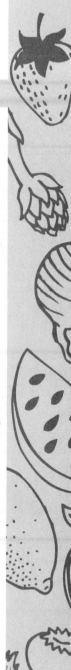

Southwestern Egg Scramble

Prep time: 15 min • **Cook time:** 8–10 min • **Yield:** 3 servings

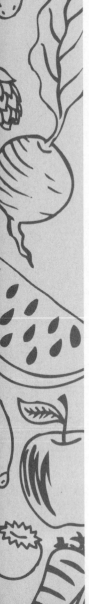

Ingredients	*Directions*
1 tablespoon canola oil **Two 5-inch-diameter corn tortillas, cut into ¼-inch strips** **½ cup finely chopped red onion** **½ green bell pepper, finely chopped** **3 eggs, plus 1 cup egg substitute, beaten to blend** **2 tablespoons chopped fresh cilantro** **⅓ cup grated or shredded cheddar cheese** **½ ripe avocado, pitted, peeled, and sliced** **1 cup salsa** **Salt and pepper to taste**	*1* Heat the oil in a 12-inch nonstick straight-side skillet over medium-high heat. Add the tortillas; sauté them until brown, about 4 to 5 minutes, turning them once. Using a slotted spoon, transfer the tortillas to a paper-towel-lined plate. Set aside about 2 tablespoons of tortilla strips for the garnish.
	2 Add the onion and pepper to the skillet; sauté over medium-high heat for 2 minutes.
	3 Add the eggs, egg substitute, and cilantro, and cook until the eggs are softly set, about 2 to 3 minutes, stirring constantly.
	4 Return the tortillas to the skillet. Mix in the cheese.
	5 Transfer the egg mixture to a platter. Top with the avocado and reserved tortilla strips. Add salt and pepper to taste, and serve with salsa.

Per serving: Calories 314 (From Fat 171); Glycemic Load 8 (Low); Fat 19g (Saturated 5g); Cholesterol 222mg; Sodium 511mg; Carbohydrate 17g (Dietary Fiber 4g); Protein 21g.

Tip: This fun recipe is the perfect solution when you feel like adding a little kick to your own breakfast meal, but you can also make it when you have guests over for brunch by doubling or tripling the recipe.

Vary It! If you want to make this dish spicy, add some cayenne pepper, chili powder, or hot sauce.

Asiago Cheese and Tomato Omelet

Prep time: 8 min • **Cook time:** 4–7 min • **Yield:** 1 serving

Ingredients	*Directions*
2 eggs 1 tablespoon lowfat milk ⅛ teaspoon salt Pepper to taste Nonstick cooking spray 2 tablespoons grated Asiago cheese 2 tablespoons diced Roma tomatoes (or large cherry tomatoes) 1 tablespoon chopped green onion 4 ripe avocado slices (approximately ¼ avocado total)	*1* Beat the eggs until frothy; whisk in the milk, salt, and pepper. *2* Heat an 8-inch nonstick skillet over medium heat. Spray the heated skillet with nonstick cooking spray, decrease the heat to low, and pour in the egg mixture. Cook the egg mixture slowly, about 3 to 5 minutes, lifting gently at the edges with a spatula to let the uncooked egg run underneath. *3* When the omelet is almost cooked and appears shiny on top, cover the skillet and continue cooking until the surface of the omelet dries, about 1 to 2 minutes. *4* Top with the cheese, tomato, green onion, and avocado; fold in half and serve.

Per serving: Calories 290 (From Fat 192); Glycemic Load 4 (Low); Fat 21g (Saturated 7g); Cholesterol 438mg; Sodium 314mg; Carbohydrate 8g (Dietary Fiber 5g); Protein 18g.

Vary It! In this omelet, we celebrate the flavor of Asiago cheese. If you can't find this cheese, you can easily substitute Parmesan or Romano.

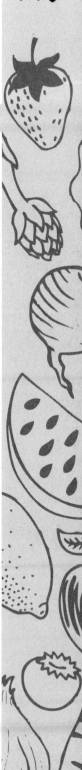

Canadian Bacon and Cheese Frittata

Prep time: 10 min • **Cook time:** 18–26 min • **Yield:** 6 servings

Ingredients	*Directions*
1 tablespoon canola oil	*1* Preheat the oven to 375 degrees.
1 cup broccoli florets	
½ small sweet onion, finely chopped	*2* In a large ovenproof skillet, heat the oil and sauté the broccoli, onions, and peppers until they begin to soften, about 4 minutes. Add the mushrooms and cook until the vegetables are tender, about 3 minutes. Add the Canadian bacon; heat through, about 1 minute. Remove the skillet from heat and keep warm.
½ red bell pepper, finely chopped	
⅔ cup sliced fresh mushrooms	
1 cup cooked Canadian bacon, slices quartered	
8 eggs	*3* In a mixing bowl, beat the eggs, water, mustard, parsley, basil, and salt until foamy. Stir in the cheddar cheese.
2 tablespoons water	
2 tablespoons Dijon mustard	*4* Pour the egg mixture over the meat-and-vegetable mixture; heat on low heat. As the eggs set, lift the edges with a spatula, letting the uncooked portion flow underneath. When the eggs are almost set (after about 3 minutes), place the skillet in the oven and bake for 5 to 10 minutes until the top is set.
¼ teaspoon dried parsley	
¼ teaspoon dried basil	
¼ teaspoon salt	
⅓ cup shredded cheddar cheese	
¼ cup grated Parmesan cheese	*5* Top with the Parmesan cheese and bake for 2 to 5 minutes longer until the cheese is warm and melting.

Per serving: Calories 203 (From Fat 125); Glycemic Load 0 (Low); Fat 14g (Saturated 5g); Cholesterol 301mg; Sodium 642mg; Carbohydrate 4g (Dietary Fiber 1g); Protein 16g.

Note: Lucky for you, Canadian bacon gives you that smoky ham taste without all the fat and calories. Just make sure you use an ovenproof skillet while cooking this recipe (shown in the color section).

Sun-Dried Tomato and Feta Egg Bake

Prep time: 8 min • **Cook time:** 34 min, plus standing time • **Yield:** 6 servings

Ingredients	*Directions*
Nonstick cooking spray 1 shallot, finely chopped	**1** Preheat the oven to 375 degrees. Spray a 9-x-13-x-2-inch glass baking dish with nonstick cooking spray.
½ cup chopped and drained oil-packed sun-dried tomatoes 2 tablespoons plus 2 tablespoons chopped fresh basil	**2** Sauté the shallots until soft, about 3 minutes. Add the sun-dried tomatoes and 2 tablespoons of basil; stir for 1 minute.
1 cup egg substitute 4 eggs ¾ cup lowfat milk	**3** In a large bowl, whisk together the egg substitute, eggs, milk, feta cheese, and salt to blend well. Add the sun-dried-tomato mixture and mix well. Pour the egg mixture into the baking dish. Bake for 20 minutes.
¼ cup crumbled feta cheese ¼ teaspoon salt ⅓ cup shredded mozzarella cheese	**4** Pull the dish out of the oven, and top with mozzarella cheese and 2 tablespoons of fresh basil. Return the casserole to the oven, and cook for another 10 minutes until the top is golden brown, the cheese is melted, and a knife inserted into the center comes out clean.
	5 Let the casserole stand for 5 minutes before serving.

Per serving: *Calories 139 (From Fat 69); Glycemic Load 2 (Low); Fat 8g (Saturated 3g); Cholesterol 153mg; Sodium 355mg; Carbohydrate 6g (Dietary Fiber 1g); Protein 12g.*

Tip: The mixture of sun-dried tomatoes and feta cheese packs a powerful punch of taste. You can leave this dish as is, or if you're craving a bit of meat with your breakfast, you can add some chicken sausage.

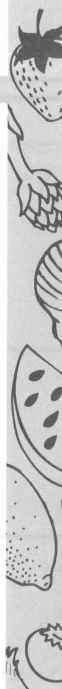

Veggie Egg Bake

Prep time: 15 min   •   **Cook time:** 25–27 min, plus standing time   •   **Yield:** 5 servings

Ingredients	Directions
1 tablespoon canola oil	*1* Preheat the oven to 375 degrees.
½ red bell pepper, seeded and finely chopped	*2* In a large ovenproof skillet, heat the canola oil over medium-high heat. Add the red pepper, zucchini, green onion, parsley, and basil. Simmer until the zucchini is tender, about 5 minutes.
2 zucchini, cut into ½-inch chunks	
2 green onions, finely chopped	
½ teaspoon parsley	*3* Stir in the mushrooms and butter until the butter is melted and mushrooms soften, about 2 minutes. Add the eggs and stir; season with salt and pepper. Cook over low heat until the eggs start to firm, about 3 to 5 minutes. Lift the pan from side to side a few times while cooking to let the wet ingredients go underneath.
½ teaspoon basil	
6 fresh mushrooms, sliced	
2 teaspoons butter	
6 eggs	
½ teaspoon salt	*4* Sprinkle with mozzarella cheese, and bake for 10 minutes.
¼ teaspoon pepper	
½ cup shredded mozzarella cheese	*5* Remove the dish from the oven. Top it with the tomato slices and Parmesan cheese. Place it back in the oven for 5 minutes until the cheese starts to melt and the tomatoes become soft and warm.
1 tomato, sliced	
3 tablespoons grated Parmesan cheese	*6* Let the dish stand for 5 minutes before cutting it into wedges.

Per serving: Calories 201 (From Fat 126); Glycemic Load 0 (Low); Fat 14g (Saturated 5g); Cholesterol 270mg; Sodium 413mg; Carbohydrate 7g (Dietary Fiber 2g); Protein 13g.

Note: Make sure you use an ovenproof skillet when making this recipe.

Chapter 9

Whipping Up Some Healthier Baked Goods

In This Chapter

▶ Warming up with freshly baked muffins

▶ Fitting quick breads into your low-glycemic diet

Although baked goods — with their white flour, butter, and sugar — aren't always the healthiest, most low-glycemic foods, we believe they're good for the soul (in moderation, of course). Not only is eating a freshly baked muffin or slice of homemade bread for breakfast or as a snack a truly wonderful experience, but taking part in the baking process itself gives you an emotional satisfaction and stress release you can't find anywhere else.

For these reasons, it's important to find some delicious baked recipes that not only feed your soul but also don't destroy your other health goals in the process. In this chapter, we bring you healthier versions of some favorite baked goods. We incorporate more whole-grain flours and less butter and sugar but keep a lot of flavor for the end product. If you have traditional baking recipes you just love, you can change them up fairly easily to make them as balanced as the ones we include here. (See the nearby sidebar "Baking treats the healthier way" for a list of tips on how to do so.)

 Health and wellness aren't just about nutrition and exercise. Laughter and joy are also important components, which is why we're passionate about finding that perfect balance where you can experience all kinds of foods for both nourishment and sheer pleasure.

Making Memorable Muffins

Our favorite thing about muffins is that you can prepare them in so many different ways. For example, you can go for the high-sugar, high-fat versions when you want a special treat, or you can make them with low-glycemic grains, nuts, and fruits for a healthy snack or quick breakfast. In this section, you find recipes for healthy muffins that taste great.

Baking treats the healthier way

Here are a few tricks to turn a high-glycemic, high-fat muffin or bread into a healthier version. Keep in mind that when changing a recipe, you always have to use a little trial and error. In other words, you may have to experiment with these tips to find the perfect fit for the recipes you're changing.

✔ Change the flour in the recipe to half all-purpose flour and half whole-grain flour, like whole wheat or oat.

✔ Add nuts and seeds for more protein and healthy fats.

✔ Add fruits for fiber, vitamins, and minerals.

✔ Replace the oil with applesauce, using the same measurement, or simply decrease the oil by one-fourth of what's called for.

✔ Add grated carrots, apples, or canned pumpkin to add more sweetness and moisture (not to mention adding a complete boost to the nutritional load!) while cutting back about one-fourth of the amount of sugar.

✔ Decrease the total amount of sugar in the recipe by one-fourth of what's called for. You may be surprised to find out that most of the time your treat is still plenty sweet.

✔ Use two egg whites in place of a whole egg.

Chocolate Chip Pumpkin Muffins

Prep time: 10 min • **Cook time:** 16–18 min • **Yield:** 15 servings

Ingredients	*Directions*
Nonstick cooking spray **1 cup all-purpose flour** **1 cup whole-wheat flour** **½ cup sugar** **1 tablespoon baking powder** **1½ teaspoons pumpkin pie spice** **¼ teaspoon salt** **1 cup canned pumpkin** **¾ cup skim milk** **1 egg plus 1 egg white, beaten** **1 teaspoon vanilla** **2 tablespoons canola oil** **⅔ cup semisweet chocolate chips**	***1*** Preheat the oven to 400 degrees, and spray two 12-cup muffin pans with nonstick cooking spray (or use paper muffin liners). ***2*** In a large bowl, combine the all-purpose and whole-wheat flours, sugar, baking powder, pumpkin pie spice, and salt, and mix well with a spoon. ***3*** In a medium bowl, combine the pumpkin, milk, eggs, vanilla, and oil, and blend well with a spoon. ***4*** Stir the pumpkin mixture into the flour mixture until the dry ingredients are just moist. Fold in the chocolate chips. ***5*** Fill 15 cups of the muffin pans ¾ full, and bake for 16 to 18 minutes, or until a toothpick inserted into the center of a muffin comes out clean.

Per serving: Calories 186 (From Fat 50); Glycemic Load 15 (Medium); Fat 6g (Saturated 2g); Cholesterol 18mg; Sodium 163mg; Carbohydrate 32g (Dietary Fiber 3g); Protein 5g.

Note: Don't make the mistake of eating these muffins warm out of the oven. Although doing so is tempting, allowing them to cool completely gives you the best flavor.

Vary It! If you're not in the mood for chocolate (it happens!), you can make this recipe with ½ cup of pumpkin seeds in place of the chocolate chips.

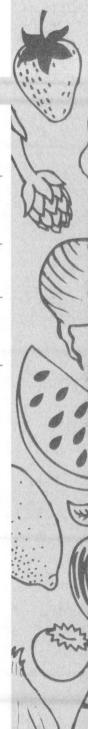

Blueberry Oatmeal Muffins

Prep time: 10 min • **Cook time:** 15–17 min • **Yield:** 12 servings

Ingredients	*Directions*
Nonstick cooking spray 1 cup oat-bran flour ½ cup all-purpose flour ½ cup quick-cooking oats 2 teaspoons baking powder ¼ teaspoon salt	**1** Preheat the oven to 400 degrees, and spray a 12-cup muffin pan with nonstick cooking spray (or use paper muffin liners).
½ teaspoon ground cinnamon ½ cup sugar 1 cup frozen blueberries, unsweetened	**2** In a large bowl, combine the oat-bran flour, all-purpose flour, quick oats, baking powder, salt, cinnamon, and sugar, and mix with a spoon. Add the frozen blueberries, and mix well.
1 cup lowfat milk	**3** In a medium bowl, combine the milk, eggs, vanilla, and oil, and blend well with a spoon.
1 egg plus 1 egg white, lightly beaten	**4** Add the milk mixture to the flour mixture, and stir until the dry ingredients are moist.
1 teaspoon vanilla 2 tablespoons canola oil	**5** Fill the cups of the muffin pan ¾ full, and bake for 15 to 17 minutes, or until a toothpick inserted into the center of a muffin comes out clean.

Per serving: Calories 156 (From Fat 40); Glycemic Load 15 (Medium); Fat 5g (Saturated 1g); Cholesterol 19mg; Sodium 73mg; Carbohydrate 25g (Dietary Fiber 2g); Protein 4g.

Note: To make these blueberry muffins (which you can see in the color section), you just add oats to a traditional recipe. The result is a wonderful, tasty muffin that's perfect as part of your breakfast or as a healthy snack. The oats, oat flour, and blueberries provide fiber, vitamins, minerals, and antioxidants that help reduce your risk of heart disease, diabetes, stroke, and cancer.

Carrot Cake Oat Muffins

Prep time: 10 min • **Cook time:** 15–17 min • **Yield:** 12 servings

Ingredients	*Directions*
Nonstick cooking spray	*1* Preheat the oven to 425 degrees, and spray a 12-cup muffin pan with nonstick cooking spray (or use paper muffin liners).
1 cup oat-bran flour	
½ cup all-purpose flour	
½ cup quick-cooking oats	*2* In a large bowl, combine the oat-bran flour, all-purpose flour, quick oats, brown sugar, baking powder, salt, and cinnamon, and mix well with a spoon.
¼ cup brown sugar	
2 teaspoons baking powder	
¼ teaspoon salt	*3* In a medium bowl, combine the milk, eggs, honey, and oil, and mix well with a spoon.
½ teaspoon ground cinnamon	
1 cup lowfat milk	*4* Add the milk mixture to the flour mixture, and mix until the dry ingredients are just moistened. Fold in the grated carrots.
1 whole egg plus 1 egg white, lightly beaten	
¼ cup honey	*5* Fill the cups of the muffin pan ¾ full, and bake until golden brown, about 15 to 17 minutes, or until a toothpick inserted into the center of a muffin comes out clean.
2 tablespoons canola oil	
1½ cups grated carrots	

Per serving: *Calories 161 (From Fat 40); Glycemic Load 15 (Medium); Fat 5g (Saturated 1g); Cholesterol 19mg; Sodium 142mg; Carbohydrate 26g (Dietary Fiber 2g); Protein 5g.*

Vary It! If you want a sweeter dessert, top off this muffin with cream cheese frosting. Keep in mind, though, that the frosting increases your glycemic load a bit.

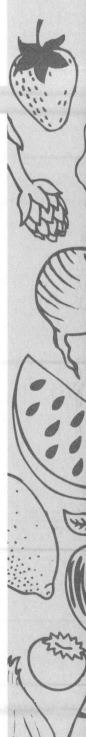

Cornbread Muffins

Prep time: 10 min • **Cook time:** 16 min • **Yield:** 12 servings

Ingredients	*Directions*
Nonstick cooking spray 1½ cups yellow cornmeal	**1** Preheat the oven to 350 degrees, and spray a 12-cup muffin pan with nonstick cooking spray.
½ cup all-purpose flour 2 teaspoons baking powder	**2** In a large bowl, combine the cornmeal, flour, baking powder, sugar, and salt, and mix well with a spoon.
¼ cup sugar ¼ teaspoon salt	**3** In a medium bowl, combine the milk, eggs, and vanilla.
1½ cups lowfat milk 1 egg plus 1 egg white, lightly beaten	**4** In a small bowl, whisk together the honey and oil. Add the honey mixture to the milk mixture, and whisk together.
1 teaspoon vanilla 1 tablespoon honey	**5** Add the milk and honey mixture to the flour mixture, and stir with a spoon until the dry ingredients are just moist (the dough will be somewhat runny).
2 tablespoons canola oil	**6** Fill the cups of the muffin pan ¾ full, and bake until golden but not browned on the top, about 16 minutes.

Per serving: Calories 145 (From Fat 31); Glycemic Load 14 (Medium); Fat 3g (Saturated 1g); Cholesterol 19mg; Sodium 138mg; Carbohydrate 25g (Dietary Fiber 1g); Protein 4g.

Tip: These muffins are the perfect standby when you're looking for a yummy, healthy accent to a hot chili or hearty stew (see Chapter 11 for some delicious chili and stew recipes). If you're like us, you may enjoy eating them as a snack, too.

Note: This recipe uses more cornmeal than the average cornbread recipe, so don't be alarmed when your final batter turns out a bit runnier compared to typical muffin batter. The thinner batter helps keep the muffins light after you cook them so they aren't too dense.

Baking Quick Breads

Baked quick breads are easy to make and can add the perfect touch of sweetness to any brunch get-together. But for many families, quick breads aren't just for brunch. In particular, they make for great snacks for kids in place of packaged cookies or other store-bought sweets.

If you're one of the many who loves quick breads anytime of day, you'll be happy to know you can make a variety of quick breads that fit perfectly into your family's low-glycemic meal plan. By following some of the tricks we offer in the earlier sidebar "Baking treats the healthier way," we've changed up some old favorites to create a couple of quick breads that are good enough to serve to guests but also healthy enough for your family to eat for breakfast or as a snack.

Banana Nut Bread

Prep time: 10 min • **Cook time:** 45 min • **Yield:** 12 servings

Ingredients	*Directions*
Nonstick cooking spray	*1* Preheat the oven to 350 degrees, and spray a 5-x-9-inch loaf pan with nonstick cooking spray.
1 cup all-purpose flour	
1 cup whole-wheat flour	*2* In a large bowl, combine the flours, baking powder, baking soda, salt, cinnamon, and nutmeg.
1½ teaspoons baking powder	
½ teaspoon baking soda	*3* On a medium-sized plate, mash the bananas with a fork until they're soft and mushy (they'll still be lumpy). Set aside.
¼ teaspoon salt	
1 teaspoon ground cinnamon	
¼ teaspoon ground nutmeg	*4* In a medium bowl, beat the sugar and egg whites together until foamy. Add the mashed bananas, orange zest, orange juice, vanilla, and yogurt, and mix until the ingredients are blended.
3 ripe bananas, peeled	
½ cup sugar	
4 egg whites	
1 teaspoon orange zest	*5* Add the banana and egg mixture to the flour mixture, and stir until the dry ingredients are just moist. Gently fold in the walnuts with a spoon.
1 tablespoon orange juice	
1 teaspoon vanilla	
¾ cup plain lowfat yogurt	*6* Fill the loaf pan with the mixture, and bake for 45 minutes, or until a toothpick inserted into the center comes out clean.
⅔ cup chopped walnuts	

Per serving: Calories 193 (From Fat 44); Glycemic Load 15 (Medium); Fat 5g (Saturated 1g); Cholesterol 1mg; Sodium 180mg; Carbohydrate 34g (Dietary Fiber 3g); Protein 6g.

Note: You don't have to use completely black bananas. You can use moderately ripened bananas as long as they're soft enough to mash with a fork.

Vary It! Feel free to make this recipe without nuts if you prefer.

Raspberry Orange Nut Bread

Prep time: 10 min • **Cook time:** 45 min • **Yield:** 12 servings

Ingredients	*Directions*
Nonstick cooking spray	*1* Preheat the oven to 350 degrees, and spray a 5-x-9-inch loaf pan with nonstick cooking spray.
¾ cup frozen raspberries, unsweetened	
1 cup all-purpose flour	*2* Chop the raspberries while they're still frozen so that they crumble into small pieces. Set them aside.
1 cup whole-wheat flour	
1½ teaspoons baking powder	*3* In a large bowl, combine the all-purpose and whole-wheat flours, baking powder, baking soda, and salt. Add the chopped raspberries and walnuts, and stir until they're coated with the flour mixture.
½ teaspoon baking soda	
¼ teaspoon salt	
⅔ cup chopped walnuts	
¾ cup orange juice	*4* In a medium bowl, mix the orange juice, orange zest, oil, sugar, and eggs with a spoon until well blended.
1 teaspoon orange zest	
2 tablespoons canola oil	*5* Add the orange juice mixture to the flour mixture, and stir until the dry ingredients are just moist.
½ cup sugar	
1 egg plus 1 egg white, lightly beaten	*6* Fill the loaf pan with the mixture, and bake for 45 minutes, or until a toothpick inserted into the center comes out clean.

Per serving: Calories 187 (From Fat 67); Glycemic Load 12 (Medium); Fat 8g (Saturated 1g); Cholesterol 18mg; Sodium 159mg; Carbohydrate 27g (Dietary Fiber 3g); Protein 5g.

Tip: This recipe makes a beautiful loaf for brunches, holiday parties, and gifts.

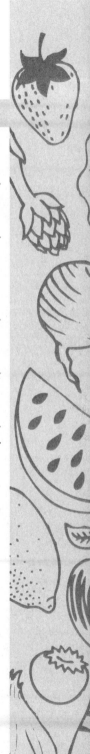

Chapter 10

Satisfying the Munchies with Scrumptious Appetizers and Snacks

In This Chapter

▶ Creating fresh and simple appetizers from the garden

▶ Spicing up any occasion with a few delicious dips

▶ Dressing up your party with some savory seafood favorites

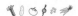
The best part of low-glycemic foods is that they aren't like typical *diet* foods that taste just okay, which means you don't have to sacrifice flavor for healthiness when you're feeding your guests and your family. You can eat (and serve) all kinds of foods that are just brimming with flavor even as you maintain a healthy diet. The trick is finding foods that are naturally low glycemic and moderately low in fat that fit into fabulous appetizers and snacks.

Whether you need some appetizers for an intimate dinner party or a New Year's Eve bash, or you just want some healthy snacks for you and your family, you've come to the right chapter. You may be surprised to find out that some of your all-time favorite snacks are already low glycemic. For instance, guacamole, salsa, and shrimp skewers are all low glycemic, low to moderate in fat content, and loaded with flavor and healthy ingredients. Keep reading if you're looking for additional ideas! You'll find everything from fresh, attractive appetizers to great dips for a family pitch-in.

Assembling Quick and Fresh Appetizers

Having guests over should be a fun event for everyone — you included. The last thing you want to do is spend hours in the kitchen making appetizers when you're already spending tons of time making the main course and dessert. However, you don't want to sacrifice visual appeal or flavor for a fast dish. At times like these, we suggest going straight to the garden — or the produce section of the grocery store — for help. You can make simple, fresh appetizers — like the ones in this section — that take only a few steps, are full of flavor, and look great on a platter.

Finding quick low-glycemic snacks for your party

We're sure you've been in a situation where you didn't have time to make an appetizer or you just wanted to serve some quick snacks for your guests or family. If you're trying to stay on the low-glycemic side, you may not be able to whip out the pretzels and potato chips, but you can find many already-prepared, low-glycemic foods in your grocery store that don't require any prep from you — other than placing them in serving dishes. The following party favorites are perfect go-to snacks when you're looking for some quick low-glycemic options to serve at your next gathering:

- Assorted nuts
- Black bean dip, refried bean dip, or salsa with tortilla chips or toasted whole-wheat tortillas
- Store-bought hummus served with whole-wheat pita bread or vegetables
- Fresh fruit, vegetable, and/or cheese platter
- Deli meats
- Smoked salmon
- Marinated olives
- Cooked shrimp with cocktail sauce

Feta-Stuffed Cherry Tomatoes

Prep time: 10 min • **Yield:** 4 servings

Ingredients	*Directions*
12 large cherry tomatoes	*1* Cut the tops off the tomatoes, and slice a thin slice off the bottoms so the tomatoes can sit upright on a dish. Scoop out the seeds with a small spoon or melon baller. Place the tomatoes on a serving dish tops up.
One 4-ounce package crumbled feta cheese	
2 tablespoons extra-virgin olive oil	
1 tablespoon minced shallot	*2* In a small bowl, toss the crumbled feta cheese with the olive oil, shallot, basil, and oregano.
1 teaspoon finely chopped fresh basil	
½ teaspoon chopped fresh oregano	*3* Use a small spoon to fill each tomato with the feta mixture, and serve.

Per serving: Calories 147 (From Fat 117); Glycemic Load 1 (Low); Fat 13g (Saturated 5g); Cholesterol 25mg; Sodium 321mg; Carbohydrate 4g (Dietary Fiber 1g); Protein 5g.

Tip: These little appetizers (shown in the color section) are great for a buffet table at a party. You can adjust the number of appetizers by doubling, tripling, or quadrupling the recipe depending on how many guests you're expecting.

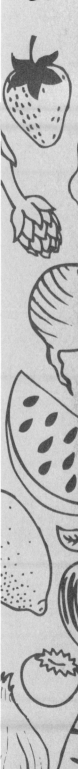

Prosciutto with Melon and Mozzarella Cheese

Prep time: 25 min • **Yield:** 9–10 servings

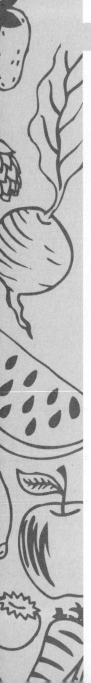

Ingredients	Directions
Twenty 1-inch chunks honeydew melon, rind removed	**1** For each appetizer, pierce 1 melon chunk, half a piece of folded prosciutto, 1 basil leaf, and 1 mozzarella cheese chunk onto a toothpick.
One 4-ounce package prosciutto ham, about 9 to 10 strips, cut in half	**2** Serve with lime wedges (if desired).
20 fresh basil leaves	
One 7-ounce package buffalo mozzarella, cut into twenty ½-inch cubes	
20 lime wedges (optional)	

Per serving: Calories 98 (From Fat 64); Glycemic Load 4 (Low); Fat 7g (Saturated 4g); Cholesterol 24mg; Sodium 278mg; Carbohydrate 3g (Dietary Fiber 0g); Protein 6g.

Tip: Find buffalo mozzarella with the specialty cheeses near the deli section of your local grocery store.

Vary It! You can use papaya or cantaloupe in place of honeydew melon in this recipe.

Dipping Your Way to Delicious Appetizers

Dips are a great way to go when you're looking for an easy party appetizer, but they also work well as everyday snacks for your family. Some dips are more appropriate for parties than others because they contain more fat and calories (and you want to eat smaller amounts of these foods at parties instead of eating more of them as snacks). Other dips are perfect for everyday eating and can actually help you reach your health goals.

Developing healthy habits can be easy when you have the right types of foods in the house, but eating all your fresh fruits and vegetables before they spoil in the fridge can be a real challenge. To help you avoid wasting fresh produce, try adding a few simple dips to your weekly menu; you may be surprised by how fast your fruits and vegetables disappear!

Dips also help you feel more satisfied when you're eating munchies and addictive foods like chips — before you eat the whole bag! For example, you can dip your chips into an 8-layer veggie dip or fresh, chunky salsa instead of just eating a bowl full of plain chips. You have a better chance of eating fewer chips when you add healthy dips because the dips slow down your eating and allow you to feel more satisfied. Plus, the dips add some healthy, low-glycemic ingredients to your not-so-healthy chips. Mixing the two is a good way to balance your diet.

In this section, you find dips that are both party appropriate and perfect for a busy family that's looking to eat some healthy snacks. The dips basically fall into two categories:

- **Tex-Mex dips:** South-of-the-border-inspired dips and salsas are not only low glycemic but also chock-full of healthy ingredients like avocadoes, black beans, tomatoes, and peppers, which offer a significant nutrient boost to your day. They're great for parties and around-the-house snacks.

- **Fruit dips:** Fruit appetizers are a wonderful accompaniment to any party, and they're a great way to get your family to eat more fruit. The mango chutney recipe we include in this section makes a really lovely appetizer for a dinner party, and the orange cream dip is a favorite for every day, especially for kids! The best part is they're both low glycemic and delicious!

Guacamole

Prep time: 8 min • **Yield:** 12 servings

Ingredients	*Directions*
3 large ripe avocadoes, pitted and peeled	**1** In a medium bowl, mash together the avocadoes, lime juice, salt, red onion, tomatoes, and garlic until all the ingredients are mixed together but still chunky.
Juice of 1 lime	
½ teaspoon salt, or to taste	**2** Stir in the ground cumin, and serve with 1 ounce of tortilla chips (about 10 chips) per serving.
⅓ cup finely chopped red onion	
2 Roma or heirloom tomatoes, diced	
½ teaspoon minced garlic	
½ teaspoon ground cumin	
12 ounces baked tortilla chips	

Per serving: Calories 200 (From Fat 70); Glycemic Load 13 (Medium); Fat 8g (Saturated 1g); Cholesterol 0mg; Sodium 302mg; Carbohydrate 32g (Dietary Fiber 6g); Protein 3g.

Note: The avocadoes provide a healthy fat, so you can enjoy this tasty snack (shown in the color section) with no guilt. Just watch how much you eat! Although avocadoes are healthy, they're also high in calories, so be sure to use only ¼ to ⅓ cup per serving for dipping.

Vary It! The beauty of guacamole is that you can vary it to fit your own tastes. If you don't like chopped tomatoes, leave them out. If you want to add a little heat to the mix, try adding some jalapeños.

Chunky Salsa with Black Beans and Tomatoes

Prep time: 10 min, plus refrigerating time • **Yield:** 12 servings

Ingredients	*Directions*
One 15-ounce can black beans, drained and rinsed	**1** In a medium bowl, mix together the black beans, corn, red onion, red pepper, serrano chiles, tomatoes, salad dressing, and garlic salt.
1 cup fresh, cooked corn or canned corn, rinsed and drained	
½ cup finely chopped red onion	**2** Cover the bowl with a lid or plastic wrap, and refrigerate it overnight, or for several hours before serving, so that the flavors blend together.
½ red pepper, finely chopped	
2 serrano chiles, finely chopped and seeded	
4 Roma tomatoes, chopped	
⅓ cup lowfat Italian salad dressing	
½ teaspoon garlic salt	

Per serving: Calories 57 (From Fat 17); Glycemic Load 3 (Low); Fat 2g (Saturated 0g); Cholesterol 0mg; Sodium 168mg; Carbohydrate 9g (Dietary Fiber 2g); Protein 2g.

Vary It! If you want a spicier salsa, add another finely chopped serrano chile or a jalapeño pepper.

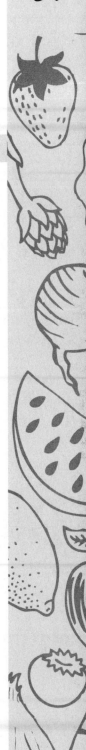

8-Layer Southwestern Dip

Prep time: 8 min • **Cook time:** 4–5 min • **Yield:** 12 servings

Ingredients	Directions
One 15-ounce can vegetarian refried beans	**1** In a medium saucepan, heat the refried beans with about 2 tablespoons of water to make a softer, dipping consistency.
2 tablespoons water	
½ teaspoon chili powder	**2** Add the chili powder and cumin, and mix until the beans are heated through, about 4 to 5 minutes.
¼ teaspoon ground cumin	
1 cup shredded cheddar cheese	**3** Spread the warm beans on the bottom of a 9-x-13-inch serving dish or glass pan. Sprinkle the shredded cheese over the beans; the cheese will melt slightly.
One 4-ounce can chopped green chiles	
¾ cup chopped fresh tomatoes	**4** On top of the cheese, layer in this order the chiles, tomatoes, avocado, sour cream, onions, and black olives.
1 ripe avocado, pitted, peeled, and cut into ½-inch chunks	
½ cup lowfat sour cream	**5** Serve immediately with 1 ounce of tortilla chips (about 10 chips) per serving.
⅓ cup chopped green onions	
One 4-ounce can sliced black olives	
12 ounces baked tortilla chips	

Per serving: Calories 243 (From Fat 80); Glycemic Load 15 (Medium); Fat 9g (Saturated 3g); Cholesterol 13mg; Sodium 512mg; Carbohydrate 35g (Dietary Fiber 6g); Protein 8g.

Note: Some people like to serve this dip cold, while others like it warm. We're in the latter camp because we think warming the beans adds more flavor to the dip. However, we don't recommend warming this dish in the oven because doing so melts the sour cream, making it inedible. So if you don't serve this dip right away, we recommend serving it cold.

Mango Chutney and Brie Bake

Prep time: 5 min • **Cook time:** 15–20 min • **Yield:** 16 servings

Ingredients	*Directions*
One 1-pound brie wheel	*1* Preheat the oven to 350 degrees.
1 cup mango chutney	
One 16-ounce package whole-grain crackers	*2* Place the brie wheel in an ovenproof dish, preferably one on which you can serve your appetizer because the cheese will soften and be difficult to move after you bake it.
	3 Spread the mango chutney over the top of the brie wheel.
	4 Place the dish in the middle of the oven. Bake for 15 to 20 minutes, or until the wheel puffs out and the cheese is soft.
	5 Remove the dish from the oven, and serve immediately with 12 small whole-grain crackers per serving.

Per serving: *Calories 234 (From Fat 125); Glycemic Load 15 (Medium); Fat 12g (Saturated 5g); Cholesterol 28mg; Sodium 281mg; Carbohydrate 20g (Dietary Fiber 1g); Protein 8g.*

Tip: You can find prepared mango chutney in your grocery store; it's usually by specialty items like jarred pesto.

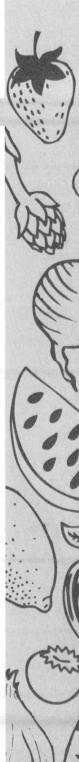

Orange Cream Fruit Dip

Prep time: 8 min • **Yield:** 12 servings

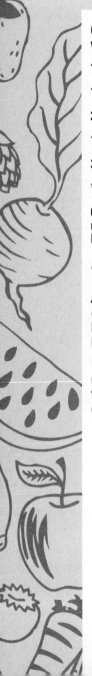

Ingredients	*Directions*
One 8-ounce package lowfat whipped cream cheese	*1* In a medium bowl, mix the cream cheese, yogurt, honey, brown sugar, vanilla, orange juice, and orange zest with a hand mixer until well blended.
1 cup lowfat plain yogurt	
1 tablespoon honey	
2 teaspoons brown sugar	*2* Serve on a plate with your favorite variety of fruits and toothpicks so your friends and family can dip the fruit; use ½ cup of fruit and ¼ cup of dip per serving.
1 teaspoon vanilla	
3 tablespoons orange juice	
½ teaspoon orange zest	
6 cups assorted fruit like melons, strawberries, bananas, or kiwi	

Per serving: Calories 98 (From Fat 33); Glycemic Load 3 (Low); Fat 4g (Saturated 2g); Cholesterol 10mg; Sodium 104mg; Carbohydrate 14g (Dietary Fiber 1g); Protein 3g.

Note: This dip is made with dairy products, so if you're serving it at a party, make sure to keep it cold for safety reasons. You can keep it cold by placing your dip container in a slightly larger bowl that's filled with ice and a small amount of water. Just make sure your larger bowl isn't so big and has so much water that your dip container floats and tips as guests try to eat it.

Tip: This dip is an ideal snack item to keep around the house — especially for kids because it's not only a good source of calcium (thanks to the yogurt) but a great way to get them to eat more fruit. When serving this dip as a snack at home, mix 1 to 2 tablespoons in a small bowl with ½ cup of fruit.

Impressing Guests with Savory Seafood Appetizers

For special occasions, you may want to serve an appetizer that's a little more substantial than veggie-based dips and finger foods. The seafood appetizers we include in this section are the perfect solution because they're quick and easy to prepare and you can use a variety of marinades, depending on your mood.

Salmon makes a wonderful appetizer and also provides the added benefit of being very high in omega-3 fatty acids. Shrimp, on the other hand, is one of those often-misconceived foods. Although it's high in cholesterol, it's also a good source of omega-3 fatty acids. As long as you don't eat it every day, it can actually be a wonderful part of a balanced diet, and because it's all protein and fat, it's naturally low glycemic.

In this section, you find a couple of really tasty shrimp dishes that you can easily pop on the grill at your next gathering. Either shrimp dish also makes for a great dinner meal when served with your favorite low-glycemic grain and vegetable side (why not try some of the recipes in Chapters 13 and 14?). As an added bonus, we also include our fabulous salmon dip, which is always a crowd-pleaser.

Smoked Salmon Dip

Prep time: 8 min • **Yield:** 10 servings

Ingredients	*Directions*
One 8-ounce block lowfat cream cheese, softened	*1* Mix the cream cheese, dill, lemon juice, and onion in a food processor until well blended. Add the salmon, and hit the pulse button a few times to mix, just until the salmon's mixed into the cream cheese mixture.
1 teaspoon fresh chopped dill	
Juice of ½ lemon	
2 tablespoons minced onion	*2* Put the salmon mixture into a small serving bowl, and garnish it with capers.
3 ounces smoked salmon	
1 teaspoon capers	*3* Serve the dip with baby carrots, celery sticks, and cucumber slices; use ½ cup of veggies and 1 ounce of dip per serving.
5 cups baby carrots, celery sticks, and cucumber slices	

Per serving: Calories 86 (From Fat 53); Glycemic Load 1 (Low); Fat 6g (Saturated 4g); Cholesterol 19mg; Sodium 292mg; Carbohydrate 5g (Dietary Fiber 1g); Protein 4g.

Note: If you don't have a food processor, you can use a hand mixer to make this dip.

Vary It! You can vary this recipe by adding more or less onion and lemon to taste.

Grilled Teriyaki Shrimp

Prep time: 5 min, plus refrigerating time • **Cook time:** 4–5 min • **Yield:** 5 servings

Ingredients	Directions
3 tablespoons olive oil	*1* In a small, shallow glass or plastic dish with a lid, use a whisk to mix the olive oil, soy sauce, lime juice, ginger, and garlic.
3 tablespoons soy sauce	
Juice of 1 lime	
1 teaspoon ground ginger	*2* Add the shrimp to the mixture. Tightly put the lid on the dish, and shake it until the shrimp are well coated. Place the dish in the refrigerator to marinate for 30 minutes.
2 cloves garlic, minced	
20 large shrimp, deveined	
	3 Spray the grill with nonstick cooking spray, and then heat the grill to medium-high heat.
	4 Thread about 10 shrimp per skewer; pierce through the thickest portion of each shrimp with the skewer. Grill the shrimp until they're cooked through, about 2½ minutes on one side and 2 minutes on the other side.
	5 Remove the shrimp from the skewers with a fork, and arrange them on a plate with toothpicks. Serve warm.

Per serving: Calories 42 (From Fat 20); Glycemic Load 0 (Low); Fat 2g (Saturated 0g); Cholesterol 43mg; Sodium 187mg; Carbohydrate 0g (Dietary Fiber 0g); Protein 5g.

Note: Teriyaki-inspired recipes always create a lot of flavor, and this one is no exception. Just be sure not to marinate your shrimp too long, or the flavor may end up being too strong.

Tip: As a general rule, always serve shrimp on a platter with toothpicks so your friends and family can place them on their plates without using their hands.

Tip: If you want to use this recipe for dinner, try serving it with ½ cup of Quinoa with Veggies and Toasted Pine Nuts (see Chapter 14 for the recipe) or plain brown rice.

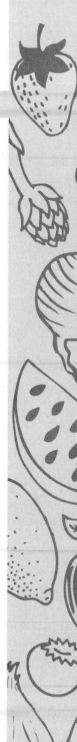

Grilled Spicy Shrimp

Prep time: 5 min, plus refrigerating time • **Cook time:** 4–5 min • **Yield:** 5 servings

Ingredients	*Directions*
3 tablespoons lime juice	*1* In a small, shallow glass or plastic dish with a lid, use a whisk to mix the lime juice, garlic, parsley, salt, black pepper, red pepper flakes, and olive oil.
2 cloves garlic, minced	
2 teaspoons dried parsley	
¼ teaspoon salt	*2* Add the shrimp to the mixture. Tightly put the lid on the dish, and shake it around until the shrimp is well coated. Place the dish in the refrigerator to marinate for 30 minutes.
⅛ teaspoon black pepper	
¼ teaspoon crushed red pepper flakes	
2 tablespoons olive oil	*3* Spray the grill with nonstick cooking spray, and then heat the grill to medium-high heat.
20 large shrimp, deveined	
	4 Thread about 10 shrimp per skewer; pierce through the thickest portion of each shrimp with the skewer. Grill the shrimp until they're cooked through, about 2½ minutes on one side and 2 minutes on the other side.
	5 Remove the shrimp from the skewers with a fork, and arrange them on a plate with toothpicks. Serve warm.

Per serving: Calories 35 (From Fat 14); Glycemic Load 0 (Low); Fat 2g (Saturated 0g); Cholesterol 43mg; Sodium 166mg; Carbohydrate 0g (Dietary Fiber 0g); Protein 5g.

Vary It! You can vary the spiciness of this recipe (which is shown in the color section) by changing the amount of red pepper flakes you add. Be warned: The recipe listed here is spicy, so don't add any more red pepper flakes until you've experimented with this recipe at least once. If you don't want any spice, feel free to omit the red pepper altogether.

Tip: If the shrimp spin around on the skewers while you're trying to cook them, you can use a second skewer to hold them in place.

Chapter 11

Warming Up with Soups, Stews, and Chilies

In This Chapter

▶ Adding variety to your menu with a few fresh and simple soups

▶ Finding a little taste of home with a few hearty stews

▶ Spicing things up with some homemade chili recipes

We don't know about you, but when we're stuck in the middle of the cold months, nothing sounds better than bundling up and eating a hot cup of soup, stew, or chili. When you're trying to maintain a low-glycemic diet, adding these one-pot meals to your dinner menu is a great idea because they're easy to cook and super healthy to eat. (After all, you can fill them with hearty vegetables, low-glycemic grains, fresh herbs, fiber-high beans, and even lean meats.) They offer you and your family many benefits, including the following:

✔ **They're economical.** The ingredients are inexpensive, and one recipe yields a plentiful amount of food. You'll have plenty of leftovers for lunches and dinners during the week.

✔ **They last a long time when you freeze them.** You can batch cook several in a day and freeze them for later meals. You can even make a fun get-together out of cooking soups with your friends.

✔ **They make convenient, quick meals for friends.** Soups and the like are perfect when you want to help out a friend or family member during a difficult or especially busy time.

✔ **They're easy to make when you don't have a lot of time to fuss over the details of cooking.** All you have to do is throw your ingredients in a bowl, heat them up, and enjoy!

This chapter gives you some of our favorite recipes for simple, delicious, and nutritious soups, stews, and chilies. Use these recipes as they are, or feel free to experiment with them by adding more spices or different vegetables according to your taste. Don't worry — you won't hurt our feelings if you decide not to follow these recipes by the book!

You can reduce the sodium of these recipes by using low-sodium broth (if the recipe doesn't already call for it).

Soup, Glorious Soup

Although some soups are a little complicated because you have to blend them to just the right consistency, many soups are so easy all you have to do is toss your ingredients into a pot, cook, and serve. One of the best parts about soups is that you can use them as either main courses or side dishes, depending on your preference. If your soup of choice is loaded with vegetables, you can even count it as your vegetable for that meal.

In this section, you find a wide variety of tasty, low-glycemic soups, from basic vegetable soups to those that include beans, lentils, nuts, and pasta. The soups in this section fall into two basic categories:

- ✔ **Vegetable soups:** Vegetable soups are a great way to add a high-nutrient, low-glycemic meal to your daily menu because they can easily include several vegetable servings. They're an especially good choice for those of you who don't enjoy the basic steamed vegetable. You may be surprised to find out that they're also quite satisfying with a lot of flavor and few calories, making them the perfect meal for people who are watching their weight.

- ✔ **Soups with beans, lentils, nuts, and pasta:** Sprucing up soups with beans, lentils, nuts, and pasta makes them more satisfying overall, so if you're looking for a soup that'll fill you up as much as a three-dish meal, you've come to the right place! Soups with these hearty ingredients also provide excellent low-glycemic, high-nutrient, and low-calorie options for those cold, winter nights when you want to fill up on something warm. Whether you're in the mood for a spicy black bean soup or a traditional lentil soup, this section provides some delicious ideas.

Vegetable Soup

Prep time: 10 min • **Cook time:** 26 min • **Yield:** 4 servings

Ingredients	Directions
1 teaspoon canola oil	**1** In a large saucepan, heat the oil over medium heat. Add the garlic, and sauté until it's soft, about 1 minute.
2 cloves garlic, minced	
Two 14-ounce cans vegetable broth	**2** Add the broth, water, carrots, cauliflower or broccoli, tomatoes, thyme, sage, and basil. Bring the mixture to a boil, reduce the heat to low, and simmer for 15 minutes, or until the vegetables begin to soften. Add the squash and continue to simmer for 10 more minutes.
1 cup water	
2 carrots, sliced	
5 ounces frozen cauliflower or broccoli	
One 14.5-ounce can diced tomatoes, undrained	**3** Add salt and pepper to taste, and serve.
½ teaspoon dried thyme	
¼ teaspoon dried sage	
½ teaspoon dried basil	
1 yellow squash, sliced	
Salt and pepper to taste	

Per serving: Calories 87 (From Fat 20); Glycemic Load 1 (Low); Fat 2g (Saturated 0g); Cholesterol 0mg; Sodium 1,150mg; Carbohydrate 16g (Dietary Fiber 5g); Protein 4g.

Tip: One of the best-kept secrets for managing your health and weight is keeping a low-calorie vegetable soup recipe on hand for those evenings when you just don't feel like having a steamed vegetable. This recipe is perfect when you want to whip up a quick and healthy soup to go with your meal. It's also a great way to get in your vegetable servings.

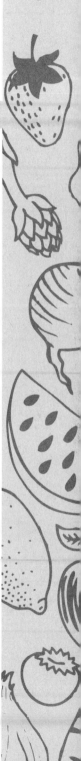

Fresh Basil Tomato Vegetable Soup

Prep time: 15 min • **Cook time:** 35 min • **Yield:** 4 servings

Ingredients	Directions
1 tablespoon extra-virgin olive oil	**1** In a large saucepan, heat the olive oil over medium-low heat. Add the celery, carrot, onion, and garlic. Cook until the mixture is very soft, about 10 minutes.
1 stalk celery, chopped	
1 small carrot, chopped	
1 medium onion, chopped	**2** Add the tomatoes, chicken broth, black pepper, bay leaf, and butter. Bring the mixture to a boil, turn down the heat, and simmer until the vegetables are very tender, about 25 minutes.
2 cloves garlic, minced	
One 28-ounce can fire-roasted, diced tomatoes, undrained	
2 cups chicken broth	**3** Add the fresh basil and parsley, and puree the mixture with an immersion blender, or blend it in a blender or food processor, until smooth. Serve.
¼ teaspoon black pepper	
1 bay leaf	
1 teaspoon butter	
¼ cup chopped fresh basil leaves	
2 tablespoons chopped fresh flat-leaf parsley	

Per serving: Calories 123 (From Fat 58); Glycemic Load 2 (Low); Fat 6g (Saturated 2g); Cholesterol 5mg; Sodium 961mg; Carbohydrate 14g (Dietary Fiber 3g); Protein 3g.

Note: For blending soup, we highly recommend using an immersion blender. If you don't have one, make sure the lid to your blender or food processor is secure so you don't burn yourself (and make a big mess in the process).

Tip: If you like a lot of texture to your soup, you can lightly blend the ingredients instead of processing until smooth.

Vary It! You can easily change this to a vegetarian soup by using vegetable broth in place of the chicken broth.

Summer Minestrone Soup

Prep time: 10 min • **Cook time:** 24–31 min • **Yield:** 6 servings

Ingredients	*Directions*
1 tablespoon extra-virgin olive oil 1 cup chopped onion 1 cup chopped carrot 1 celery stalk, chopped 2 cloves garlic, minced 1 teaspoon dried thyme ½ teaspoon dried oregano 6 cups low-sodium chicken broth One 8-ounce can tomato sauce 1 bay leaf 1½ teaspoons salt 1 cup fresh green beans, ends trimmed and cut into ½-inch pieces 1 yellow squash, diced 2 tomatoes, diced ½ cup elbow macaroni 4 tablespoons grated Parmesan cheese	***1*** In a large saucepan, heat the olive oil over medium heat. Add the onion, carrot, celery, and garlic, and sauté until the vegetables are soft, about 3 to 5 minutes. ***2*** Stir in the thyme and oregano, and cook for about 1 minute. Add the chicken broth, tomato sauce, bay leaf, salt, and green beans. Mix the ingredients together with a spoon, and cook for about 10 minutes to blend the flavors. ***3*** Add the squash, tomatoes, and pasta, and cook for another 10 to 15 minutes, or until the pasta is cooked through. ***4*** Ladle the soup into serving bowls, and sprinkle each serving with 2 teaspoons of Parmesan cheese.

Per serving: Calories 147 (From Fat 48); Glycemic Load 7 (Low); Fat 5g (Saturated 2g); Cholesterol 7mg; Sodium 960mg; Carbohydrate 19g (Dietary Fiber 4g); Protein 8g.

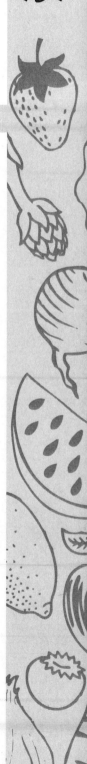

Spicy Black Bean Soup

Prep time: 10 min • **Cook time:** 3–4 hr • **Yield:** 6 servings

Ingredients	*Directions*
1 medium onion, chopped	*1* In a 5-quart slow cooker, stir together the onion, carrot, garlic, cumin, chili powder, black pepper, chipotle pepper, beans, tomatoes, and chicken broth. Cook on high for 3 to 4 hours.
1 carrot, chopped	
2 cloves garlic, minced	
2 teaspoons ground cumin	
½ teaspoon chili powder	*2* Before serving, add the lime juice and cilantro to the soup, and mix well. Ladle the soup into bowls, and serve with 1 ounce of tortilla chips (about 10 chips) per serving (if desired).
¼ teaspoon black pepper	
1 teaspoon finely chopped chipotle pepper, canned in adobo sauce	
Two 15-ounce cans black beans, undrained	
One 15-ounce can diced tomatoes with juice	
2 cups chicken broth	
Juice of 1 lime	
2 tablespoons chopped fresh cilantro	
6 ounces tortilla chips (optional)	

Per serving: Calories 168 (From Fat 24); Glycemic Load 6 (Low); Fat 3g (Saturated 0g); Cholesterol 2mg; Sodium 950mg; Carbohydrate 26g (Dietary Fiber 9g); Protein 9g.

Note: You can easily make this soup on the stove top if you don't have a slow cooker (or don't want to use it). All you have to do is sauté your vegetables in a little olive oil in a large saucepan, add the rest of the ingredients, and simmer for about 30 minutes.

Vary It! You can substitute vegetable broth for the chicken broth to make this soup vegetarian.

Hearty Lentil Soup

Prep time: 8 min • **Cook time:** 23–35 min • **Yield:** 6 servings

Ingredients	*Directions*
1 tablespoon extra-virgin olive oil	*1* In a large saucepan, heat the olive oil over medium heat. Add the cumin and coriander, and stir until fragrant, about 20 seconds.
1 teaspoon ground cumin	
1 teaspoon ground coriander	*2* Add the onion, carrot, and garlic, and cook until soft, about 3 to 5 minutes.
1 medium onion, chopped	
1 carrot, chopped	
2 cloves garlic, minced	*3* Add the broth, lentils, tomato sauce, tomato paste, salt, pepper, red pepper flakes, and thyme. Cook for 20 to 30 minutes, or until the lentils are cooked.
2 quarts low-sodium vegetable broth	
2 cups red or brown lentils, washed	*4* Stir in the balsamic vinegar, and serve.
1 cup tomato sauce	
2 tablespoons tomato paste	
1½ teaspoons salt	
½ teaspoon black pepper	
¼ teaspoon crushed red pepper flakes	
6 sprigs of fresh thyme	
2 tablespoons balsamic vinegar	

Per serving: Calories 310 (From Fat 35); Glycemic Load 3 (Low); Fat 4g (Saturated 0g); Cholesterol 0mg; Sodium 1,458mg; Carbohydrate 52g (Dietary Fiber 18g); Protein 19g.

Note: Red lentils cook quicker than brown lentils (20 minutes compared to 30 minutes), so be sure to adjust the cooking time according to which lentil you use.

Vary It! If you're not a fan of vinegar, you can replace it with the juice of 1 lemon.

Tip: The best part about this soup is that it tastes even better the day after you make it when all the flavors have had time to blend together.

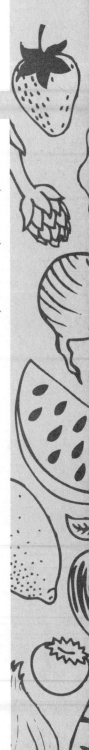

Curried Butternut Squash and Cashew Soup

Prep time: 15 min • **Cook time:** 43 min • **Yield:** 6 servings

Ingredients	*Directions*
½ cup unsalted cashews	**1** Preheat the oven to 350 degrees.
1 tablespoon canola oil	
1 cup diced onion	**2** Place the cashews on a baking sheet, and roast them in the oven until golden brown, about 10 minutes. Put them in a small bowl and set aside.
3 cloves garlic, minced	
6 cups butternut squash (about 2 pounds), peeled and cubed	**3** In a large saucepan, heat 1 tablespoon of oil over medium-high heat, and sauté the onion and garlic until tender, about 3 minutes.
2 teaspoons curry powder	
1½ teaspoons cardamom	**4** Add the squash, curry powder, cardamom, cumin, and vegetable broth, and bring to a boil. Reduce the heat, and simmer the mixture for 20 minutes, or until the squash is tender.
1 teaspoon ground cumin	
6 cups vegetable broth	
Salt to taste	**5** Add the cashews, and puree the squash-cashew mixture with an immersion blender until smooth, or remove it from the saucepan in batches to blend it in a blender or food processor.
6 tablespoons plain lowfat yogurt (optional)	
	6 Return the blended soup to the saucepan (if you removed it to blend it together), and bring it to a boil. Reduce the heat and simmer for 10 minutes. Add salt to taste.
	7 Ladle the soup into bowls, and add 1 tablespoon of yogurt per serving if you want a creamier texture and taste.

Per serving: Calories 182 (From Fat 83); Glycemic Load 4 (Low); Fat 9g (Saturated 1g); Cholesterol 0mg; Sodium 1,106mg; Carbohydrate 25g (Dietary Fiber 6g); Protein 6g.

Note: For blending soup, we highly recommend using an immersion blender. If you don't have one, make sure the lid to your blender or food processor is secure so you don't burn yourself (and make a big mess in the process).

Tip: To provide even more texture, simply reduce the time you spend pureeing the nuts in this soup (which is shown in the color section).

Tortellini Soup

Prep time: 10 min • **Cook time:** 20–25 min • **Yield:** 6 servings

Ingredients	*Directions*
1 tablespoon extra-virgin olive oil 1 cup chopped onion 1 cup chopped carrots 2 cloves garlic, minced 4 cups chicken broth 2½ cups water 1 cup tomato sauce 1 teaspoon dried basil 1 teaspoon dried parsley ½ teaspoon dried oregano ¼ teaspoon smoked paprika (optional) 1½ cups zucchini, diced One 8-ounce package cheese tortellini 1 cup spinach 2 tablespoons grated Parmesan cheese	*1* In a large saucepan, heat the olive oil over medium heat. Sauté the onion, carrots, and garlic until soft, about 5 minutes. *2* Add the broth, water, tomato sauce, basil, parsley, oregano, and paprika (if desired). Bring the mixture to a boil, and simmer for about 5 minutes. *3* Add the zucchini and tortellini, and cook until the tortellini is cooked through, about 10 to 15 minutes. *4* Add the spinach, and cook until it's just wilted. Ladle the soup into bowls, and serve with 1 teaspoon of Parmesan cheese per serving.

Per serving: Calories 172 (From Fat 66); Glycemic Load 17 (Medium); Fat 7g (Saturated 2g); Cholesterol 11mg; Sodium 1,031mg; Carbohydrate 21g (Dietary Fiber 4g); Protein 7g.

Vary It! Because the tortellini is the star ingredient of this soup, you have quite a few options for making this soup your own. We've tried it with both chicken and beef broth, and you can easily substitute vegetable broth to make a vegetarian version. In addition, you can keep the smoked paprika for a smoky flavor, as we do here, or you can omit it if you want a lighter flavor.

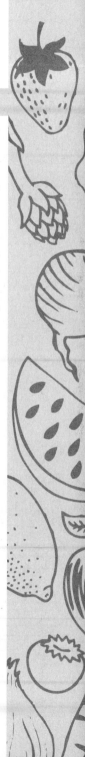

Mir what? Starting your soup with chopped veggies

One of the most important first steps in making any soup is making your *mirpoix*. Don't panic if you're thinking "Mir what?" because that's exactly what Meri thought when she heard the term for the first time. She was in a small restaurant asking the chef how she made a particularly delicious soup, and she started rambling on about starting with your mirpoix and moving on from there.

The term may sound complicated, but *mirpoix* is simply the cut-up vegetables you use as the base in a soup. It typically consists of some combination of chopped onions, carrots, and celery and is used as a flavor enhancer. So don't worry if you're not crazy about cooked carrots and the recipe for the soup you want to make calls for them. The carrots are just a part of the *mirpoix;* they help create a more abundant flavor for the overall dish (in other words, they aren't the main vegetable in the pot).

If you hate chopping the vegetables every time you make a soup, check out the produce section of your local grocery store. Somewhere near the fruit plates and other prepared produce items, you may just find a container of *mirpoix* all ready to go. Or, at the very least, you'll find a container of chopped onions. Although they may cost more, they also save you time in the kitchen!

Homemade Stews: Comfort Food at Its Best

Nothing says comfort and warmth like a good stew. Lucky for you, stews are just as easy to make as the soups in the preceding section. The stews you find here make perfect low-glycemic meals on cold winter days — or anytime you're in the mood for a little warming up.

Now if you're like a lot of people, you like eating your stew with lots of bread. Having a slice of bread is fine, but if you're trying to maintain a low-glycemic diet, try eating your stew with no bread, a lower-glycemic cornmeal muffin (see Chapter 9 for a great recipe), or a slice of whole-grain bread.

Chicken and Hominy Stew

Prep time: 15 min • **Cook time:** 21–22 min • **Yield:** 8 servings

Ingredients	Directions
1 tablespoon canola oil	**1** In a large saucepan, heat the oil over medium-high heat. Add the onion and bell pepper, and cook until they're both soft and the onion is golden, about 5 minutes.
1 large sweet onion, chopped	
1 red bell pepper, stemmed, seeded, and chopped	
2 cloves garlic, minced	**2** Add the garlic, chili powder, cumin, and oregano, and continue to cook until fragrant, 1 to 2 more minutes.
1 teaspoon chili powder	
½ teaspoon ground cumin	
1 teaspoon dried oregano	**3** Add the tomatoes, broth, and hominy, and cook until boiling. Reduce the heat to low, cover, and simmer to blend flavors, about 10 minutes.
One 14.5-ounce can diced tomatoes, undrained	
One 14.5-ounce can low-sodium chicken broth	**4** Add the rotisserie chicken, and continue to simmer until heated through, about 5 minutes.
2 cups canned hominy, rinsed and drained	
3 cups rotisserie chicken (breast and thigh meat), pulled into large pieces and skin removed	**5** Add salt and pepper to taste, stir in the cilantro, and serve.
Salt and pepper to taste	
¼ cup minced fresh cilantro	

Per serving: *Calories 166 (From Fat 64); Glycemic Load 4 (Low); Fat 7g (Saturated 2g); Cholesterol 39mg; Sodium 544mg; Carbohydrate 12g (Dietary Fiber 3g); Protein 15g.*

Note: If you've never cooked with hominy (which consists of dried maize kernels), it's time to give it a try! With its corn-like features, hominy adds great flavor and texture to stews and soups and is low to medium glycemic, depending on how much you eat in one sitting. You can find canned hominy at your local grocery store. It's usually stashed in the aisle with other canned veggies or sometimes in the Southern-inspired section where you find collard greens.

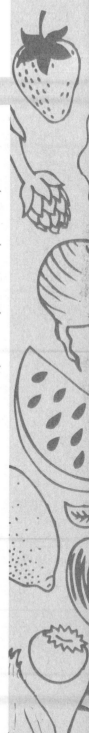

Chicken and Vegetable Stew

Prep time: 15 min • **Cook time:** 55 min • **Yield:** 6 servings

Ingredients

1 tablespoon canola oil

4 boneless, skinless chicken breasts, cut into 1-inch pieces

3 new potatoes, quartered

1½ cups sliced carrots

1 cup zucchini, cut into ½-inch chunks

1 medium onion, chopped

1½ teaspoons garlic powder

½ teaspoon turmeric

½ teaspoon ground cumin

½ teaspoon dried oregano

½ teaspoon black pepper

1½ teaspoons salt

3 tablespoons tomato paste

Three 14-ounce cans low-sodium chicken broth

¼ cup all-purpose flour

½ cup water

Directions

1 In a small stockpot, heat the oil over medium-high heat. Add the chicken, and cook until browned on both sides, about 5 minutes.

2 Add the potatoes, carrots, zucchini, onion, garlic powder, turmeric, cumin, oregano, black pepper, salt, tomato paste, and chicken broth. Bring the mixture to a boil, cover, reduce heat to low, and simmer for 45 minutes, or until the chicken is cooked through.

3 Combine the flour and water in a small bowl, and stir with a whisk until smooth. Add the flour mixture to the broth mixture and bring to a boil. Cook the stew for about 5 minutes to thicken it. Serve.

Per serving: Calories 241 (From Fat 54); Glycemic Load 9 (Low); Fat 6g (Saturated 2g); Cholesterol 46mg; Sodium 751mg; Carbohydrate 24g (Dietary Fiber 4g); Protein 23g.

Tip: This recipe is easy to throw together on short notice because you can change up the vegetables with whatever you have on hand. Here, we include some medium-glycemic new potatoes because, let's face it, potatoes are great in stews!

Beef Barley Stew

Prep time: 15 min • **Cook time:** About 5 hr • **Yield:** 8 servings

Ingredients	*Directions*
2 teaspoons plus 1 teaspoon canola oil **¾ cup chopped onion** **1½ cups chopped carrots** **1 cup chopped celery** **4 cloves garlic, minced** **1 cup sliced shiitake or porcini mushrooms**	**1** In a medium skillet, heat 2 teaspoons of oil over medium-high heat. Add the onions, carrots, celery, garlic, and mushrooms, and sauté until the vegetables are tender, about 6 minutes. Transfer the entire vegetable mixture with liquid into a 5-quart slow cooker.
1 pound boneless beef short ribs **¼ teaspoon salt** **¼ teaspoon black pepper** **3 cups beef broth**	**2** Sprinkle the beef with the salt and pepper. In the same skillet you used in Step 1, heat 1 teaspoon of oil over medium-high heat. Add the beef, and cook for 4 minutes on each side. Add the beef to the slow cooker.
1½ cups plus ½ cup water **One 15-ounce can stewed tomatoes in juice** **¾ cup pearl barley** **1 teaspoon dried thyme** **2 teaspoons dried marjoram**	**3** In the slow cooker, stir in the beef broth, 1½ cups of water, tomatoes with juice, barley, thyme, and marjoram. Cover and cook on high until the beef is cooked through and the barley is tender, about 4½ hours.
6 ounces green beans, trimmed and cut into ½-inch pieces **1 zucchini, diced** **2 tablespoons red wine**	**4** Remove the beef from the slow cooker, and let it cool for about 5 to 10 minutes so you can shred it without burning yourself. Shred the meat with your fingers, and then return it to the slow cooker. Add the green beans, zucchini, and red wine to the slow cooker. Cover and cook until the beans are tender, about 15 minutes.
¼ cup all-purpose flour **Salt to taste**	**5** In a small bowl, use a whisk to mix together the flour and ½ cup of water. Stir the flour mixture into the slow cooker to thicken the stew, and cook for an additional 5 minutes.
	6 Ladle the stew into bowls, season with salt to taste, and serve.

Per serving: Calories 339 (From Fat 169); Glycemic Load 12 (Medium); Fat 19g (Saturated 7g); Cholesterol 36mg; Sodium 574mg; Carbohydrate 31g (Dietary Fiber 6g); Protein 13g.

Vary It! Feel free to use your favorite mushrooms; there's no rule that you have to use shiitake or porcini. Feel free to leave out the mushrooms entirely if you're not a big fan of them.

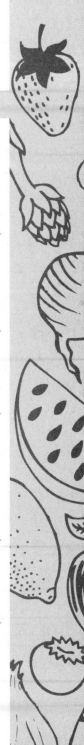

Getting skinny with the help of soup?

New research shows that eating soup may be helpful for your waistline. A 2007 study through Penn State University found that subjects who ate a bowl of soup before their lunch entree ate 20 percent fewer calories for the day compared to those who didn't eat soup. The types of soups tested in the study included

✔ Broth-based soup (like French onion soup without the cheese)

✔ Broth-based soup with chunky vegetables (like vegetable soup)

✔ Chunky, pureed vegetable soup (like chunky tomato bisque)

✔ Smooth, pureed vegetable soup (like tomato soup)

So you think you're ready to test this study in your own life? Go for it! Just keep in mind that the researchers used versions of the preceding styles of soup that are low in calories, not those that are high in calories, like corn chowder or cream soups. So if you want to experiment to see if you benefit from eating soup before lunch or dinner, be sure to stick with the actual styles of soups tested.

Chili Recipes to Warm Up Those Chilly Nights

Anytime we hear the word *chili,* we picture a warm, spicy meal topped off with a piece of delicious cornbread. If you have similar imaginings, you're sure to love the recipes we include in this section. (And why not try the cornbread muffin recipe we provide in Chapter 9?)

Although chili typically uses pinto beans, we've never been a huge fan of eating them in our chili, so we don't include them in the recipes included here. For many of you chili purists out there, we may have crossed a line with that bold statement. But with so many different beans to choose from and combinations of flavors to create, we just can't help exploring the infinite chili-no-pinto-bean possibilities! If you're like us or if you're just looking for a few more options for chili night, try out the following healthy chili recipes using white beans, kidney beans, and black beans.

Turkey and White Bean Chili

Prep time: 10 min • **Cook time:** 35 min • **Yield:** 4 servings

Ingredients	*Directions*
1 tablespoon canola oil	*1* In a large saucepan, heat the oil over medium-high heat. Add the onion and bell pepper, and sauté until they're soft, about 5 minutes. Add the garlic, and cook for an additional 2 minutes.
1 medium onion, chopped	
1 medium red bell pepper, chopped	
2 cloves garlic, minced	*2* Add the ground turkey to the pan, and sprinkle it with the salt, cumin, chili powder, oregano, and bay leaf. Stir the turkey and spices together, and cook until the turkey is browned and cooked through, about 8 minutes.
½ pound lean ground turkey	
1 teaspoon salt	
½ teaspoon ground cumin	
1 teaspoon chili powder	
1 teaspoon dried oregano	*3* Add the green chilies, beans, and chicken broth, and bring the mixture to a boil. Reduce the heat and simmer for 20 minutes.
1 bay leaf	
One 4-ounce can green chiles	*4* Stir in the lime juice and cilantro just before serving. Ladle the chili with 1½ tablespoons of salsa on top of each serving. Add salt and pepper to taste.
Two 15-ounce cans northern white beans, undrained	
One 15-ounce can low-sodium chicken broth	
2 tablespoons fresh lime juice	
2 tablespoons chopped fresh cilantro	
6 tablespoons salsa	
Salt and pepper to taste	

Per serving: Calories 208 (From Fat 48); Glycemic Load 4 (Low); Fat 5g (Saturated 1g); Cholesterol 39mg; Sodium 660mg; Carbohydrate 19g (Dietary Fiber 7g); Protein 20g.

Vary It! If you prefer more spice in your chili, add a tablespoon of minced jalapeño when you add the onion and red bell pepper.

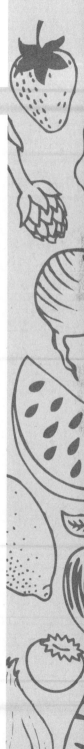

Chipotle, Chicken, and Black Bean Chili

Prep time: 15 min • **Cook time:** 43–45 min • **Yield:** 8 servings

Ingredients	*Directions*
1 tablespoon canola oil	**1** In a large pot, heat the oil over medium heat. Add the onion, garlic, green bell pepper, and yellow bell pepper, and sauté until the vegetables begin to soften, about 3 to 5 minutes. Pour in the water, and continue cooking until about half of the liquid has evaporated, about 10 minutes.
1 small onion, chopped	
2 cloves garlic, minced	
1 green bell pepper, chopped	
1 yellow bell pepper, chopped	
1 cup water	
One 15-ounce can kidney beans, undrained	**2** Stir in the kidney beans, black beans, diced tomatoes, corn, chicken, chili powder, cumin, chipotle pepper, adobo sauce, cayenne pepper, and oregano.
One 15-ounce can black beans, undrained	
One 15-ounce can diced tomatoes, undrained	
One 11-ounce can corn, drained and rinsed	**3** Reduce the heat to low, and mix in the chicken broth and tomato paste. Simmer for 30 minutes, or until the stew has thickened, stirring occasionally.
3 cups rotisserie chicken, cut into ½-inch chunks and skin removed	
1 tablespoon chili powder	**4** Ladle the chili into bowls, and top each serving with about 1 teaspoon of cilantro, or to taste. Add salt and pepper to taste, and serve.
1 tablespoon ground cumin	
1 chipotle pepper in adobo sauce, finely chopped	
1 teaspoon adobo sauce	
½ teaspoon ground cayenne pepper	
½ teaspoon dried oregano	
2½ cups chicken broth	
2 tablespoons tomato paste	
8 teaspoons chopped fresh cilantro	
Salt and pepper to taste	

Per serving: Calories 208 (From Fat 43); Glycemic Load 5 (Low); Fat 5g (Saturated 1g); Cholesterol 43mg; Sodium 871mg; Carbohydrate 24g (Dietary Fiber 7g); Protein 19g.

Chapter 12

Greening Up Your Diet with Salads

In This Chapter

▶ Adding a little green to your meals with side salads

▶ Freshening things up with fruit salads

▶ Creating healthy, low-glycemic meals with entree salads

*F*illing up your plate with healthy greens and fruits is one of the easiest ways to incorporate low-glycemic foods into your diet. Fiber, vitamins, minerals, and powerful antioxidants make salads a great meal strategy for achieving all your wellness goals. The only problem with salads is that you can easily get stuck in a rut when you eat the same old lettuce and dressing with every meal. Lucky for you, this chapter is all about how to spruce up the basic salad to add a little variety to the green part of your diet. Here, we share some unique ways to add low-glycemic greens, fruits, vegetables, nuts, and cheese to take your salads from super boring to excitingly delicious!

Field of Greens: Savoring Side Salads

Having a side salad every day with lunch or dinner definitely isn't a bad habit to start. In fact, doing so adds more vegetables to your plate and helps you feel full so you don't overeat the more calorie-heavy parts of your meal, like your entrees and starchy sides. The salad-a-day strategy offers many benefits, including the following:

✔ Helps you eat fewer calories and stay full longer so you can lose weight or manage your current weight

✔ Keeps your blood sugar balanced

✔ Increases your fiber intake to help with weight loss, blood sugar control, and heart health

✔ Increases your overall servings of fruits and vegetables each day to reduce your risk of certain cancers, heart disease, and diabetes

✔ Optimizes your antioxidant intake to help reduce the risk of chronic diseases

✔ Gives you an extra boost in hydration, which is great if you find it hard to drink enough water during the day

✔ Takes your vitamin and mineral intake up a notch so your body gets the important nutrients it needs for overall health and well-being

Follow these basic steps to create a variety of side salads using your favorite ingredients:

1. **Start with your bed of greens.**

   Here are just some of your green options: romaine, iceberg, baby greens, spinach, Boston, Bibb, endive, cabbage, radicchio, arugula, dandelion greens, and chard. Use just one in your salad, or combine two or more for different flavors. Keep in mind that the darker the leaf, the more nutrition, so go beyond iceberg!

2. **Add some texture with toppings.**

   Here are just a few topping choices: beans (kidney, garbanzo, and so on), lentils, chopped vegetables (bell peppers, tomatoes, cucumbers, and so on), cheese (feta, mozzarella, or goat cheese), olives, artichoke hearts, avocados, nuts, and fruit.

   Keep your portion sizes in mind when making your salads. Too much cheese can start to increase your calorie level and glycemic load. Keep your cheese to 1 ounce per salad, and try to stay away from starchy toppings like croutons. If you really love croutons, use them sparingly. Using ½ to 1 ounce of croutons gives you some nice crunch while keeping you in a lower-glycemic range.

3. **End with your dressing.**

   When it comes to maintaining a healthy diet, vinaigrettes are usually better than creamy salad dressings because they're lower in saturated fat and calories; however, you can certainly use what you like. Just be mindful of how much you use. Don't use more than a tablespoon of salad dressing per serving so you don't overdo it in calories.

If you're using a vinaigrette dressing (especially something like Italian dressing), try squeezing some fresh lemon juice on your salad to mix with the dressing. The lemon juice brings out big flavors so you don't have to use as much salad dressing.

The following sections show you some different ways to use the preceding ingredients as well as some homemade salad dressings to create refreshingly tasty salads for any occasion. We hope you not only find some favorites among the veggie and nut options we offer here, but also get some ideas for how to create your own yummy salad concoctions.

Wilted Spinach Salad with Feta

Prep time: 5 min   •   **Cook time:** 4–5 min   •   **Yield:** 4 servings

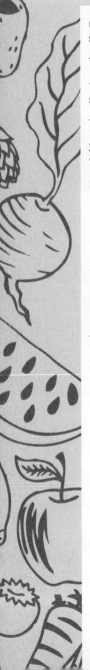

Ingredients	*Directions*
One 9-ounce bag baby spinach	**1** In a large bowl, mix the spinach and feta cheese; set aside.
¼ cup crumbled feta cheese	
1 tablespoon plus 1 table-spoon extra-virgin olive oil	**2** In a small skillet, heat 1 tablespoon of oil over medium-high heat. Add the onion, and sauté it until it's softened and starting to brown, about 4 to 5 minutes. Pour the oil-onion mixture over the spinach and feta.
½ sweet onion, sliced	
2 tablespoons balsamic vinegar	**3** Remove the skillet from heat, and add the vinegar and the remaining tablespoon of oil; whisk together.
Salt and pepper to taste	
	4 Pour the oil-vinegar dressing over the spinach mixture, and toss to coat everything evenly (the spinach will wilt slightly). Season the salad with salt and pepper to taste; then serve.

Per serving: Calories 121 (From Fat 79); Glycemic Load 1 (Low); Fat 9g (Saturated 2g); Cholesterol 8mg; Sodium 130mg; Carbohydrate 10g (Dietary Fiber 3g); Protein 3g.

Note: You may want to add less than the prepared amount of dressing to the salad, depending on your taste.

Fresh Garden Salad with Avocado and Lemon Vinaigrette

Prep time: 10 min • **Yield:** 4 servings

Ingredients	Directions
¼ cup extra-virgin olive oil	**1** In a small bowl, whisk together the olive oil, lemon juice, mustard, thyme, parsley, garlic salt, and pepper.
2 tablespoons lemon juice	
½ teaspoon Dijon mustard	
½ teaspoon dried thyme	**2** In a large serving bowl, mix the salad greens, tomatoes, and sugar snap peas. Pour about 1 tablespoon of the oil-mustard dressing over the salad mixture, and continue to add more dressing to taste; toss to coat everything evenly.
¼ teaspoon dried parsley	
¼ teaspoon garlic salt	
⅛ teaspoon black pepper	
8 cups torn or cut mixed salad greens	**3** Arrange the avocado slices on top of the salad, and serve.
3 medium Roma tomatoes, chopped	
½ cup sugar snap peas	
1 large avocado, pitted, peeled, and cut into slices	

Per serving: Calories 246 (From Fat 187); Glycemic Load 1 (Low); Fat 21g (Saturated 3g); Cholesterol 0mg; Sodium 114mg; Carbohydrate 15g (Dietary Fiber 8g); Protein 4g.

Note: You may want to add less than the prepared amount of dressing to the salad, depending on your taste. This one is tangy, so a little goes a long way!

Vary It! If you aren't a fan of sugar snap peas, you can always replace them with cucumbers, or you can add them both.

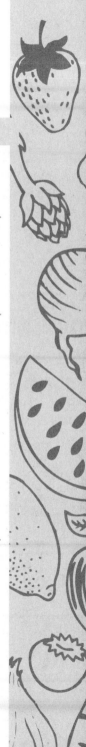

Cranberry Walnut Salad

Prep time: 10 min • **Cook time:** 5–8 min • **Yield:** 4 servings

Ingredients	*Directions*
½ cup walnut halves	*1* Preheat the oven to 400 degrees. Lay out the walnut pieces on a nonstick cookie sheet, and bake until lightly toasted, fragrant, and just starting to brown, about 5 to 8 minutes. Pour the nuts into a bowl and set aside.
¼ cup extra-virgin olive oil	
3 tablespoons balsamic vinegar	
1 teaspoon Dijon mustard	*2* In a small bowl, whisk together the oil, vinegar, mustard, honey, salt, and pepper until well blended.
½ tablespoon honey	
½ teaspoon salt	
⅛ teaspoon black pepper	*3* In a large serving bowl, mix the walnuts, salad greens, cranberries, and onion. Add the oil-vinegar dressing, and toss to coat everything evenly.
8 cups mixed salad greens	
½ cup dried cranberries	
¼ medium sweet onion, thinly sliced	*4* Add the crumbled Gorgonzola cheese, and toss lightly. Serve immediately.
¼ cup crumbled Gorgonzola cheese	

Per serving: Calories 308 (From Fat 217); Glycemic Load 8 (Low); Fat 24g (Saturated 4g); Cholesterol 6mg; Sodium 449mg; Carbohydrate 22g (Dietary Fiber 4g); Protein 5g.

Note: You may want to add less than the prepared amount of dressing to the salad, depending on your taste.

Tangerines, Pistachios, and Feta over Mixed Greens

Prep time: 10 min • **Cook time:** 5–8 min • **Yield:** 4 servings

Ingredients	Directions
½ cup pistachio pieces	**1** Preheat the oven to 400 degrees. Lay out the pistachio pieces on a nonstick cookie sheet, and bake until lightly toasted, fragrant, and just starting to brown, about 5 to 8 minutes. Pour the pistachios into a small bowl and set aside.
2 tablespoons extra-virgin olive oil	
1 tablespoon balsamic vinegar	
1 tablespoon low-sodium soy sauce	**2** In a small bowl, whisk together the olive oil, vinegar, soy sauce, mustard, honey, lemon juice, and orange juice until well blended.
2 teaspoons Dijon mustard	
1 tablespoon honey	
3 tablespoons lemon juice	**3** In a large serving bowl, toss together the salad greens, tangerines, onion, and about ¼ cup of the oil-vinegar dressing until well coated.
1 cup orange juice	
8 cups mixed salad greens	
2 large seedless tangerines, peeled and sectioned	**4** Add the pistachios and cheese to the salad. Serve immediately.
½ cup sliced sweet onion	
¼ cup crumbled feta cheese	

Per serving: Calories 259 (From Fat 152); Glycemic Load 7 (Low); Fat 17g (Saturated 3g); Cholesterol 8mg; Sodium 414mg; Carbohydrate 23g (Dietary Fiber 6g); Protein 8g.

Note: You may want to add less than the prepared amount of dressing to this salad (which is shown in the color section), depending on your taste. Start with ¼ cup, then add more to taste.

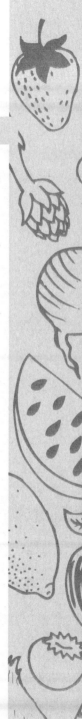

Tangy Cabbage Slaw with Peanuts

Prep time: 10 min, plus standing time • **Yield:** 12 servings

Ingredients	*Directions*
½ **teaspoon ground cumin**	*1* In a small bowl, whisk together the cumin, honey, lime juice, salt, olive oil, vinegar, ginger, black pepper, and red pepper.
2 **teaspoons honey**	
1 **tablespoon lime juice**	
½ **teaspoon salt**	*2* In a large serving bowl, toss the onions, tomatoes, cabbage, and cilantro.
1 **tablespoon extra-virgin olive oil**	
¼ **cup rice vinegar**	*3* Add the honey-vinegar dressing to the cabbage mixture, and toss to coat everything evenly.
½ **teaspoon ground ginger**	
¼ **teaspoon black pepper**	*4* Cover and refrigerate for 2 hours to let the flavors blend together. When ready to serve, gently mix in the peanuts.
⅛ **teaspoon crushed red pepper**	
¾ **cup thinly sliced green onions**	
2 **cups grape tomatoes, halved**	
8 **cups thinly sliced green cabbage**	
¼ **cup chopped fresh cilantro**	
⅓ **cup chopped dry-roasted peanuts**	

Per serving: Calories 63 (From Fat 30); Glycemic Load 0 (Low); Fat 3g (Saturated 1g); Cholesterol 0mg; Sodium 109mg; Carbohydrate 7g (Dietary Fiber 2g); Protein 2g.

Note: This recipe creates a tangy lime flavor rather than the typical mayonnaise-based taste of most slaws. Quick and easy to make, this recipe gives you a tasty way to incorporate cabbage into your diet.

Vary It! You can replace the cilantro with parsley if you want a different flavor in your slaw. You can also add leftover baked or grilled chicken to make it a full meal.

Note: You may want to add less than the prepared amount of dressing to the salad, depending on your taste.

Fresh and Fabulous: Fixing Fruit Salads

Fruit is a delicious and healthy snack on its own, but sometimes you may get tired of the same old fruit options in your refrigerator. You may also have a hard time getting your family to eat a lot of fresh fruit before it goes bad. One way to mix things up a bit — and get people to eat fruit like it's going out of style — is to whip up a tasty fruit salad. On those days when you just aren't in the mood for vegetable side dishes for lunch or dinner or when you need a fun yet healthy side for a family picnic, try your hand at creating one of the fruit salads we describe in this section. Then think about your family's favorite fruits, and come up with a few more fresh salad recipes.

Fruit salads make great sweet treats for kids in the afternoon; instead of giving your kids packaged cookies when they crave a sugary snack, give them a healthy but delicious fruit salad.

Fresh Fruit Salad with Orange Yogurt Dressing

Prep time: 10 min, plus standing time • **Yield:** 6 servings

Ingredients	Directions
½ cup lowfat plain yogurt	**1** In a small bowl, mix together the yogurt, orange juice, orange zest, vanilla, and sugar.
¼ cup orange juice	
1 teaspoon orange zest	**2** In a large bowl, combine the kiwis, tangerines, and bananas. Cover the yogurt dressing and the fruit separately, and chill until you're ready to serve them, up to 6 hours.
1 teaspoon vanilla	
1 teaspoon sugar	
2 kiwis, peeled and cut into 1-inch chunks	
2 seedless tangerines, peeled, seeded, and sectioned	**3** Before serving, mix the yogurt dressing with the fruit mixture. Let the salad stand for 15 minutes to blend flavors; then serve.
2 medium bananas, sliced	

Per serving: Calories 87 (From Fat 5); Glycemic Load 8 (Low); Fat 1g (Saturated 0g); Cholesterol 0mg; Sodium 16mg; Carbohydrate 20g (Dietary Fiber 3g); Protein 2g.

Vary It! If you don't have the exact fruits called for on hand, mix in some others. Trust us: You can't go wrong when adding fresh fruit to this recipe (which is shown in the color section).

Tip: Slice the bananas right before serving so they don't brown.

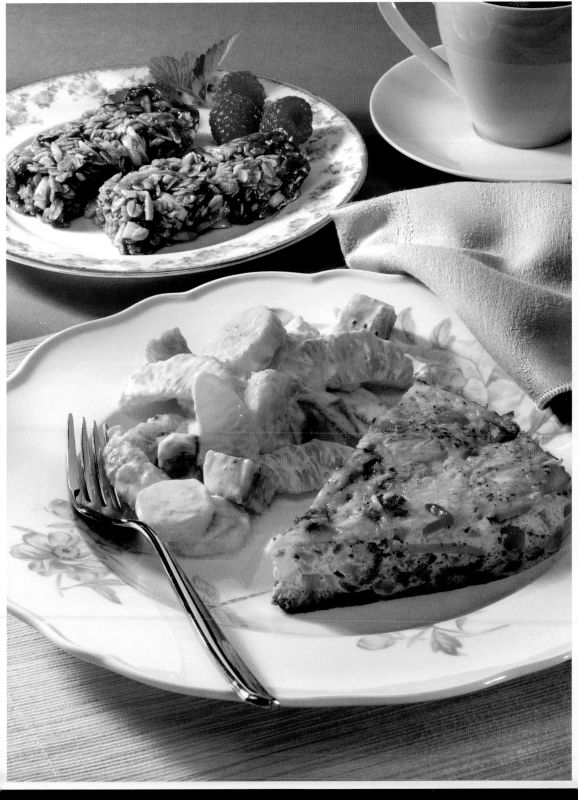

Oatmeal Raspberry Bars (Chapter 8); Fresh Fruit Salad with Orange Yogurt Dressing (Chapter 12);

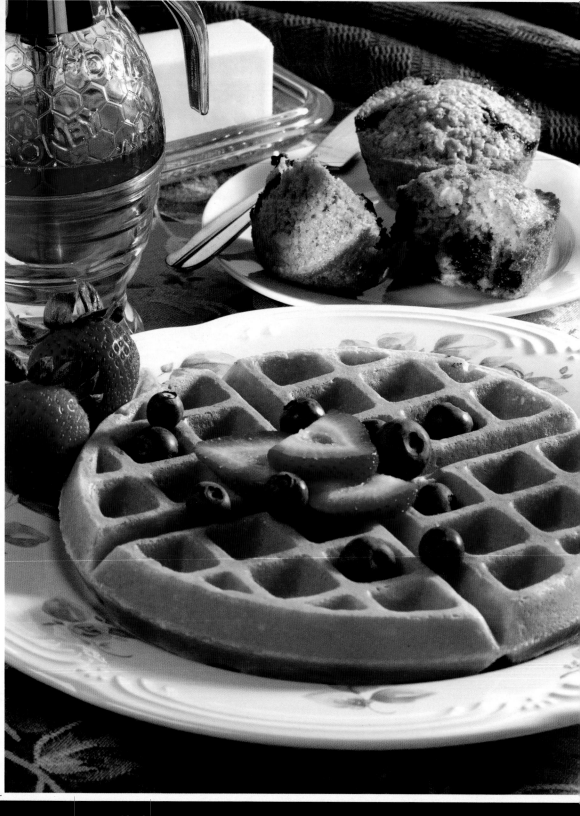

Blueb

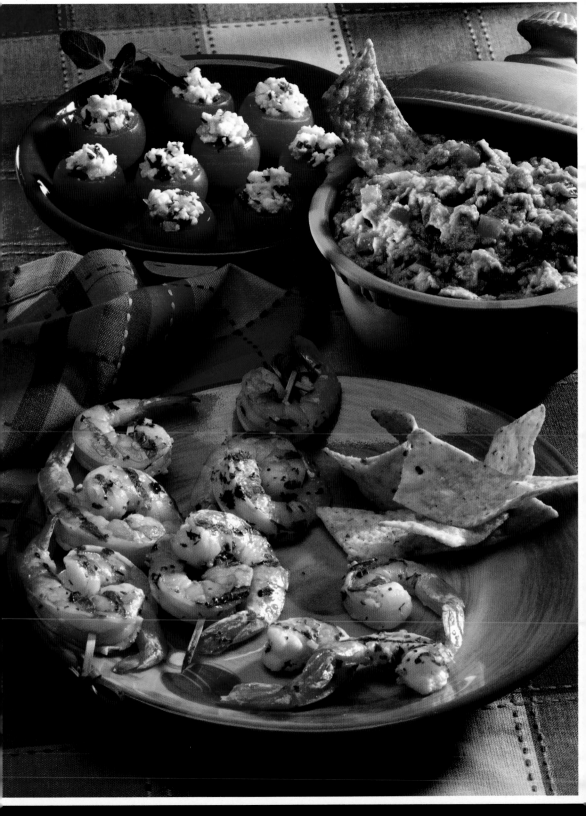

Feta-Stuffed Cherry Tomatoes (Chapter 10); Guacamole (Chapter 10); Grilled Spicy Shrimp (Chapter 10)

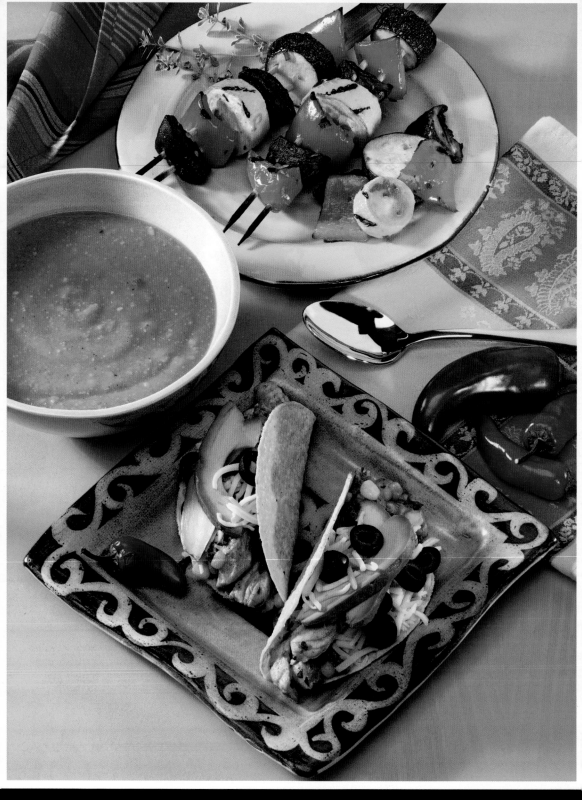

Spicy Grilled Veggie Skewers (Chapter 13); Curried Butternut Squash and

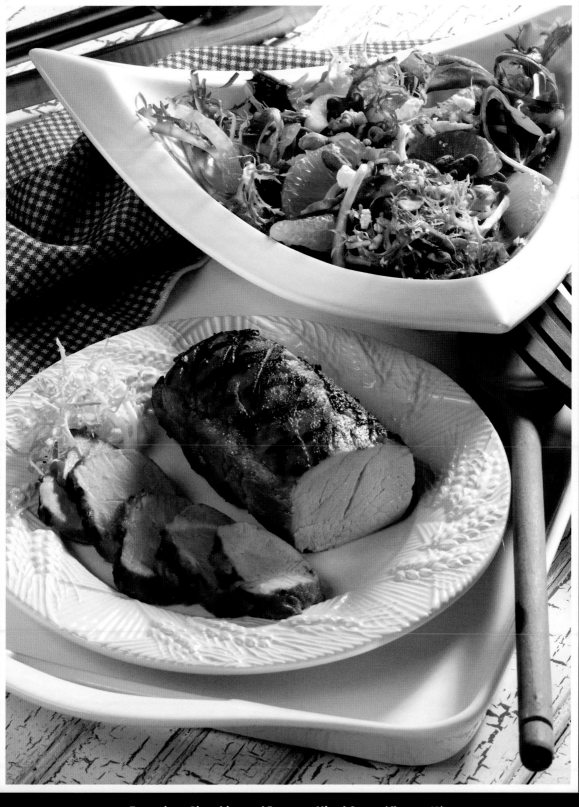

Tangerines, Pistachios, and Feta over Mixed Greens (Chapter 12);
Marinated Grilled Pork Tenderloin (Chapter 16)

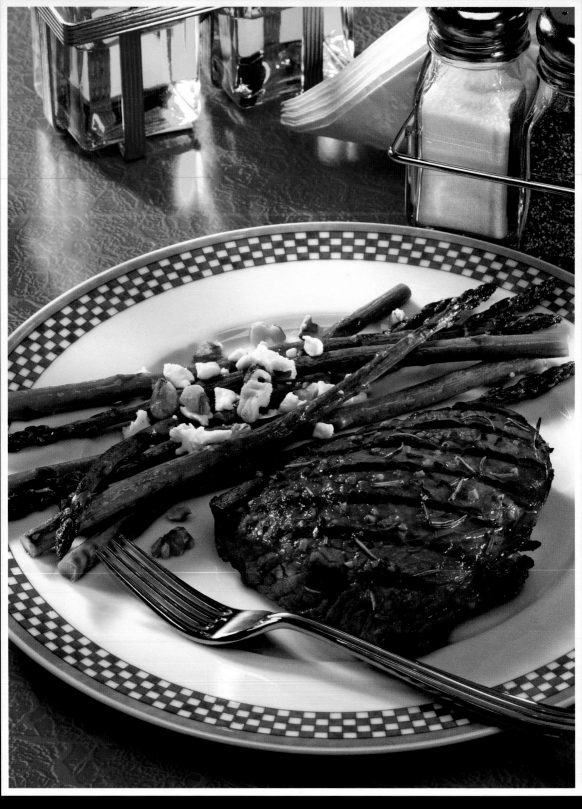

**Asparagus with Goat Cheese and Toasted Walnuts (Chapter 13);
Marinated Sirloin Steak (Chapter 16)**

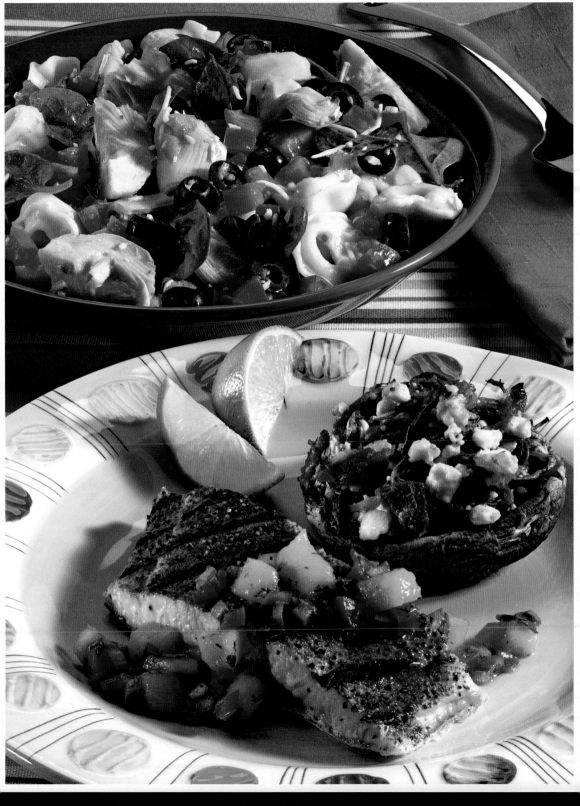

Fresh Spinach and Tomato Tortellini Salad (Chapter 14); Stuffed Portobello Mushrooms

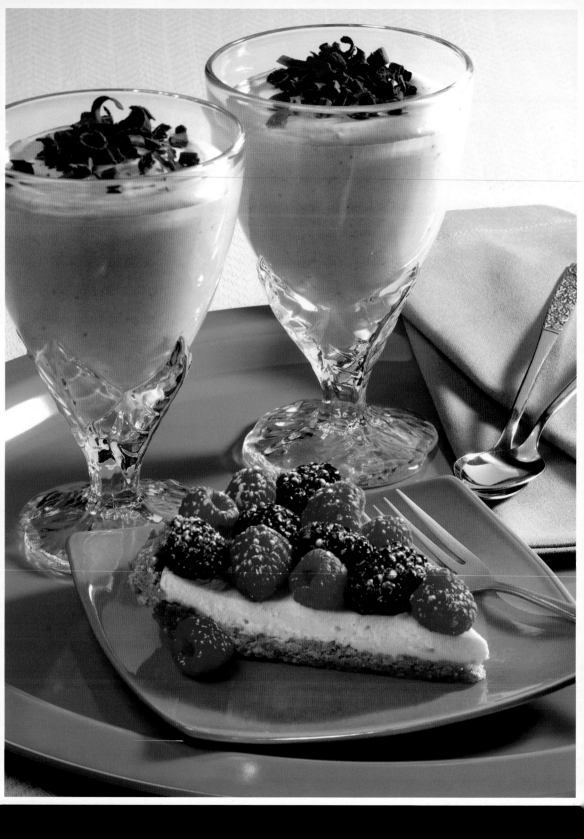

Summer Melon Salad with Lime Dressing

Prep time: 10 min • **Yield:** 6 servings

Ingredients	Directions
½ cup lowfat plain yogurt	**1** In a small bowl, mix the yogurt, lime juice, lime zest, and honey until blended; set aside.
¼ cup lime juice	
1 teaspoon lime zest	**2** Combine the cantaloupe, honeydew melon, grapes, and strawberries in a large bowl. Cover the yogurt dressing and the fruit separately, and chill until you're ready to serve them, up to 6 hours.
2 teaspoons honey	
1 cup cantaloupe, peeled and cut into 1-inch chunks	
1 cup honeydew melon, peeled and cut into 1-inch chunks	**3** Serve the fruit in bowls, about ¾ cup per serving, and top with 2 to 3 tablespoons of the yogurt dressing.
1 cup seedless red or green grapes	
1 cup halved, hulled strawberries	

Per serving: Calories 70 (From Fat 7); Glycemic Load 6 (Low); Fat 1g (Saturated 0g); Cholesterol 1mg; Sodium 21mg; Carbohydrate 16g (Dietary Fiber 1g); Protein 2g.

Vary It! If you aren't a lime fan, don't abandon this ship just yet! You can substitute another juice (like orange juice) for the lime juice in this recipe.

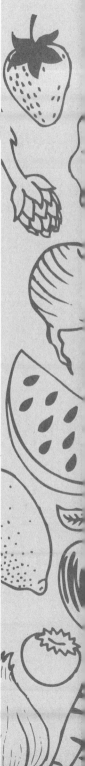

Fruit and Vegetable Salad

Prep time: 10 min • **Yield:** 4 servings

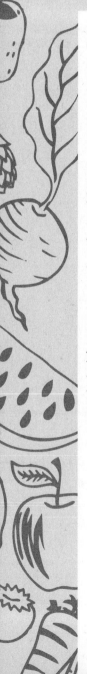

Ingredients	*Directions*
½ fresh, cored pineapple, chopped into ½-inch chunks	**1** In a large bowl, combine the chopped pineapple, pepper, cucumber, celery, tomatoes, and basil. (See Figure 12-1 if you need help with peeling and coring a pineapple.)
1 large orange or yellow pepper, seeded and chopped	
½ cucumber, peeled and chopped	**2** In a small bowl, whisk together the pineapple juice, lime juice, and cinnamon. Pour this dressing over the fruit to taste, and toss to coat everything evenly. Serve immediately after tossing.
1 celery stalk, chopped	
1 cup cherry tomatoes, halved	
2 tablespoons chopped fresh basil	
¼ cup pineapple juice from fresh or canned pineapple	
Juice of 1 lime	
1 teaspoon ground cinnamon	

Per serving: Calories 69 (From Fat 5); Glycemic Load 5 (Low); Fat 1g (Saturated 0g); Cholesterol 0mg; Sodium 19mg; Carbohydrate 17g (Dietary Fiber 2g); Protein 2g.

Note: The combination of flavors in this salad may seem a bit odd when you first read through the recipe, but as soon as you try it, you'll see why we've included it here. It's the perfect combo for a light, refreshing summer salad. The mix of fruits and vegetables provides lots of texture and flavor, and the citrus-pineapple-cinnamon dressing brings everything together.

Tip: If you're in a hurry, you can replace the fresh pineapple with 1 can of cut pineapple tidbits in natural juice. Just be sure to drain them before you use them.

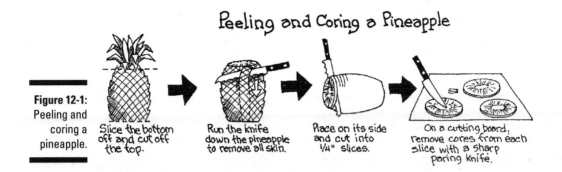

Figure 12-1: Peeling and coring a pineapple.

Peeling and Coring a Pineapple

Slice the bottom off and cut off the top.

Run the knife down the pineapple to remove all skin.

Place on its side and cut into 1/4" slices.

On a cutting board, remove cores from each slice with a sharp paring knife.

All in One: Enjoying Salad Entrees

Salad makes an easy, tasty, and healthy lunch or dinner for any day of the week. By adding a protein source, such as lean meats, eggs, tofu, beans, cheese, or nuts, you create a balanced meal that's low glycemic, too. As an added bonus, incorporating hearty toppings like chopped vegetables and beans into your salad helps you feel more satisfied. In fact, you can feel fuller and more satisfied from a loaded salad entree than from a burger and fries, with about half the calories to boot.

If you're ready to make salads a part of your low-glycemic menu, don't skip this section. Here, we offer you some delicious salad recipes that include a significant source of protein, making them ideal entrees for lunch or dinner. We've split the recipes into three categories: chicken, salmon, and pork.

To have a salad on the go, simply keep your veggies and other toppings separate from your dressings and mix them up at work or wherever your busy schedule takes you.

Grilled Chicken Caesar Salad

Prep time: 10 min • **Cook time:** 6–8 min • **Yield:** 4 servings

Ingredients	*Directions*

1 tablespoon plus 2 teaspoons extra-virgin olive oil

1 tablespoon Worcestershire sauce

1 pound boneless, skinless chicken breasts (about 2 medium breasts)

¼ teaspoon salt

⅛ teaspoon plus ⅛ teaspoon black pepper

Nonstick cooking spray

¼ cup reduced-fat plain yogurt

2 tablespoons fresh lemon juice

2 teaspoons water

1 teaspoon capers

¼ teaspoon garlic powder

1 teaspoon Dijon mustard

12 cups romaine lettuce, torn into bite-size pieces

4 to 8 teaspoons grated Parmesan cheese

4 lemon wedges

1 In a small bowl, mix together 1 tablespoon of the olive oil and the Worcestershire sauce; then brush the mixture onto both sides of the chicken breasts. Sprinkle the chicken with the salt and ⅛ teaspoon of the pepper.

2 Spray the grill with nonstick cooking spray, and then heat it to medium-high heat. Grill the chicken for 3 to 4 minutes on each side, or until it's cooked through and the juices run clear. Remove the chicken from the grill, cool, and cut into 1-inch strips.

3 Combine the remaining ⅛ teaspoon of black pepper, yogurt, lemon juice, water, the remaining 2 teaspoons of olive oil, capers, garlic powder, and mustard in a blender or food processor; blend until smooth.

4 Put the lettuce in a large bowl, and pour the blended dressing over it; toss to coat the lettuce evenly.

5 Divide the salad mixture onto 4 plates, top each serving with ¼ of the chicken strips, and sprinkle with 1 to 2 teaspoons of Parmesan cheese, depending on your taste. Serve with lemon wedges.

Per serving: Calories 237 (From Fat 94); Glycemic Load 1 (Low); Fat 11g (Saturated 3g); Cholesterol 68mg; Sodium 412mg; Carbohydrate 8g (Dietary Fiber 3g); Protein 29g.

Tip: To make this meal even faster, just buy a bottle of low-fat Caesar dressing at the store and skip Step 3 altogether!

Note: You may want to add less than the prepared amount of dressing to the salad, depending on your taste.

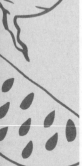

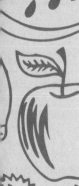

Grilled Chicken and Berry Salad with Toasted Almonds

Prep time: 10 min, plus refrigerating time • **Cook time:** About 20 min • **Yield:** 4 servings

Ingredients	Directions
1 pound boneless, skinless chicken breast halves	*1* Preheat the oven to 400 degrees.
1 to 2 cups barbeque sauce	*2* Place the chicken breasts in a shallow container with a lid. Add your favorite barbeque sauce to coat the chicken evenly, and cover and marinate it in the refrigerator for 30 minutes.
½ cup slivered almonds	
2 teaspoons yellow mustard	
1 tablespoon honey	*3* Place the almonds on a nonstick cookie sheet, and bake them until just toasted and lightly browned, about 5 to 8 minutes. Put them in a small bowl and set aside.
1 tablespoon balsamic vinegar	
2 tablespoons extra-virgin olive oil	
3 tablespoons orange juice	*4* In a medium bowl, whisk together the mustard, honey, vinegar, olive oil, and orange juice. Set aside.
Nonstick cooking spray	
12 cups mixed baby lettuce	*5* Spray the grill with nonstick cooking spray, and then heat it to low heat. Grill the chicken over indirect heat for 13 minutes on one side. Turn it over and cook for 7 more minutes on the other side, or until it's cooked through and the juices run clear. Remove the chicken from the heat, cool, and then slice into 1-inch strips.
1 cup sliced fresh strawberries	
½ cup fresh blackberries	
1 cup sugar snap peas	
	6 In a large bowl, toss together the almonds, chicken, lettuce, strawberries, blackberries, and sugar snap peas. Pour the mustard dressing over the salad mixture, and toss to mix all the ingredients together and coat everything evenly. Serve immediately after tossing.

Per serving: Calories 467 (From Fat 177); Glycemic Load 16 (Medium); Fat 20g (Saturated 3g); Cholesterol 96mg; Sodium 671mg; Carbohydrate 31g (Dietary Fiber 9g); Protein 44g.

Note: You may want to add less than the prepared amount of dressing to the salad, depending on your taste.

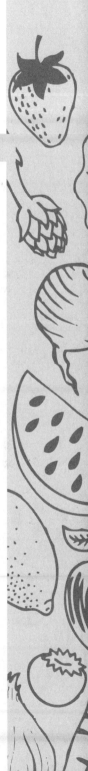

Grilled Salmon with Asparagus Tips and Mixed Greens

Prep time: 10 min • **Cook time:** About 12 min • **Yield:** 4 servings

Ingredients	Directions
¼ cup balsamic vinegar	**1** In a small bowl, whisk together the vinegar, olive oil, shallot, dry mustard, ½ teaspoon of salt, and ⅛ teaspoon of pepper; set aside.
2 tablespoons extra-virgin olive oil	
1 tablespoon shallot, minced	**2** Add water to a pot with a steamer basket so that the water level is just below the steamer basket; bring it to a boil. Add the asparagus tips to the steamer, and cook until just tender, about 1 to 2 minutes. Remove from heat, and rinse under cold water to stop the cooking. Set aside.
½ teaspoon dry mustard	
½ teaspoon salt plus salt to taste	
⅛ teaspoon black pepper plus black pepper to taste	
1 pound thin asparagus, washed and stalks cut off and discarded	**3** Heat the grill to high heat. Take a piece of aluminum foil twice the size of the fish and spray it with nonstick cooking spray. Rinse the salmon, and set it on the sheet of foil.
Nonstick cooking spray	
1 pound salmon filet	**4** In a small bowl, blend together the brown sugar, cumin, coriander, paprika, and salt and pepper to taste. Rub the mixture onto both sides of the salmon until it's well coated. Close up all sides of the foil to package the salmon.
2 teaspoons brown sugar	
1 teaspoon ground cumin	
1 teaspoon ground coriander	
1 teaspoon paprika	**5** Place the salmon package on the grill, and cook with the lid closed and vents open for about 5 minutes on each side, or until the salmon is flaky. Remove from grill and set aside to cool. Cut the salmon into 4 even pieces.
10 cups (about 18 ounces) mixed salad greens	
1 cup chopped Roma tomatoes	
4 lime wedges	

6 In a large bowl, mix together the asparagus tips, mixed greens, and tomatoes. Pour the vinegar-oil dressing over the salad mixture, and toss to coat everything evenly.

7 Divide the salad onto 4 plates, and top each serving with ¼ of the salmon. Serve with lime wedges.

Per serving: *Calories 280 (From Fat 109); Glycemic Load 1 (Low); Fat 12g (Saturated 2g); Cholesterol 65mg; Sodium 424mg; Carbohydrate 16g (Dietary Fiber 5g); Protein 29g.*

Vary It! If you aren't a fish fan, you can always replace the salmon with chicken or pork.

Note: You may want to add less than the prepared amount of dressing to the salad, depending on your taste.

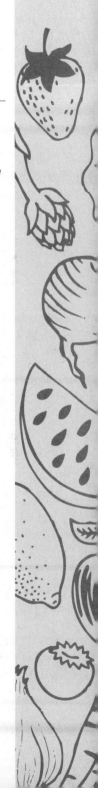

BBQ Pork with Grilled Pineapple and Mixed Greens

Prep time: 15 min • **Cook time:** 10–12 min • **Yield:** 4 servings

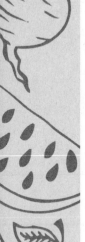

Ingredients	*Directions*
3 thickly cut pork chops (at least 1-inch thick; about 12 ounces total), cubed into 1-inch chunks	*1* Thread the cubed pork onto 2 skewers, about 6 to 8 pieces per skewer, and set aside. Wash your hands, and then thread the pineapple onto 2 or 3 skewers, about 5 to 6 chunks of pineapple per skewer; set aside. Pour the barbeque sauce into a small bowl for basting.
2 cups fresh pineapple, peeled, cored, and cut into 1-inch chunks	
1 to 2 cups barbecue sauce	*2* Spray the grill with nonstick cooking spray, and then heat it to low heat. Cook the pork skewers for about 2 minutes; baste the pork with about ⅓ of the barbeque sauce, or enough to coat one side of the skewers. Turn the pork skewers over, and continue to baste, cooking them for 4 to 5 more minutes, or until they're cooked through. Set aside.
Nonstick cooking spray	
12 cups mixed greens	
16 cherry tomatoes	
2 tablespoons balsamic vinegar	*3* Place the pineapple skewers on the grill, and cook for 4 to 5 minutes, or until they're browned and heated. Remove the pork and pineapple chunks from the skewers.
2 tablespoons extra-virgin olive oil	
1 tablespoon honey	*4* In a large serving bowl, mix together the pork, grilled pineapple chunks, mixed greens, and tomatoes.
½ tablespoon Dijon mustard	
½ teaspoon chili powder	*5* In a medium bowl, whisk together the vinegar, olive oil, honey, Dijon mustard, chili powder, and salt.
½ teaspoon salt	
1 avocado, peeled, pitted, and cut into thin slices	*6* Pour the dressing over the salad mixture, and toss to coat everything evenly.
	7 Place the sliced avocado on top of the salad, and serve.

Per serving: Calories 372 (From Fat 132); Glycemic Load 8 (Low); Fat 15g (Saturated 3g); Cholesterol 52mg; Sodium 801mg; Carbohydrate 33g (Dietary Fiber 5g); Protein 28g.

Note: You may want to add less than the prepared amount of dressing to the salad, depending on your taste.

Tip: You know the pork is cooked through when the internal temperature reads 155 degrees with a meat thermometer.

Tip: Refer to Figure 12-1 if you need help with peeling and coring a pineapple.

Chapter 13

Reinventing Vegetable Sides the Low-Glycemic Way

In This Chapter

▶ Giving new life to steamed and boiled vegetables

▶ Adding extra flavor to your meals with sautéed vegetables

▶ Roasting vegetables the easy and flavorful way

▶ Grilling delicious vegetables that everyone will love

*Y*ou've probably been hearing the message that vegetables are good for you since you were a child. Now that you're an adult, you see the same message across the Internet, television, and newspapers: vegetables, vegetables, vegetables! Well, we're here to tell you that you may want to start listening to this message if you're trying to develop a healthier lifestyle. After all, this one food group can

✔ Help you lose weight even as you eat a large volume of food

✔ Help you feel full longer

✔ Decrease your risk of chronic diseases like heart disease, diabetes, and some cancers

✔ Help you reverse some issues like high blood pressure and high cholesterol

✔ Provide the proper nutrients your body needs to feel great

With all these benefits, why are Americans still not eating the recommended 2 to 3 cups of vegetables a day? Many people confess that they don't eat them strictly because they don't like their taste or don't know how to cook them. However, we believe there may be another reason.

Vegetables can be pretty boring to eat if you don't know how to spruce them up. And it seems that most people in the United States — where the most common way to prepare vegetables is to warm them out of a can either by boiling or steaming them — don't know how to make them more exciting. Yes, steaming can be a healthier way to cook vegetables, but what good is it if you never eat them?

In this chapter, our goal is to show you some different ways to cook vegetables to add a little more flavor while keeping it easy. We show you how to add some punch to steamed and boiled veggies and how to tap into even more flavor by sautéing, roasting, and grilling them instead.

Steaming and Boiling Veggies with a Twist

Steaming is one of the healthiest ways to cook vegetables because it retains all their nutrients. Unfortunately, though, the traditional steaming method doesn't lend itself to adding seasonings and spices, which often means your steamed veggies are less than flavorful, or shall we say boring?

Although boiling isn't necessarily unhealthy, when you boil vegetables in water, you often lose many of the nutrients in the water itself. When you discard the water, you also discard most of the nutritional content. Thus, the key to boiling veggies is cooking them in a liquid that you can eat afterward or that reabsorbs into the vegetable.

Instead of just adding butter and salt to your bland veggies after you steam or boil them, why not throw the veggies in a pan and coat them with some great ingredients while you cook them? In this section, we challenge you to throw out all the old rules about steaming and boiling and try some new ways. We promise you won't be disappointed!

Garlic Green Beans with Almonds and Parmesan

Prep time: 5 min • **Cook time:** 5–7 min • **Yield:** 4 servings

Ingredients	*Directions*
1 pound green beans, ends trimmed	*1* Steam the green beans in a medium saucepan with a steamer basket until they're still crisp but beginning to cook, about 2 to 3 minutes. Remove from heat and set aside.
1 teaspoon extra-virgin olive oil	
2 cloves garlic, minced	*2* In a large skillet, heat the olive oil over medium-high heat. Add the steamed beans and garlic, and cook for about 1 minute, stirring continuously. Add the vegetable broth, and cook until the liquid from the broth has evaporated, about 1 more minute.
2 tablespoons vegetable broth	
⅓ cup sliced almonds	
¼ cup grated Parmesan cheese	
	3 Stir in the almonds and Parmesan, and cook until the cheese is warm and coats the beans, about 1 to 2 minutes. Serve warm.

Per serving: Calories 120 (From Fat 63); Glycemic Load 2 (Low); Fat 7g (Saturated 2g); Cholesterol 4mg; Sodium 128mg; Carbohydrate 11g (Dietary Fiber 5g); Protein 6g.

Note: The key to this recipe is steaming the beans first and then adding them to a skillet to blend in other flavors. Trust us, this steam-skillet duo is the new way to steam!

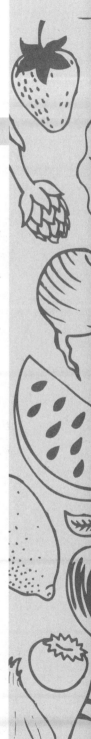

Curried Cauliflower

Prep time: 5 min • **Cook time:** About 8 min • **Yield:** 4 servings

Ingredients	Directions
2 cups cauliflower florets, washed	*1* Steam the cauliflower in a medium pot with a steamer basket until it's just tender, about 5 minutes. Drain and set aside.
1½ teaspoons curry powder	
1 teaspoon all-purpose flour	*2* Heat a medium-sized nonstick skillet over medium heat, add the curry powder and flour, and whisk them together for about 15 seconds.
¼ cup vegetable broth	
1 tablespoon honey	
¼ cup lowfat plain yogurt	*3* Whisk the broth and honey into the flour mixture over medium-high heat, and boil until thick, about 2 minutes, whisking continuously. Add the cauliflower, and toss to coat evenly. Turn off the heat, and stir in the yogurt until it's creamy and warm. Serve immediately.

Per serving: Calories 43 (From Fat 5); Glycemic Load 4 (Low); Fat 1g (Saturated 0g); Cholesterol 1mg; Sodium 82mg; Carbohydrate 9g (Dietary Fiber 2g); Protein 2g.

Note: If the yogurt doesn't seem warm enough after you mix it with the cauliflower, you can turn the heat on low and continue to stir until it's warm enough to eat. Just be sure you don't bring it to a boil, or you'll scorch the yogurt!

Vary It! If you enjoy a lot of spice, by all means, add some chili powder along with the curry!

Wilted Spinach with Lemon and Pine Nuts

Prep time: 5 min • **Cook time:** 3–4 min • **Yield:** 4 servings

Ingredients	Directions
2 tablespoons extra-virgin olive oil	**1** In a small bowl, whisk together the olive oil, lemon juice, thyme, Dijon mustard, and vinegar. Set aside.
Juice of 1 lemon (about 2 to 4 tablespoons)	
½ teaspoon dried thyme	**2** In a large saucepan with a steamer basket, steam the spinach over water, put the lid on, and turn the heat up to medium-high. Cook until the spinach just wilts, about 3 to 4 minutes. (You don't want soggy spinach, so make sure you take it out as soon as it starts to wilt.)
¼ teaspoon Dijon mustard	
1 teaspoon balsamic vinegar	
One 10-ounce bag prewashed baby spinach	
¼ cup pine nuts	**3** Use a pair of tongs to remove the spinach from the steamer, and place it in a medium serving bowl; gently toss the spinach with the lemon-oil dressing until it's coated evenly. Add the pine nuts, salt to taste, and serve.
Salt to taste	

Per serving: Calories 142 (From Fat 100); Glycemic Load 0 (Low); Fat 11g (Saturated 2g); Cholesterol 0mg; Sodium 126mg; Carbohydrate 10g (Dietary Fiber 4g); Protein 4g.

Note: You may not need to add all the dressing; the lemon flavor is strong.

Vary It! You can use pistachios in place of the pine nuts — they're also delicious.

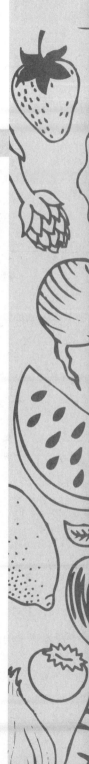

Broccoli with Red Peppers

Prep time: 10 min • **Cook time:** 4–6 min • **Yield:** 4 servings

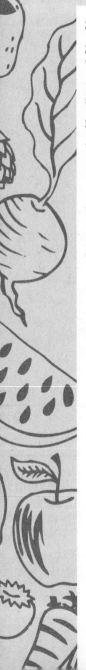

Ingredients	*Directions*
2 teaspoons butter	*1* In a medium skillet, heat the butter over medium-high heat until melted. Add the broccoli, bell pepper, and shallots; toss to coat everything evenly.
2 cups broccoli florets, washed	
1 red bell pepper, cut into thin strips	*2* Add the vegetable broth. Bring it to a boil, turn down the heat, and simmer with the lid on for 3 to 4 minutes. Remove the lid, and cook, stirring often, for 1 to 2 more minutes, or until the broth is evaporated and the broccoli is crisp but tender enough to pierce with a fork. Serve warm.
3 shallots, sliced	
¼ cup vegetable broth	

Per serving: Calories 47 (From Fat 19); Glycemic Load 1 (Low); Fat 2g (Saturated 1g); Cholesterol 5mg; Sodium 75mg; Carbohydrate 7g (Dietary Fiber 2g); Protein 2g.

Vary It! You can easily replace the broccoli with asparagus or green beans if you prefer those veggies.

Italian Tomatoes with Green Beans

Prep time: 5 min • **Cook time:** 10–15 min • **Yield:** 4 servings

Ingredients	*Directions*
One 15-ounce can whole tomatoes, undrained	*1* In a small bowl, crush the tomatoes into smaller chunks with a spoon.
2 cups green beans, trimmed and cut into 1-inch pieces	*2* In a medium saucepan, mix together the green beans, basil, oregano, crushed tomatoes, wine, and capers. Bring the mixture to a boil over medium-high heat.
½ teaspoon dried basil	
¼ teaspoon dried oregano	
2 tablespoons white wine or cooking sherry	*3* Turn the heat down to low, and simmer until the beans are tender enough to pierce with a fork, about 10 to 15 minutes. Serve warm.
1 tablespoon capers	

Per serving: Calories 41 (From Fat 3); Glycemic Load 3 (Low); Fat 0g (Saturated 0g); Cholesterol 0mg; Sodium 223mg; Carbohydrate 9g (Dietary Fiber 3g); Protein 2g.

Tip: When you start gathering the ingredients for this recipe, we encourage you to find a high-quality canned tomato (such as Cento San Marzano tomatoes) because the taste of your canned tomatoes really makes or breaks this dish.

Vary It! If you have fresh basil on hand, add about 1 tablespoon of chopped fresh basil in place of the dried basil.

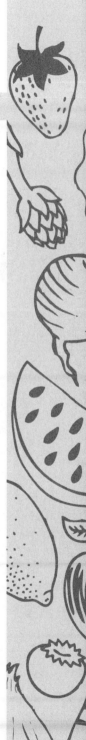

Serving Sautéed Specialties

The next step up from steaming and boiling vegetables is sautéing them. You may be surprised by how much you can do with a little oil, some vegetables, and a few spices. In this section, we show you some simple ways to dress up your veggies on the stove top. You don't have to be throwing a dinner party to eat these delicious veggie sides, although they are worthy of any event!

You don't necessarily need a recipe to sauté veggies; for example, you can sauté some asparagus or spinach in a little oil and just sprinkle a little salt on top. The trick is to avoid going overboard with the oil, or you'll end up with a boatload of calories. Limit your oil to a few teaspoons for veggies.

Broccoli with Garlic, Lemon, and Parmesan

Prep time: 5 min • **Cook time:** 6–7 min • **Yield:** 4 servings

Ingredients	Directions
1 tablespoon extra-virgin olive oil 3 cups broccoli florets, washed 2 cloves garlic, minced 2 teaspoons lemon juice 2 tablespoons grated Parmesan cheese Salt to taste	**1** In a medium nonstick skillet, heat the olive oil over medium-high heat. Add the broccoli, and cook for 4 minutes. **2** Add the garlic and lemon juice, and cook until the broccoli is crisp but tender enough to pierce with a fork, about 2 to 3 minutes (the broccoli will start to brown). **3** Place the broccoli in a serving dish, and toss with the Parmesan cheese. Add salt to taste, and serve.

Per serving: Calories 59 (From Fat 39); Glycemic Load 2 (Low); Fat 4g (Saturated 1g); Cholesterol 2mg; Sodium 53mg; Carbohydrate 4g (Dietary Fiber 2g); Protein 3g.

Tip: After you make this recipe a time or two, you may find you like more lemon flavor or more garlic; feel free to play with the ingredient amounts to make it your own. Go easy on the cheese, though, so you don't overdo it with calories and fat.

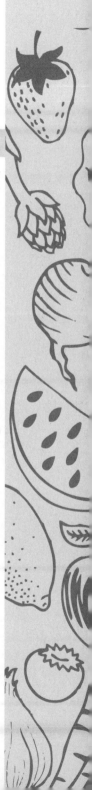

Sautéed Carrots with Rosemary Honey Glaze

Prep time: 2 min • **Cook time:** 14 min • **Yield:** 4 servings

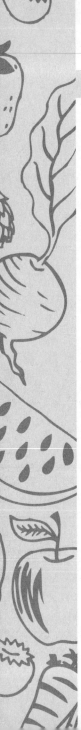

Ingredients	Directions
1 teaspoon extra-virgin olive oil	**1** In a large skillet, heat the olive oil over medium-high heat. Add the carrots, and sprinkle them with salt and pepper to taste. Sauté the carrots until they begin to brown at the edges, about 12 minutes.
1 pound baby carrots	
Salt and pepper to taste	
1 teaspoon butter	**2** Add the butter, rosemary, thyme, and honey to the sautéed carrots, and toss to coat them evenly. Cook over medium heat, stirring continuously, until the carrots are glazed and tender enough to pierce with a fork, about 2 minutes.
1 teaspoon chopped fresh rosemary	
1 teaspoon chopped fresh thyme	
1 tablespoon honey	**3** Season the glazed carrots with more salt and pepper to taste (if desired) and serve.

Per serving: Calories 93 (From Fat 21); Glycemic Load 3 (Low); Fat 2g (Saturated 0g); Cholesterol 0mg; Sodium 46mg; Carbohydrate 17g (Dietary Fiber 3g); Protein 2g.

Note: When you're craving a butter flavor, you can certainly add a little butter to your veggie dish; just remember that you don't need to add much to achieve the flavor you crave. By using only the amount of butter called for here, you keep your vegetable dish on the healthy side instead of loading it up with fat and high-glycemic sugars.

Sautéed Spinach with Caramelized Onions

Prep time: 10 min • **Cook time:** 11–13 min • **Yield:** 6 servings

Ingredients	*Directions*
1 tablespoon extra-virgin olive oil 1 teaspoon butter 1 large sweet onion, chopped 1 clove garlic, minced ½ teaspoon ground cumin ¼ teaspoon ground coriander 1 tablespoon vegetable broth 2 pounds fresh baby spinach, rinsed and patted dry Salt and pepper to taste	*1* In a large nonstick skillet, heat the olive oil and butter over medium-high heat. Add the chopped onion, reduce the heat to medium-low, and sauté the onion for about 3 to 4 minutes. Add the garlic, cumin, and coriander, and continue cooking until the onion is golden brown, about 4 to 5 minutes. Remove from heat and set aside. *2* Add the vegetable broth to the hot skillet, and heat it on medium heat for about 30 seconds. Add the fresh spinach to the broth, and stir until wilted, about 3 minutes. Add salt and pepper to taste. *3* Transfer the spinach to a serving bowl, and place the cooked onions on top. Serve immediately.

Per serving: Calories 100 (From Fat 27); Glycemic Load 1 (Low); Fat 3g (Saturated 1g); Cholesterol 2mg; Sodium 51mg; Carbohydrate 19g (Dietary Fiber 8g); Protein 4g.

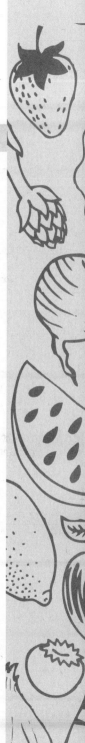

Roasting Vegetables to Perfection

Roasting is a great way to cook vegetables because you don't have to add a lot of fat via oil and cheese to add flavor. The roasting method itself really brings out the flavors of the actual vegetables. The trick is to add enough moisture through oil, broth, wine, or juice to keep the veggies from drying out while cooking. Many vegetables, like asparagus or mushrooms, release enough of their own juices during roasting that you don't have to add more moisture during roasting. Others, like broccoli, need a little added moisture for the tastiest results.

The best part about roasting veggies is that you don't even need a recipe to do it. Just throw some veggies in a roasting pan, add a little salt and moisture, and roast until they're softened! If you prefer a little more direction or you're just aching to try something new, check out the fun recipes we offer in this section. Get ready to combine a little moisture and a few seasonings to give veggie sides a whole new twist!

Asparagus with Goat Cheese and Toasted Walnuts

Prep time: 5 min • **Cook time:** 7–12 min • **Yield:** 4 servings

Ingredients	Directions
½ cup chopped walnuts	**1** Preheat the oven to 400 degrees. Put the walnuts in a small pie tin, and bake them for about 3 to 4 minutes. Pour them into a small bowl and set aside.
1 pound fresh asparagus, rinsed and dried, ½ inch of thick part of bottoms trimmed	**2** Arrange the asparagus spears in a single layer in a shallow baking dish lined with a sheet of tin foil. Drizzle the olive oil over the asparagus, and roll the spears to coat them evenly. Sprinkle the asparagus lightly with salt.
1 tablespoon extra-virgin olive oil	
Salt to taste	
⅓ cup crumbled goat cheese	**3** Roast the asparagus in the oven until it's crisp but tender enough to pierce with a fork, about 4 to 8 minutes, depending on the thickness of the spears (thin spears take much less time than thick ones).
	4 Divide the asparagus among four plates, and sprinkle them with the goat cheese and roasted walnuts; then allow the asparagus to cool slightly. Serve at room temperature for best flavor.

Per serving: Calories 167 (From Fat 138); Glycemic Load 0 (Low); Fat 15g (Saturated 3g); Cholesterol 4mg; Sodium 54mg; Carbohydrate 5g (Dietary Fiber 2g); Protein 6g.

Note: If you're serving an elegant dinner, you may want to consider this recipe for one of your veggie sides (see it for yourself in the color section). Although it's easy to make, the combination of goat cheese and toasted walnuts creates an amazing flavor that's sure to awe your guests. Plus, it looks beautiful on your plate!

Tip: You can bake your asparagus at the same time that you bake the walnuts if you want to speed up the cook time. Just watch the walnuts closely to make sure they don't burn!

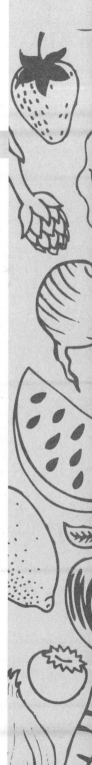

Roasted Mixed Vegetables with Caramelized Shallots

Prep time: 12 min • **Cook time:** 15–20 min • **Yield:** 6 servings

Ingredients	Directions
1 small yellow squash, cut into 1-inch round slices	*1* Preheat the oven to 450 degrees. In a large bowl, combine the squash, zucchini, asparagus, bell pepper, and shallots.
1 small zucchini, cut into 1-inch round slices	
½ pound asparagus, ½ inch of thick part of bottoms trimmed	*2* In a small bowl, stir together the thyme, rosemary, olive oil, vinegar, and salt and pepper to taste. Add this mixture to the vegetables, and toss until they're evenly coated. Spread the vegetables evenly on the bottom of a large roasting pan.
1 red bell pepper, seeded and sliced into 1-inch strips	
3 shallots, peeled and cut in half	
1 teaspoon dried thyme	*3* Roast for 15 to 20 minutes, or until the vegetables are cooked through and browned, stirring every 5 minutes.
1 teaspoon dried rosemary	
2 tablespoons extra-virgin olive oil	
1 tablespoon balsamic vinegar	
Salt and pepper to taste	

Per serving: Calories 68 (From Fat 43); Glycemic Load 1 (Low); Fat 5g (Saturated 1g); Cholesterol 0mg; Sodium 2mg; Carbohydrate 6g (Dietary Fiber 2g); Protein 1g.

Vary It! This recipe is more like a template for you to work from than a specific map to follow. You can mix in any vegetables you want and change up the seasonings for different flavors. Let your imagination — and your stomach — be your guide!

Taking Veggies to the Grill

We're leaving the best for last because, in our opinion, grilling vegetables is the tastiest way to go. Grilling really brings out the flavors of the vegetables, so you can either start simple by just tossing your veggies on the grill with a little salt or add a lot of flavor by marinating your veggies before grilling them. Grilled veggies are a great option when you're already grilling other foods in your meal, and the best part is that cleanup is a snap!

In this section, we share a couple of veggie marinades, one with a light buttery flavor that doesn't include too much fat and another that's spicy and full of flavor. Choose the one that sounds best to you, and fire up that grill!

Grilled Summer Squash and Zucchini

Prep time: 10 min • **Cook time:** 10 min • **Yield:** 4 servings

Ingredients	*Directions*
1 medium zucchini, cut into ½-inch sticks	**1** In a large bowl, mix together the zucchini, squash, and shallots. Spread the mixture on the top half of a large sheet of heavy-duty aluminum foil.
1 medium yellow squash, cut into ½-inch sticks	
2 shallots, peeled and halved	**2** Drizzle the veggies with the white wine, and top them with the butter. Add salt and pepper to taste. Top the veggies with the fresh rosemary.
4 tablespoons white wine	
2 teaspoons butter	
Salt and pepper to taste	**3** Take the foil and fold it like you would fold a piece of paper in half. Then fold the sides and top over — kind of like an envelope — so that you're left with a sealed rectangle.
2 sprigs fresh rosemary	
	4 Heat the grill to medium-high heat, and place the foil packet on the grill. Cook until the veggies are tender enough to pierce with a fork, about 10 minutes, flipping the packet at least once with a pair of tongs before they're done. Serve warm.

Per serving: Calories 60 (From Fat 19); Glycemic Load 1 (Low); Fat 2g (Saturated 1g); Cholesterol 5mg; Sodium 2mg; Carbohydrate 6g (Dietary Fiber 2g); Protein 2g.

Spicy Grilled Veggie Skewers

Prep time: 12 min, plus refrigerating time • **Cook time:** 8–10 min • **Yield:** 6 servings

Ingredients	*Directions*
1 teaspoon ground ginger	*1* In a large, shallow container with a lid, mix together the ginger, shallot, soy sauce, vinegar, oil, lime juice, and red pepper.
2 tablespoons shallot, minced	
¼ cup low-sodium soy sauce	
1 teaspoon rice vinegar	*2* Place the zucchini, squash, mushrooms, and bell pepper in the container, put the lid on tightly, and shake the container until the vegetables are well coated. Let the veggies marinate for 10 to 20 minutes in the refrigerator.
3 tablespoons canola oil	
1 tablespoon lime juice	
¼ teaspoon crushed red pepper	
1 medium zucchini, cut into 1-inch round slices	*3* Skewer the vegetables onto 6 skewer sticks, alternating veggies as you go. For example, start with a piece of red pepper, and then add a piece of mushroom, a piece of zucchini, and a piece of squash; then repeat until each skewer has about 8 veggies on it. After you skewer all the vegetables, save the marinade for basting.
1 medium yellow squash, cut into 1-inch round slices	
2 portobello mushrooms, stems cut off and quartered into 1-inch pieces	
1 red bell pepper, cut into 1-inch chunks	*4* Spray the grill with nonstick cooking spray, and then heat it to medium-high. Grill the vegetables until they're browned and soft, about 8 to 10 minutes, turning frequently. Baste the veggies with the leftover marinade frequently throughout cooking. Serve warm.
Nonstick cooking spray	

Per serving: *Calories 101 (From Fat 64); Glycemic Load 1 (Low); Fat 7g (Saturated 1g); Cholesterol 0mg; Sodium 235mg; Carbohydrate 7g (Dietary Fiber 2g); Protein 3g.*

Note: Looking for a lot of flavor and a little heat? Well then, this recipe's for you (you can check it out in the color section to see what it looks like). The marinade makes any vegetable taste amazing, so feel free to mix in whatever your heart desires. We highly recommend mushrooms and zucchini, though, because they turn out especially great.

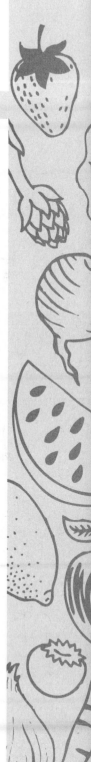

Chapter 14

On the Side: Grains, Pasta, and Potatoes

In This Chapter

▶ Creating tasty sides with low-glycemic grains

▶ Finding pasta recipes that work as part of a low-glycemic diet

▶ Discovering recipes using the forbidden high-glycemic food: potatoes

A lthough this book is chock-full of helpful, recipe-heavy chapters just waiting to guide you toward a tasty, low-glycemic meal plan, this one may be the most important. Why? Because when you think about side dishes, you likely think more about rice, pasta, and potatoes than anything else. These three foods are not only the most common sides eaten by people in the United States, but also members of one of the higher-glycemic food categories.

Don't panic if rice, pasta, and potatoes make up a large chunk of your weekly meal plan. Our goal in this chapter is to offer you some great side dish recipes using lower-glycemic grains and to show you how to incorporate those medium-glycemic favorites like pasta and potatoes the healthy way. Although the lower-glycemic alternatives we use here may seem strange at first and you may not know how to cook them just yet, after reading this chapter, you'll be a pro at eating (and making) starchy sides the low-glycemic way!

You're more likely to stick with diet changes if they work in your lifestyle. If you can't find some old favorite sides that are low glycemic or you're afraid to try out a few new recipes, chances are you'll give up pretty quickly. Let's face it: You're busy and the last thing you want to think about is how to serve barley as a side dish with the grilled chicken you're serving for dinner. Even so, don't pull out that bag of russet potatoes just yet! All you have to do is find a few new standby sides to replace the old rice, pasta, and potato dishes you may have turned to in the past.

Exploring New Grains

It's easy to become dependent on rice as your primary grain, but although you don't have to omit it entirely from your diet, you may have to explore some new grains if you want to make a low-glycemic meal plan work for your lifestyle. After all, you certainly don't want to feel limited in your meal choices; if you do, your new meal plan probably won't last very long.

Barley, polenta, and quinoa are three low- to medium-glycemic grains that you can cook with on a regular basis. You can create all kinds of side dishes out of these grains that taste just as good as, if not better than, your old standby rice. Don't know where to start? No worries. This section offers you a variety of recipes that can help you broaden your recipe box to include low-glycemic grain sides that everyone (including you) will enjoy. Here's additional info about these grains:

- ✔ *Barley* is a cereal grain with a wonderful nutty flavor and a pasta-like texture. *Whole-grain barley* refers to barley with the *hull* (an inedible part of the grain) removed. Whole-grain barley is low glycemic and contains more fiber and nutrients, but the downside is that it is harder to find in the grocery store. *Pearl barley* has the hull and much of the bran removed as well. Although it doesn't have quite the amount of nutrients of whole-grain barley, pearl barley is still a wonderful, low-glycemic source of fiber that you can easily find in most stores. Not only is it a great grain to eat in soups, but it also makes a nice creamy side dish.

- ✔ *Polenta* is basically just cooked cornmeal. It's an Italian dish that used to be considered "peasant food" and now, ironically, is found in high-end restaurants around the world. Although it has some fiber and a small amount of B vitamins, the best part of polenta is its sweet corn flavor and the fact that cooked cornmeal is low glycemic.

- ✔ *Quinoa* is an ancient grain once considered "the gold of the Incas," yet it's certainly not an item most people find in their pantry. Quinoa is a protein-rich grain that has a creamy texture and a nutty taste. It cooks as easily as rice and is one of the only plant-based foods that provide a *complete protein* (including all nine essential amino acids). Half a cup of quinoa has a glycemic load of around 9, making it a great and tasty low-glycemic option.

Parmesan and Mushroom Barley Pilaf

Prep time: 5 min • **Cook time:** 35–40 min • **Yield:** 8 servings

Ingredients	Directions
2 cups chicken broth 1 cup pearl barley 1 tablespoon extra-virgin olive oil 1 small sweet onion, minced 3 cloves garlic, pressed 2 cups sliced mushrooms 2 teaspoons dried basil, or to taste 2 tablespoons chopped fresh parsley ¼ cup grated Parmesan cheese Salt and pepper to taste	***1*** In a medium saucepan, bring the chicken broth and barley to a boil over medium-high heat. Reduce the heat to low, and simmer, covered, until the liquid is absorbed, about 35 to 40 minutes.
	2 While the barley is cooking, heat the oil in a medium skillet over medium heat. Add the onion and garlic, and cook, stirring frequently, until both are softened, about 3 minutes.
	3 Add the sliced mushrooms to the onion and garlic mixture, and cook, stirring frequently, until they become soft, about 6 minutes. Turn off the heat and set the mixture aside until the barley is finished cooking.
	4 Once the barley is done cooking, add the mushroom mixture, basil, parsley, and Parmesan to the barley, and mix well. Add salt and pepper to taste, and serve.

Per serving: Calories 131 (From Fat 29); Glycemic Load 10 (Low); Fat 3g (Saturated 1g); Cholesterol 3mg; Sodium 150mg; Carbohydrate 22g (Dietary Fiber 4g); Protein 5g.

Vary It! You can replace the chicken broth with vegetable broth to create a vegetarian version.

Tip: Because barley is such a hearty grain, this particular pilaf goes great with a light meal like grilled fish or chicken.

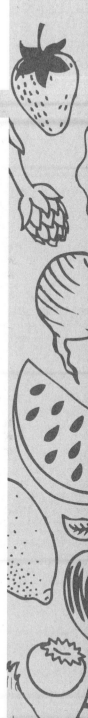

Barley with Zucchini, Tomatoes, and Basil

Prep time: 20 min • **Cook time:** 45–50 min • **Yield:** 8 servings

Ingredients	Directions
1 teaspoon plus 2 teaspoons extra-virgin olive oil	*1* In a medium saucepan, heat 1 teaspoon of the oil over moderately high heat until hot. Add half of the chopped onion, and cook until it begins to soften, about 2 minutes. Add the cumin, coriander, salt, black pepper, and garlic powder, and stir until fragrant, about 1 minute.
1 medium onion, chopped and divided in half	
1½ teaspoons ground cumin	
½ teaspoon ground coriander	
¼ teaspoon salt	*2* Add the barley to the oil and onion mixture, and stir until the barley is well coated, about 2 minutes.
¼ teaspoon black pepper	
¼ teaspoon garlic powder	*3* Add the broth, and bring it to a boil over medium-high heat. Reduce the heat to low, and simmer, covered, until all the liquid is absorbed and the barley is tender, about 35 to 40 minutes. Remove from heat and let stand, covered, for 5 minutes.
1 cup pearl barley	
2 cups low-sodium chicken broth	
1 zucchini, cut into ½-inch cubes	*4* While the barley is cooking, heat 2 teaspoons of the oil in a medium skillet over medium-high heat. Add the remainder of the onions, and cook until they're soft, about 2 minutes. Add the zucchini and mushrooms, and cook until the vegetables are soft, about 8 minutes, stirring frequently.
¾ cup sliced shiitake or cremini mushrooms	
1 cup cherry tomatoes, halved	
1 tablespoon lime juice	*5* After the barley has stood for 5 minutes, add the vegetable mixture to the barley and mix well. Add the tomatoes, lime juice, and fresh basil, and mix until well blended. Serve.
½ cup chopped fresh basil	

Per serving: Calories 127 (From Fat 24); Glycemic Load 10 (Low); Fat 3g (Saturated 1g); Cholesterol 1mg; Sodium 106mg; Carbohydrate 23g (Dietary Fiber 5g); Protein 4g.

Vary It! Feel free to replace the chicken broth with vegetable broth if you're looking for a vegetarian recipe.

Basic Polenta

Prep time: 5 min • **Cook time:** 35 min • **Yield:** 8 servings

Ingredients	Directions
7 cups water 2½ teaspoons salt 1⅔ cups coarse yellow cornmeal	**1** In a small stockpot, bring the water to a boil over medium-high heat. Add the salt, and slowly whisk in the cornmeal. As you add the cornmeal, continue to whisk.
	2 Reduce the heat to medium-low, and stir continuously until the mixture becomes thick, forms a mass, and pulls away from the pan, about 35 minutes.
	3 If you're cooking a meal with the polenta, serve promptly. To store it for use later in the week, spread the polenta about 1 to 2 inches thick on a nonstick baking sheet; cool completely. Cut the polenta into 2-x-2-inch squares (approximately half a cup of polenta per square), and store in the refrigerator.

Per serving: Calories 129 (From Fat 4); Glycemic Load 9 (Low); Fat 0g (Saturated 0g); Cholesterol 0mg; Sodium 727mg; Carbohydrate 28g (Dietary Fiber 0g); Protein 3g.

Note: Polenta isn't too difficult to make, but it does take some time — and gives your arm a workout since you have to stir for about 30 minutes!

Vary It! Add 2 teaspoons of butter to give your polenta a creamier flavor.

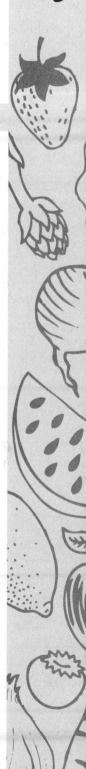

Baked Polenta with Tomatoes

Prep time: 5 min • **Cook time:** 10–15 min • **Yield:** 6 servings

Ingredients	*Directions*
Nonstick cooking spray **Six 1-inch-round slices polenta (½ cup each)** **1 tablespoon extra-virgin olive oil**	*1* Preheat the oven to 400 degrees, and spray a cookie sheet with nonstick cooking spray. Place the polenta slices on the cookie sheet, and brush each slice with about ½ teaspoon of olive oil. Bake the polenta for 5 minutes.
1 heirloom or 2 Roma tomatoes, cut into 6 slices **6 fresh basil leaves**	*2* Remove the polenta from the oven, and layer each slice with 1 tomato slice, 1 basil leaf, and 1 teaspoon of Parmesan.
2 tablespoons grated Parmesan cheese	*3* Bake for an additional 5 to 10 minutes, or until the tomatoes soften and the cheese is melted. Serve warm.

Per serving: Calories 161 (From Fat 29); Glycemic Load 9 (Low); Fat 3g (Saturated 1g); Cholesterol 1mg; Sodium 760mg; Carbohydrate 29g (Dietary Fiber 1g); Protein 4g.

Note: You can use premade polenta you buy at the grocery store or homemade polenta that you make using the Basic Polenta recipe earlier in this chapter.

Baked Polenta with Wild Mushrooms

Prep time: 5 min • **Cook time:** About 15 min • **Yield:** 6 servings

Ingredients	*Directions*
Nonstick cooking spray **Six 1-inch-round slices polenta (½ cup each)** **1 tablespoon extra-virgin olive oil**	*1* Preheat the oven to 400 degrees, and spray a cookie sheet with nonstick cooking spray. Place the polenta slices on the cookie sheet, and brush each slice with about ½ teaspoon of olive oil. Bake for 5 minutes; set aside.
1 cup sliced cremini and shiitake mushrooms **2 tablespoons chopped fresh flat-leaf parsley**	*2* While the polenta is baking, spray a medium nonstick skillet with nonstick cooking spray, and heat over medium-high heat. Add the mushrooms and sauté them until they're soft, about 6 minutes. Stir in the parsley, and heat until it's fragrant and wilted.
2 tablespoons grated Parmesan cheese	*3* Spoon ⅙ of the mushroom mixture onto each polenta slice, and sprinkle each slice with 1 teaspoon of Parmesan cheese. Bake the mushroom-topped polenta for an additional 5 to 10 minutes, or until the cheese softens. Serve warm.

Per serving: *Calories 160 (From Fat 29); Glycemic Load 9 (Low); Fat 3g (Saturated 1g); Cholesterol 1mg; Sodium 759mg; Carbohydrate 29g (Dietary Fiber 1g); Protein 4g.*

Note: You can use premade polenta you buy at the grocery store or homemade polenta that you make using the Basic Polenta recipe earlier in this chapter.

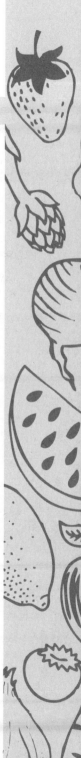

Cheesy Quinoa with Spinach

Prep time: 10 min • **Cook time:** 22–28 min • **Yield:** 6 servings

Ingredients	*Directions*
¼ cup pine nuts	**1** Preheat the oven to 400 degrees. Spread the pine nuts on a cookie sheet, and bake for about 2 minutes; give them a quick stir, and then cook an additional 3 minutes or until lightly browned. Remove the nuts from the oven, place them into a small bowl, and set aside.
1 teaspoon extra-virgin olive oil	
1 shallot, chopped	
1¾ cups vegetable broth	
¼ cup water	**2** In a small skillet, heat the oil over medium heat. Add the shallot, and cook until it's softened, about 2 to 3 minutes. Set aside.
1 cup quinoa, rinsed	
1 cup fresh spinach leaves	**3** In a medium saucepan, bring the broth and water to a boil over medium-high heat. Add the quinoa, turn down the heat to low, and simmer, covered, until the quinoa is tender and the liquid has been absorbed, about 15 to 20 minutes. Remove from heat.
2 teaspoons lemon juice	
¼ cup crumbled goat cheese	
Salt and pepper to taste	
	4 Add the shallot, spinach, lemon juice, and toasted pine nuts to the quinoa, and stir until the spinach is just wilted. Add the goat cheese, and mix until melted. Salt and pepper to taste, and serve immediately.

Per serving: Calories 175 (From Fat 62); Glycemic Load 9 (Low); Fat 7g (Saturated 2g); Cholesterol 4mg; Sodium 214mg; Carbohydrate 23g (Dietary Fiber 3g); Protein 7g.

Quinoa with Veggies and Toasted Pine Nuts

Prep time: 10 min • **Cook time:** About 20 min • **Yield:** 6 servings

Ingredients	*Directions*
⅓ cup pine nuts 2 cups vegetable broth 1 cup quinoa, rinsed 1 tablespoon extra-virgin olive oil 3 cloves garlic, minced 1 red bell pepper, chopped ½ cup diced zucchini ½ cup chopped onion 1 teaspoon dried basil 1 teaspoon dried parsley 1 teaspoon dried oregano Salt and pepper to taste 3 green onions, chopped 6 lemon wedges	**1** Preheat the oven to 400 degrees. Spread the pine nuts on a cookie sheet, and bake for about 2 minutes; give them a quick stir, and then cook an additional 3 minutes or until lightly browned. Remove the nuts from the oven, place them into a small bowl, and set aside. **2** In a medium saucepan, bring the broth to a boil over medium-high heat and add the quinoa. Reduce the heat to medium-low, and simmer, covered, until the quinoa is tender and the liquid is absorbed, about 15 to 20 minutes. **3** While the quinoa is cooking, heat the olive oil in a medium saucepan over medium heat. Stir in the garlic, and cook until the garlic browns, about 30 seconds. **4** Add the red bell pepper, zucchini, and onions to the garlic-oil mixture, and continue cooking over medium heat until the vegetables soften, about 5 minutes. Add the basil, parsley, oregano, and salt and pepper to taste, and cook for 1 more minute. Then stir in the cooked quinoa, green onions, and pine nuts. **5** Divide the quinoa on 6 plates to serve, and squeeze the juice of one lemon wedge onto each serving.

Per serving: Calories 199 (From Fat 72); Glycemic Load 9 (Low); Fat 8g (Saturated 1g); Cholesterol 0mg; Sodium 260mg; Carbohydrate 27g (Dietary Fiber 4g); Protein 7g.

Tip: For the best outcome, chop all the vegetables the same size.

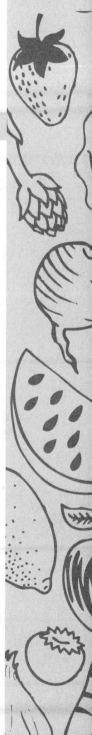

Cooking Pasta Favorites the Low-Glycemic Way

Pasta is one of the toughest foods to incorporate into a low-glycemic diet because most pastas fall into the high-glycemic category. As an Italian, coauthor Meri can't even imagine life without pasta, so, of course, she has discovered more than one way to make pasta work in a low-glycemic meal plan.

Here are just a few tricks for incorporating pasta into a low-glycemic diet:

- ✔ Use low- to medium-glycemic pastas like whole-wheat spaghetti, tortellini, and vermicelli in place of some of the higher-glycemic choices like penne, linguini, and fusilli.

- ✔ Add vegetables and lean protein sources to your pasta so you eat less pasta per serving.

- ✔ Enjoy high-glycemic pasta in moderation while balancing out the rest of your day with low-glycemic food choices.

When you're ready to give these tricks a try, check out the recipes in this section. They show you how to use lower-glycemic pasta in your meals and which foods to add to your pasta so you eat less per serving.

Fresh Spinach and Tomato Tortellini Salad

Prep time: 5 min • **Cook time:** About 12 min • **Yield:** 6 servings

Ingredients	*Directions*
One 9-ounce package cheese tortellini 1 cup fresh spinach 2 Roma tomatoes, chopped One 4-ounce can sliced black olives, drained ½ cup artichoke hearts, drained and chopped 1 tablespoon grated Parmesan cheese ¼ cup lowfat Italian salad dressing	*1* In a medium saucepan, cook the tortellini according to the package directions. After you cook the tortellini, use a colander to drain the water out, and place the tortellini in a medium serving bowl. *2* Add the spinach to the tortellini while the pasta is hot, and stir until the spinach is wilted. Mix in the tomatoes, black olives, artichoke hearts, and Parmesan. *3* Add the Italian dressing, and toss the salad to coat everything evenly. Either serve the salad warm immediately, or refrigerate it to serve it cold later.

Per serving: Calories 146 (From Fat 55); Glycemic Load 12 (Medium); Fat 6g (Saturated 2g); Cholesterol 7mg; Sodium 475mg; Carbohydrate 19g (Dietary Fiber 3g); Protein 6g.

Tip: This salad (which is shown in the color section) is great warm, but it works well cold, too, if you prefer cold pasta salads.

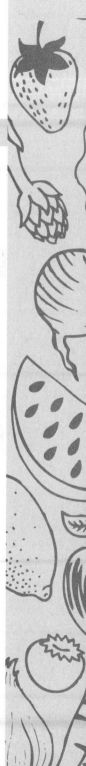

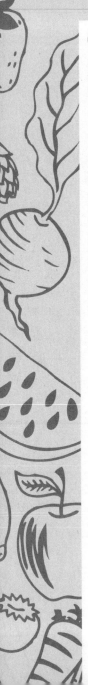

Summer Pasta Salad

Prep time: 10 min • **Cook time:** About 10 min • **Yield:** 8 servings

Ingredients	*Directions*
6 quarts of water One 16-ounce package whole-wheat or regular spaghetti	*1* In a large saucepan, bring the water to a boil over medium-high heat. Add the spaghetti, reduce the heat to low, and cook the pasta until it's tender, about 8 to 10 minutes. Drain and set aside.
1 cup broccoli florets 1 cup cherry tomatoes, halved 1 large orange or yellow bell pepper, chopped	*2* While the pasta is cooking, steam the broccoli in a separate pan until it's just tender, about 5 minutes. Set aside.
½ cup chopped onion ¼ cup chopped fresh basil Italian-style lowfat salad dressing to taste	*3* In a large bowl, combine the spaghetti, broccoli, tomatoes, bell pepper, onion, and basil. Stir in about ¼ cup of the salad dressing, gradually adding more to taste until everything's well coated. Either serve warm or refrigerate and serve cold later.

Per serving: Calories 244 (From Fat 41); Glycemic Load 18 (Medium); Fat 5g (Saturated 1g); Cholesterol 0mg; Sodium 130mg; Carbohydrate 46g (Dietary Fiber 8g); Protein 9g.

Pasta with Sun-Dried Tomatoes and Olives

Prep time: 5 min • **Cook time:** 36 min • **Yield:** 6 servings

Ingredients	Directions
1 tablespoon extra-virgin olive oil	**1** In a medium saucepan, heat the oil over medium heat. Break the vermicelli in half and add it to the pan, tossing it in the oil until it's golden brown in color, about 3 minutes. Remove the vermicelli from the pan; set aside.
8 ounces vermicelli	
½ cup chopped onion	
2 cloves garlic, minced	**2** Add the onion and garlic to the same saucepan you used to cook the vermicelli, and cook them until they're softened, about 3 minutes.
½ cup sun-dried tomatoes, packaged in oil, drained and chopped	
¼ cup kalamata olives, pitted and halved	**3** Add the sun-dried tomatoes, olives, and broth, and bring to a boil over medium-high heat. Add the vermicelli to the boiling broth mixture, reduce the heat to low, cover, and simmer until the pasta has soaked up the liquid, about 30 minutes. Serve warm.
2 cups low-sodium chicken broth	

Per serving: Calories 208 (From Fat 53); Glycemic Load 18 (Medium); Fat 6g (Saturated 1g); Cholesterol 1mg; Sodium 144mg; Carbohydrate 33g (Dietary Fiber 2g); Protein 7g.

Tip: Add some chicken to this dish and you have a complete meal!

Tip: Keep your eye on the broth level. You may need to add ½ cup more if it gets too low and the pasta starts to stick.

Vary It! If you're looking for a vegetarian pasta side, use vegetable broth in place of the chicken broth.

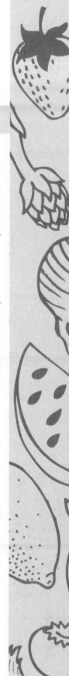

Spaghetti with Roasted Tomatoes and Bell Peppers

Prep time: 5 min • **Cook time:** 23–30 min • **Yield:** 8 servings

Ingredients	*Directions*
1 tablespoon extra-virgin olive oil	*1* Preheat the oven to 425 degrees.
3 cloves garlic, minced 6 Roma tomatoes, halved lengthwise 1 orange or yellow bell pepper, seeded, cored, and sliced julienne style 1 large onion, cut into 1-inch wedges Salt and pepper to taste	*2* In a medium bowl, toss the oil with the garlic, tomatoes, bell peppers, and onions; season them with salt and pepper to taste. Place the vegetables on a nonstick cookie sheet and bake for about 10 minutes; then remove the garlic and bake the vegetables for an additional 5 to 10 minutes until browned, turning occasionally.
6 quarts of water	*3* Remove the vegetables from the oven and allow to cool. Coarsely chop the tomatoes, and toss them in a large bowl with the onions, peppers, and garlic to mix everything together.
12 ounces spaghetti 2 tablespoons grated Parmesan cheese ½ cup coarsely chopped fresh basil	*4* Boil the water and cook the spaghetti until tender, about 8 to 10 minutes. Reserve ¼ cup of the water, and drain the rest. Mix together the reserved water, the vegetable mixture, the Parmesan, and the basil. Toss with the spaghetti and serve warm.

Per serving: Calories 189 (From Fat 27); Glycemic Load 18 (Medium); Fat 3g (Saturated 1g); Cholesterol 1mg; Sodium 102mg; Carbohydrate 34g (Dietary Fiber 3g); Protein 6g.

Vary It! We use tomatoes, bell peppers, and onions in this recipe, but you can play around with other veggies like broccoli or green beans, too.

Creating Low-Glycemic Potato Dishes (Seriously!)

So you've looked at the glycemic load list in Appendix A and noticed that baked potatoes tend to be among the forbidden foods when you're trying to maintain a low-glycemic diet. Does that mean you can't ever eat a potato again? Of course not! Although russet potatoes have one of the highest glycemic loads of any plant-based food, potatoes in general are also loaded with healthy nutrients like fiber and vitamin C. Like pasta, you just need to know how to eat your potatoes to make them a little lower in the glycemic department.

By using medium-glycemic potatoes like *new potatoes* (the little red, white, and purple thin-skinned varieties you see in the stores) in place of russet potatoes or by reducing the number of potatoes in your dish and increasing the number of other ingredients, you can smile while you enjoy your low-glycemic lifestyle *and* eat potatoes. Check out the recipes in this section for inspiration.

Roasted Sweet Potatoes

Prep time: 10 min • **Cook time:** 25 min • **Yield:** 6–8 servings

Ingredients	Directions
4 sweet potatoes, peeled and sliced into ½-inch slices	**1** Preheat the oven to 400 degrees.
2 tablespoons extra-virgin olive oil Salt to taste	**2** Place the potatoes in a 9-x-11-inch glass baking dish. Drizzle the potatoes with the olive oil, and salt them to taste.
	3 Bake the potatoes for 25 minutes, or until golden and tender, turning them over after 10 minutes so they cook evenly. Serve warm.

Per serving: Calories 148 (From Fat 62); Glycemic Load 10 (Low); Fat 5g (Saturated 1g); Cholesterol 0mg; Sodium 43mg; Carbohydrate 29g (Dietary Fiber 4g); Protein 2g.

Roasted Red-Skinned Potatoes with Shallots

Prep time: 10 min • **Cook time:** 45 min • **Yield:** 5 servings

Ingredients	*Directions*
1 tablespoon butter 1 tablespoon extra-virgin olive oil 1 teaspoon chopped fresh rosemary	*1* Preheat the oven to 350 degrees. In a small saucepan, melt the butter over medium heat, and stir in the olive oil and rosemary.
1½ pounds red new potatoes (larger sized), peeled and cut into quarters	*2* Place the potatoes in a large baking dish, and pour the butter mixture over them; toss to coat the potatoes evenly.
8 shallots, peeled and halved	*3* Add the shallots to the baking dish, and cook for 45 minutes, or until a fork pierces through the potato easily, stirring after about 20 minutes so they brown evenly. Serve warm.

Per serving: Calories 188 (From Fat 47); Glycemic Load 18 (Medium); Fat 5g (Saturated 2g); Cholesterol 6mg; Sodium 15mg; Carbohydrate 32g (Dietary Fiber 3g); Protein 4g.

Tip: Try out this recipe when you're looking for something yummy and easy to have for dinner; it goes well with almost any meal.

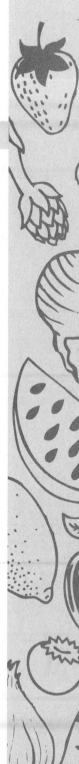

Potato and Squash Gratin

Prep time: 20 min • **Cook time:** About 1 hr, plus standing time • **Yield:** 6 servings

Ingredients	Directions
2 teaspoons chopped fresh thyme	*1* Preheat the oven to 375 degrees. In a small bowl, combine the thyme and rosemary. Set aside.
2 teaspoons fresh rosemary, stems removed, chopped	
Nonstick cooking spray	*2* Spray a 9-x-13-inch glass baking dish with nonstick cooking spray. Place the squash, potatoes, and onions in the baking dish, and mix well. Sprinkle the veggies with the thyme and rosemary, and toss to coat evenly. Add salt and pepper to taste.
1 butternut squash, peeled and sliced into ½-inch cubes	
4 large new potatoes, peeled and cut into ½-inch round slices	
1 medium onion, finely chopped	*3* Firmly press down on the squash and potatoes with a large spatula to evenly disperse them in the pan. Slowly pour the half-and-half over the top and down the sides of the dish, adding just enough to barely cover the vegetables so that you still see just their tops — you may need less than 2 cups.
Salt and pepper to taste	
2 cups fat-free half-and-half	
⅓ cup coarsely grated Jarlsberg or Emmentaler cheese	*4* Cover the baking dish with foil, and bake for 45 to 50 minutes. Remove the foil, and sprinkle with the cheese. Continue to bake, uncovered, for 10 to 20 more minutes, or until the vegetables are tender, the cream is nearly absorbed, and the top is lightly browned.
	5 Let the veggies au gratin stand for about 10 minutes before serving.

Per serving: Calories 278 (From Fat 18); Glycemic Load 18 (Medium); Fat 2g (Saturated 1g); Cholesterol 4mg; Sodium 211mg; Carbohydrate 54g (Dietary Fiber 6g); Protein 9g.

Vary It! We like to use white potatoes in this recipe, but any new variety will work fine.

Vary It! If you can't find either Jarlsberg or Emmentaler cheese, you can use a basic Swiss.

Part IV
Making Memorable Main Dishes and Desserts

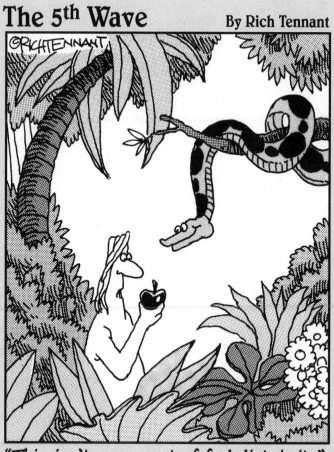

The 5th Wave   By Rich Tennant

"This isn't some sort of fad diet, is it?"

In this part . . .

The nice thing about following a low-glycemic diet is that no protein sources are off-limits because they don't contain — or contain very few — carbohydrates, but we encourage you to stick to what you know about low-fat cooking techniques and use lean, lower-fat meats in your main dishes. In this part, you find new and tasty ways to prepare poultry, beef, pork, and seafood in everyday entrées as well as those you can serve to guests. We also show you how to use low-glycemic ingredients to make flavorful vegetarian entrées.

Let's not forget about dessert! In this part, we include recipes for treats that are low- to medium-glycemic and also lower in fat and calories than typical desserts, showing you that you can satisfy your sweet tooth without ruining your progress toward your health goals.

Chapter 15

Poultry Dishes That'll Make People Flock to Your Table

Skinless, white-meat poultry is a great source of lean protein with minimal fat, and it works well in a low-glycemic diet. However, cooking chicken breasts can be a little boring and bland. Baking a plain, lightly seasoned chicken breast may be okay once in a while, but we're sure you sometimes wish for more flavor and variety. Over the years, we've heard many clients complain that they know they should eat more chicken but that it can just be so tasteless and dry. Well, it's time to break out of that rut — this chapter celebrates variety and taste with chicken!

So you want to add more turkey to your diet to break up the monotony of chicken or whatever else you eat, but you can't seem to do so without having to make an entire Thanksgiving meal. To help keep your meals simple (and delicious, of course), you can use turkey cutlets, tenderloins, or just the breast in place of a whole turkey.

With so many ways to cook poultry — including grilling, sautéing, stir-frying, and baking — the only thing you need to decide is what seasonings and spices you want to add tonight! You can eat poultry four nights a week and still have completely different types of meals like Mexican, French, Italian, and Asian. This chapter explores many ways to cook up chicken and turkey in new and tasty ways that'll keep your family asking for more!

Poultry does come with a risk of food-borne illness from a bacteria called *salmonella,* so you want to make sure it's completely cooked before you eat it. Although you can look to see whether the juices run clear as an indicator, the best way to know for certain whether your meat is cooked is to use a meat thermometer. Place it in the thickest part of your poultry, without hitting any bones, and look for a reading of 165 degrees Fahrenheit. Then you know it's done!

Grilling Chicken for a Quick and Tasty Meal

Grilling chicken is a simple way to create a low-glycemic meal with a lot of flavor, and it's perfect for serving guests on a nice summer day. Plus, cleanup's a snap! One of the biggest problems with grilled chicken, however, is that it can dry out fast if you don't use enough moisture. Although you can easily slather your favorite barbeque sauce on a few chicken breasts and grill them, you may want to experiment with some different marinades and rubs for a bit of variety. This section shows you a couple of ways to grill up some very flavorful chicken as alternatives to basic barbeque sauce.

Prepare your grill by cleaning it with a grill brush and spraying with nonstick cooking spray prior to heating to avoid any dangerous flames.

Garlic and Lime Grilled Chicken

Prep time: 10 min, plus refrigerating time • **Cook time:** 12 min • **Yield:** 4 servings

Ingredients	*Directions*
¼ cup low-sodium soy sauce 2 tablespoons lime juice 1 tablespoon honey ¼ cup onion, minced 2 medium cloves garlic, minced	*1* In an 8-x-8-inch glass baking dish, whisk together the soy sauce, lime juice, honey, onion, garlic, and ginger. Add the chicken, cover it, and refrigerate the dish for 2 hours, turning the chicken over after 1 hour.
1 teaspoon ground ginger 4 boneless, skinless chicken breast halves Nonstick cooking spray	*2* Spray the grill with nonstick cooking spray, and heat it to medium. *3* Place the chicken on the grill, discarding the extra marinade. Grill until it's cooked through, about 6 minutes on each side.

Per serving: Calories 138 (From Fat 24); Glycemic Load 4 (Low); Fat 3g (Saturated 1g); Cholesterol 63mg; Sodium 357mg; Carbohydrate 3g (Dietary Fiber 0g); Protein 24g.

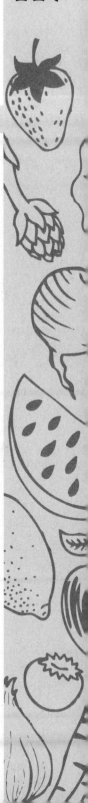

Grilled Jerk Chicken

Prep time: 10 min, plus refrigerating time • **Cook time:** 12 min • **Yield:** 4 servings

Ingredients	*Directions*
3 scallions, chopped	*1* Blend the scallions, garlic, onions, chiles, lime juice, Worcestershire sauce, olive oil, brown sugar, thyme, coriander, nutmeg, allspice, salt, black pepper, and cinnamon in a blender until smooth. (If you need help with seeding a hot pepper before you start blending, check out Figure 15-1; make sure to wear gloves!)
4 large cloves garlic	
1 small onion, chopped	
2 to 4 serrano chiles, stemmed and seeded	
¼ cup lime juice	*2* Divide the chicken and marinade between 2 sealable plastic bags. Seal the bags, pressing out the excess air; turn the bags over several times to cover the chicken evenly with the marinade. Put the bags of chicken in a shallow pan and refrigerate for 8 to 9 hours, turning the bags over once or twice.
2 tablespoons Worcestershire sauce	
3 tablespoons extra-virgin olive oil	
1 tablespoon packed brown sugar	*3* Remove the chicken from the bag and discard the marinade.
1 teaspoon dried thyme	
1 teaspoon ground coriander	*4* Spray the grill with nonstick cooking spray; then heat it to medium. Grill the chicken until it's cooked through, about 6 minutes on each side. Serve warm.
¼ teaspoon ground nutmeg	
2 teaspoons ground allspice	
½ teaspoon salt	
1 teaspoon black pepper	
1 teaspoon ground cinnamon	
4 boneless, skinless chicken breast halves, cut crosswise	
Nonstick cooking spray	

Per serving: Calories 174 (From Fat 56); Glycemic Load 2 (Low); Fat 6g (Saturated 1g); Cholesterol 63mg; Sodium 172mg; Carbohydrate 6g (Dietary Fiber 1g); Protein 23g.

Tip: If you have a milder palate, use fewer chiles.

Vary It! If you want more spice, you can replace the serrano chiles with jalapeño chiles.

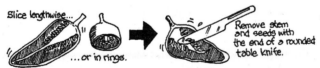

Figure 15-1:
Seeding a
hot pepper.

Seeding a Hot Pepper

Slice lengthwise...

...or in rings.

Remove stem
and seeds with
the end of a rounded
table knife.

CAREFUL!
Always wear gloves
when you handle
hot peppers!

Mixing Up Sautés and Stir-Fries

What we love about sautéing and stir-frying is that you can add so many
ingredients and flavors to your meal with just a little time and prep work.
Sautéing is the ideal way to sear or brown foods significantly to bring out
their flavors. It's also a great way to cook when you don't have a lot of time.
Stir-frying is using high heat and a small amount of oil while stirring your
ingredients continuously until cooked. The faster cooking and constant stirring make it a bit different from sautéing. All you need for these techniques is
a good sauté pan or wok and a little oil. The following recipes show you how
to incorporate low-glycemic ingredients to make fast, tasty meals on your
stove top.

Lemon Chicken

Prep time: 5 min   •   **Cook time:** 9–14 min   •   **Yield:** 4 servings

Ingredients	*Directions*
2 teaspoons canola oil	*1* In a large nonstick skillet, heat the canola oil over high heat. Sprinkle the chicken breast halves with salt and pepper to taste.
4 boneless, skinless chicken breast halves	
Salt and pepper to taste	
1 cup chicken broth	*2* Add the chicken breast halves to the hot pan, and cook them until browned, about 2 minutes on each side (the chicken isn't cooked through at this point).
1 tablespoon lemon juice	
½ teaspoon lemon zest	*3* Turn the heat down to medium-high, and stir in the chicken broth, lemon juice, lemon zest, garlic, and butter. Simmer until the chicken is cooked through, about 5 to 10 minutes. Serve warm.
2 medium cloves garlic, minced	
1 teaspoon butter	

Per serving: Calories 164 (From Fat 62); Glycemic Load 0 (Low); Fat 7g (Saturated 2g); Cholesterol 67mg; Sodium 450mg; Carbohydrate 1g (Dietary Fiber 0g); Protein 23g.

Tip: Lemon chicken is a great recipe to have on hand because it's so versatile. You can eat the chicken as it is, or you can cook it in batches and use some of it later in the week on salads or in a light pasta dish with Italian-style dressing.

Chicken Caesar Wraps

Prep time: 13–15 min • **Cook time:** 10–12 min • **Yield:** 8 servings

Ingredients	*Directions*
4 boneless, skinless chicken breast halves 2 teaspoons extra-virgin olive oil Salt and pepper to taste 1 tablespoon canola oil Eight 6-inch low-carb or whole-wheat wraps 1 cup coarsely chopped romaine lettuce 1 cup chopped Roma tomatoes 3 green onions, chopped 8 tablespoons lowfat Caesar salad dressing	*1* Brush the chicken with olive oil, and sprinkle it with salt and pepper to taste. Heat the canola oil in a large nonstick pan over medium heat. Cook the chicken until it's cooked through, about 10 to 12 minutes, turning the chicken after 5 minutes. *2* Remove the chicken from the pan, transfer it to a clean cutting board, and let it cool for 3 to 5 minutes. Slice the chicken into thin, ¼-inch strips. *3* Place each wrap on a small plate. Top each wrap with ⅛ of the chicken, chopped lettuce, tomatoes, and onions. Drizzle each serving with 1 tablespoon of Caesar dressing. *4* Roll up each wrap, folding up from the bottom and then folding over one side and then the other to tuck in the wrap.

Per serving: Calories 210 (From Fat 67); Glycemic Load 12 (Medium); Fat 8g (Saturated 1g); Cholesterol 32mg; Sodium 380mg; Carbohydrate 17g (Dietary Fiber 9g); Protein 19g.

Vary It! If you're running short on time, just use leftover grilled chicken in this recipe.

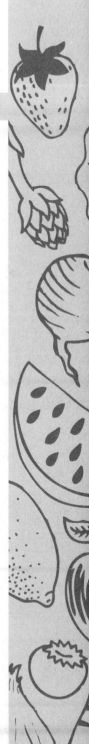

Ginger Chicken and Broccoli Stir-Fry

Prep time: 10 min, plus refrigerating time • **Cook time:** 8 min • **Yield:** 4 servings

Ingredients	Directions
¼ cup low-sodium soy sauce	*1* In a large bowl, whisk together the soy sauce, sherry, honey, garlic, ginger, and orange zest. Add the chicken, and toss to coat evenly. Cover the bowl and refrigerate for 2 hours, turning the chicken over after 1 hour.
¼ cup dry sherry or white wine	
1 tablespoon honey	
2 medium cloves garlic, minced	*2* Boil the broccoli in a large pot of water for 2 minutes; drain. Rinse the broccoli under cold water to stop its cooking, and drain well. Set aside.
1 teaspoon ground ginger	
1 teaspoon grated orange zest	*3* Heat the oil in a large, heavy wok or skillet over high heat. Drain the chicken well, keeping the leftover marinade for later.
4 boneless, skinless chicken breast halves cut diagonally into thin strips	
1 large head broccoli, cut into florets	*4* Add the chicken to the wok, and stir-fry it until almost cooked through, about 2 minutes. Add the broccoli and stir-fry the mixture until the broccoli is still crisp but tender enough to pierce with a fork, about 2 minutes.
1 tablespoon canola oil	
2 cups cooked brown rice or cooked quinoa	*5* Add the reserved marinade mixture to the skillet, and boil until the sauce thickens, about 2 minutes, stirring constantly and coating the chicken and broccoli evenly. Serve the chicken-broccoli mixture over half a cup of brown rice or quinoa per serving, and add salt and pepper to taste.
Salt and pepper to taste	

Per serving: Calories 312 (From Fat 66); Glycemic Load 14 (Medium); Fat 7g (Saturated 1g); Cholesterol 63mg; Sodium 830mg; Carbohydrate 33g (Dietary Fiber 4g); Protein 29g.

Vary It! You can always switch up this recipe by replacing the broccoli with 2 cups of sliced zucchini.

Garlic Chicken and Vegetables over Polenta Cakes

Prep time: 15 min • **Cook time:** 19–23 min • **Yield:** 4 servings

Ingredients	Directions
2 teaspoons extra-virgin olive oil 3 boneless, skinless chicken breast halves, cut into 1-inch chunks Salt to taste 1 large orange or yellow bell pepper, seeded and cut into 2- to 3-inch strips 1 sweet onion, cut into thin strips 3 medium cloves garlic, minced 1 cup zucchini, sliced diagonally in ¼-inch slices 1 cup yellow squash, sliced diagonally in ¼-inch slices ¼ teaspoon dried parsley ¼ teaspoon black pepper ¼ cup chopped fresh basil 2 tablespoons balsamic vinegar ½ cup sun-dried tomatoes, packed in oil, drained and sliced Eight ½-inch rounds of precooked polenta	**1** Heat the oil in a nonstick wok over medium heat. Add the chicken, salt to taste, and stir-fry until the chicken is cooked through, about 10 to 12 minutes. Remove chicken from the pan and set aside. **2** Add the bell pepper and onion, and stir-fry for 3 to 4 minutes. Add the garlic, and stir-fry for 1 minute. (If you need help seeding the bell peppers, refer to Figure 15-1.) **3** Add the zucchini, yellow squash, parsley, and black pepper. Stir-fry so the vegetables stay crisp, about 4 minutes. Remove from the heat, add the basil, vinegar, and sun-dried tomatoes, and toss to coat everything evenly. **4** Meanwhile, microwave the polenta rounds in a covered container for 1 to 2 minutes, or until hot throughout. Place 2 polenta rounds on each plate, and top them with the stir-fried chicken and vegetables.

Per serving: Calories 240 (From Fat 61); Glycemic Load 11 (Medium); Fat 7g (Saturated 1g); Cholesterol 55mg; Sodium 412mg; Carbohydrate 22g (Dietary Fiber 3g); Protein 23g.

Vary It! We use bell peppers, zucchini, and squash, but you can use whatever fresh veggies you have on hand to mix it up a bit.

Tip: You can buy precooked polenta or cook your own from scratch — see Chapter 14 for a recipe.

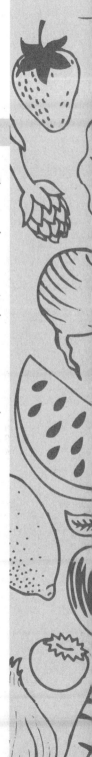

Sautéed Chicken with Tomatoes and Olives

Prep time: 15 min • **Cook time:** 30 min • **Yield:** 6 servings

Ingredients	*Directions*
1 tablespoon canola oil 4 chicken breasts, each cut lengthwise into three pieces Salt and pepper to taste	**1** In a large skillet, heat the oil over medium-high heat. Add the chicken pieces, salt and pepper to taste, and brown the chicken, about 3 minutes on each side. Remove the chicken from the pan, and set aside.
1 cup chopped onion 2 medium cloves garlic, minced	**2** Add the onions to the hot skillet and sauté until soft, about 3 minutes. Add the garlic, and sauté for 1 minute.
One 15-ounce can diced, peeled tomatoes with juices One 14½-ounce can low-sodium chicken broth ½ cup dry white wine 2 teaspoons dried thyme 1 bay leaf	**3** Add the tomatoes, broth, wine, thyme, bay leaf, and chicken. Bring to a boil; turn down the heat to low, and simmer for about 15 minutes.
½ cup kalamata olives, pitted and halved ½ cup canned artichoke hearts, drained and cut in half ½ cup sliced fresh basil 3 cups cooked regular or whole-wheat spaghetti	**4** Add the olives, artichoke hearts, and basil, and cook for another 5 minutes. Serve over half a cup of cooked spaghetti per serving.

Per serving: Calories 287 (From Fat 77); Glycemic Load 14 (Medium); Fat 8g (Saturated 2g); Cholesterol 45mg; Sodium 539mg; Carbohydrate 30g (Dietary Fiber 4g); Protein 23g.

Tip: Using whole-wheat spaghetti lowers your glycemic load to 8.

Reinventing Baked Chicken

If you're looking for some new (and low-glycemic!) ways to bake chicken, you've come to the right place. Instead of settling on the plain old piece of chicken breast baked with a little salt and pepper, try exploring the variety of flavors we offer you in the following recipes. Depending on the spices you add, you can create several different kinds of easy, oven-friendly chicken entrees.

Baked Chicken with Herbes de Provence

Prep time: 5 min • **Cook time:** 35–45 min • **Yield:** 4 servings

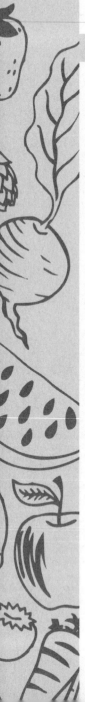

Ingredients	Directions
Nonstick cooking spray 8 bone-in chicken thighs, skin removed 2½ tablespoons herbes de Provence 2 tablespoons extra-virgin olive oil 1 lemon, sliced	**1** Preheat the oven to 350 degrees. Spray a 9-x-13-inch glass baking dish with nonstick cooking spray.
	2 Rinse the chicken thighs under cold water and place them in the bottom of the baking dish. Sprinkle the chicken with the herbes de Provence, and drizzle the olive oil on top.
	3 Arrange the lemon slices over the chicken thighs and bake in the oven until the chicken is lightly browned and cooked through, about 35 to 45 minutes. Serve warm.

Per serving: Calories 283 (From Fat 163); Glycemic Load 0 (Low); Fat 18g (Saturated 4g); Cholesterol 99mg; Sodium 93mg; Carbohydrate 2g (Dietary Fiber 1g); Protein 27g.

Note: Herbes de Provence is a wonderful mix of herbs that typically contains savory, fennel, basil, and thyme, with thyme being the dominant flavor. In the United States, you may even find a little lavender added to the mix.

Vary It! You can replace the chicken thighs with chicken breasts to decrease the fat content a little.

Teriyaki Chicken Thighs

Prep time: 5 min • **Cook time:** 45 min • **Yield:** 3 servings

Ingredients	*Directions*
6 bone-in chicken thighs, skins removed	*1* Preheat the oven to 350 degrees. Place the chicken in a bowl with the soy sauce, and mix until well coated. Spray a 9-x-13-inch glass baking dish with nonstick cooking spray, and arrange the chicken thighs in the bottom of the dish.
2 tablespoons low-sodium soy sauce	
Nonstick cooking spray	
½ teaspoon garlic powder	*2* Sprinkle all the chicken pieces with garlic powder and ground ginger. Bake the chicken in the oven until it's crisp and cooked through, about 45 minutes.
1 teaspoon ground ginger	

Per serving: Calories 228 (From Fat 102); Glycemic Load 0 (Low); Fat 11g (Saturated 3g); Cholesterol 99mg; Sodium 495mg; Carbohydrate 1g (Dietary Fiber 0g); Protein 28g.

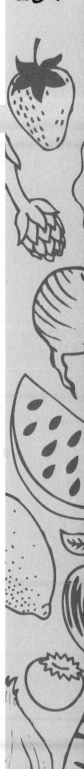

Cooking South-of-the-Border Chicken

Love Mexican food? We do, too. Experimenting with new ways to make some old, spicy favorites such as tacos, enchiladas, and burritos is always fun because you can get pretty inventive with your favorite ingredients. This section offers a few south-of-the-border standards with a new, low-glycemic twist!

We use rotisserie chicken in a few of the recipes in this section simply as a timesaver. You can also use any leftover baked or grilled chicken you have on hand.

Chicken Tacos with Poblano Chiles

Prep time: 12 min • **Cook time:** 7–8 min • **Yield:** 6 servings

Ingredients	*Directions*
1 tablespoon canola oil 3 medium fresh poblano chiles, seeded and chopped (about 1½ cups)	**1** In a large nonstick skillet, heat the oil over medium-high heat. Add the poblano chiles and sauté until they begin to soften, about 3 minutes. (If you're not sure how to seed the chiles, refer to Figure 15-1.)
1½ pounds boneless, skinless chicken breast halves, cut into ½-inch-thick strips 2 teaspoons ground cumin 1 teaspoon chili powder Salt and pepper to taste	**2** Add the chicken, cumin, and chili powder, and sprinkle with salt and pepper to taste. Sauté until the chicken is almost cooked through, about 2 to 3 minutes. Mix in the taco sauce, and cook for 1 minute.
¾ cup bottled red or green taco sauce 2 cups frozen corn kernels, thawed and patted dry ⅓ cup lowfat sour cream 2 tablespoons fresh chopped cilantro	**3** Stir in the corn and sauté until it's heated through, about 1 minute. Turn the heat down to low, and mix in the sour cream and cilantro until mixed and just heated, making sure the mixture doesn't boil. Remove from heat.
6 soft corn tortillas ¾ cup grated four-cheese Mexican blend or queso fresco One 4-ounce can sliced black olives 2 ripe avocados, peeled, pitted, and sliced thinly	**4** Spoon the chicken mixture in a strip down the center of each tortilla; top each tortilla with 1 tablespoon of cheese, ⅙ of the black olives, and 2 avocado slices.

Per serving: Calories 431 (From Fat 153); Glycemic Load 16 (Medium); Fat 18g (Saturated 6g); Cholesterol 89mg; Sodium 544mg; Carbohydrate 35g (Dietary Fiber 6g); Protein 36g.

Vary it! If you really want more heat to your tacos, add one seeded, chopped jalapeño when you add your poblano chile. You can also use hard corn taco shells with this recipe (which we show in the color section).

Tip: To eliminate some extra calories, simply skip the sour cream.

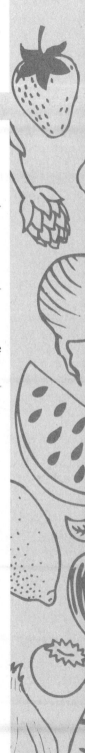

Chicken Chipotle Burritos

Prep time: 15 min • **Cook time:** 4 min • **Yield:** 8 servings

Ingredients	*Directions*
2 teaspoons canola oil	*1* In a large skillet, heat the oil over medium-high heat. Add the shallot and bell pepper and sauté until they start to soften, about 3 minutes. Add the chipotle chile and cumin; stir until well mixed and aromatic, about 1 minute.
1 shallot, chopped	
1 orange or yellow bell pepper, chopped	
1 chipotle chile, canned in adobo sauce, finely chopped	*2* Turn the heat down to medium. Add the tomato paste, broth, shredded chicken, and black beans, and mix well. Remove the chicken mixture from heat.
1 teaspoon ground cumin	
One 6-ounce can tomato paste	
1 cup chicken broth	*3* Heat the tortillas in the microwave oven for 10 seconds.
2 cups precooked rotisserie chicken, white meat, skin removed, shredded	*4* For each tortilla, spread about ¼ cup of the chicken mixture down the center of the tortilla. Add 1 tablespoon of shredded cheese, 1 tablespoon of tomatoes, 1 tablespoon of lettuce, and 1 avocado slice to each tortilla. Roll the tortillas, and serve warm.
One 15-ounce can black beans, rinsed and drained	
Eight 8-inch flour tortillas	
2 cups Monterey Jack cheese, shredded	
½ cup diced tomatoes	
½ cup shredded iceberg lettuce	
1 ripe avocado, peeled, pitted, and sliced	

Per serving: Calories 259 (From Fat 128); Glycemic Load 14 (Medium); Fat 14g (Saturated 6g); Cholesterol 53mg; Sodium 520mg; Carbohydrate 14g (Dietary Fiber 5g); Protein 20g.

Chicken Enchiladas

Prep time: 25 min • **Cook time:** 25 min • **Yield:** 10 servings

Ingredients	*Directions*
1 tablespoon canola oil	*1* In a large skillet, heat the oil over medium-high heat. Add the shallots and bell peppers, and sauté until they begin to soften, about 4 minutes. Add the cumin, chili powder, and oregano, and stir until mixed well, about 30 seconds.
1 shallot, chopped	
1 small green bell pepper, seeded and chopped	
1 teaspoon ground cumin	
½ teaspoon chili powder	*2* Turn the heat down to medium, and add the tomato paste and chicken broth; stir until well blended.
½ teaspoon dried oregano	
3 tablespoons tomato paste	*3* Add the shredded chicken, and mix everything together until well blended; remove the chicken mixture from heat.
⅔ cup chicken broth	
2 cups white meat rotisserie chicken, skin removed, shredded	*4* Pour ½ cup of enchilada sauce in the bottom of a 9-x-13-inch glass baking dish. For each tortilla, spread about 3 tablespoons of the chicken mixture down the center of the tortilla.
One 12-ounce bottle enchilada sauce	
Ten 8-inch flour tortillas	*5* Top each tortilla with 1 tablespoon of grated cheese; roll the tortilla and place it in the baking dish seam side down. Repeat until all the filling and tortillas are used.
1¼ cup grated Mexican four-cheese blend	
10 tablespoons lowfat sour cream	*6* Pour the remainder of the enchilada sauce over the filled enchiladas. Sprinkle the top of the tortillas with the remainder of the cheese.
	7 Bake uncovered for 20 minutes, or until the cheese is melted and the sauce is well heated. Serve 1 enchilada per serving with 1 tablespoon of lowfat sour cream.

Per serving: *Calories 325 (From Fat 116); Glycemic Load 14 (Medium); Fat 13g (Saturated 5g); Cholesterol 40mg; Sodium 639mg; Carbohydrate 36g (Dietary Fiber 2g); Protein 16g.*

Vary It! You can use grated cheddar or Monterey Jack cheese in place of the Mexican four-cheese blend.

Vary It! We like to add a little more spice to enchiladas by using cumin and chili powder, but feel free to omit the spices from this recipe if you want something more traditional.

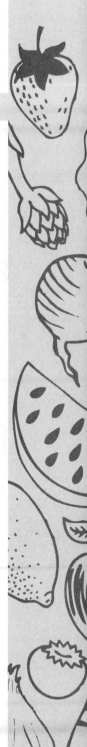

Beyond Thanksgiving: Adding a Twist to Turkey

You may be one of those people who cooks with turkey often, or you may struggle to even think of turkey ideas that don't include a whole roasted turkey. Good news: The breast of turkey is a great lean-protein source and is super tasty! Using turkey cutlets, turkey tenderloins, and ground turkey are our favorite ways to cook this lean meat non-Thanksgiving style. Incorporating turkey into your diet really opens up the door to more lean-meat variety; that way, you don't have to eat chicken every day. Check out the low-glycemic recipes in this section to get started. Our recipes fall into two basic categories:

✔ **Turkey cutlets and tenderloins:** Turkey cutlets are a great alternative to chicken. You can find them easily in most stores and can cook them like chicken cutlets. The *turkey tenderloin* is the small strip of white meat found under the breast and is a very tender cut of poultry. Just like chicken breasts, turkey cutlets and tenderloins are a lean source of protein and provide a delicious flavor.

✔ **Ground turkey:** Ground turkey (including ground turkey breast) is a great alternative to ground beef because it's lower in fat and still has great flavor. However, because turkey is such a lean meat, it can often turn out dry. The trick is to add ingredients like onions and vegetables that release moisture into the meat.

Honey Mustard Turkey Tenderloin

Prep time: 10 min, plus refrigerating time • **Cook time:** About 8 min • **Yield:** 4 servings

Ingredients	*Directions*
1 pound turkey tenderloin	*1* Place the turkey in a sealable plastic bag, and set aside.
1 tablespoon extra-virgin olive oil	
1 tablespoon balsamic vinegar	*2* In a small bowl, combine the oil, vinegar, soy sauce, mustard, rosemary, and marjoram. Pour the oil-vinegar mixture over the turkey, seal the bag, and shake to coat the turkey evenly. Put the turkey in the refrigerator, and let it marinate for 1 to 4 hours, shaking the bag once or twice during that time.
2 tablespoons low-sodium soy sauce	
1 tablespoon honey mustard	
1 tablespoon chopped fresh rosemary	*3* Preheat the oven on the broiler setting, and spray a broiler pan with nonstick cooking spray. Remove the turkey from the marinade, and place it on the rack in the broiler pan.
¼ teaspoon dried marjoram	
Nonstick cooking spray	
	4 Broil the turkey 4 inches from the heat for 3 to 4 minutes on each side, or until the meat is cooked through (thermometer reads 165 degrees) and the juices run clear when you pierce the turkey with a fork. Cook an additional 30 seconds on each side if it still needs browning.
	5 Remove the turkey from the oven, and let it sit for 3 to 5 minutes. Slice and serve.

Per serving: Calories 134 (From Fat 15); Glycemic Load 0 (Low); Fat 2g (Saturated 0g); Cholesterol 74mg; Sodium 125mg; Carbohydrate 1g (Dietary Fiber 0g); Protein 27g.

Vary It! You can trade in the rosemary for fresh sage to change up the flavors a bit.

Tip: If you want only a little flavor, marinate for the shorter amount of time.

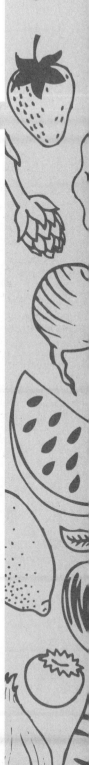

Parmesan Turkey Cutlets

Prep time: 20 min • **Cook time:** About 12 min • **Yield:** 5 servings

Ingredients	Directions
20 ounces turkey cutlets (about 5 cutlets)	**1** Place the turkey cutlets between 2 sheets of plastic wrap; gently pound the cutlets with a flat meat pounder or a rolling pin until they're ¼-inch thick.
1 egg	
2 tablespoons lowfat milk	**2** In a shallow bowl, beat the egg and milk together. In a separate bowl, mix together the salt, pepper, garlic powder, Parmesan cheese, bread crumbs, and parsley.
¼ teaspoon salt plus salt to taste	
¼ teaspoon black pepper plus black pepper to taste	**3** Heat the oil in a 12-inch nonstick skillet over medium-high heat. Working quickly, dip each cutlet in the egg mixture and then in the dry ingredients to coat both sides; add each cutlet to the skillet (2 to 3 at a time), making sure not to crowd them in the skillet so you can easily flip them with a spatula.
¼ teaspoon garlic powder	
½ cup finely grated Parmesan cheese	
½ cup bread crumbs	
2 tablespoons chopped fresh flat-leaf parsley	**4** Cook the cutlets until they're golden and just cooked through, about 4 minutes total, turning them over after about 2 minutes. Add salt and pepper to taste. Serve each cutlet with a lemon wedge.
1 tablespoon extra-virgin olive oil	
5 lemon wedges	

Per serving: Calories 231 (From Fat 58); Glycemic Load 0 (Low); Fat 6g (Saturated 2g); Cholesterol 81mg; Sodium 410mg; Carbohydrate 10g (Dietary Fiber 1g); Protein 32g.

Turkey Burgers

Prep time: 12 min • **Cook time:** 8 min • **Yield:** 4 servings

Ingredients	_Directions_
1 pound lean ground turkey	_1_ In a large bowl, use your hands to mix together the turkey, garlic powder, salt, Worcestershire sauce, salsa, and cilantro until well mixed.
¼ teaspoon garlic powder	
½ teaspoon salt	
1 tablespoon Worcestershire sauce	_2_ Using your hands, roll the turkey mixture into balls and flatten them into four 4-ounce patties. Set aside.
¼ cup chunky black bean and corn salsa	_3_ Spray the grill with nonstick cooking spray; then heat it to high. Cook the burgers until they're completely cooked through (no pink in the middle), about 4 minutes on each side. When you have about 1 minute left on your cooking time, add 1 slice of cheese to the top of each burger.
¼ cup chopped fresh cilantro	
Nonstick cooking spray	
4 slices provolone cheese	
4 whole-wheat hamburger buns	_4_ Serve the burgers on whole-wheat buns with your favorite toppings.
Toppings of your choice	

**Per serving:** Calories 346 (From Fat 92); Glycemic Load 16 (Medium); Fat 10g (Saturated 5g); Cholesterol 94mg; Sodium 928mg; Carbohydrate 25g (Dietary Fiber 3g); Protein 38g.

**Tip:** Add any of your favorite burger toppings like lettuce, tomatoes, and pickles — all are low glycemic, so you're good to go!

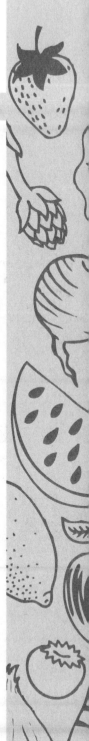

Turkey-Stuffed Peppers with Mozzarella Cheese

Prep time: 15 min • **Cook time:** About 1 hr • **Yield:** 8 servings

Ingredients	Directions
Nonstick cooking spray	**1** Preheat the oven to 350 degrees. Spray a 9-x-13-inch glass baking dish with nonstick cooking spray. Cut a small slice off the bottom of each pepper so it can sit upright, and place the peppers in the dish so that the open sides are up.
8 green bell peppers, tops cut off, cored and seeded	
1 tablespoon extra-virgin olive oil	
1 pound lean ground turkey	**2** Heat the oil in a large skillet with a lid over medium heat. Add the ground turkey, break it into small chunks with a spoon, and cook until it's cooked through, about 8 minutes.
1 medium onion, chopped	
½ cup button mushrooms, sliced	
One 15-ounce can hominy, rinsed and drained	**3** Add the onions and mushrooms, and cook until they're soft, about 4 minutes. Add the hominy, tomatoes, garlic powder, black pepper, thyme, rosemary, and cumin; stir everything together.
4 Roma tomatoes, chopped	
¼ teaspoon garlic powder	
¼ teaspoon black pepper	**4** Pour in the broth, and bring it to a boil. Turn the heat down to low, cover, and simmer for 15 minutes. Stir in the basil until it's wilted.
1½ teaspoons dried thyme	
1½ teaspoons dried rosemary	**5** For each pepper, fill it ⅓ full with the turkey mixture, sprinkle about 2 teaspoons of mozzarella cheese on top, add another layer of the turkey mixture to fill it completely, and top with another 2 teaspoons of cheese.
½ teaspoon ground cumin	
1 cup chicken broth	
¼ cup chopped fresh basil	
1 cup grated mozzarella cheese	**6** Cover the stuffed peppers with aluminum foil, and bake them in the oven until they're softened, about 35 to 40 minutes.

Per serving: Calories 192 (From Fat 57); Glycemic Load 2 (Low); Fat 6g (Saturated 2g); Cholesterol 49mg; Sodium 281mg; Carbohydrate 16g (Dietary Fiber 4g); Protein 19g.

Chapter 16

Adding Variety with Some Healthy Beef and Pork Entrees

In This Chapter

▶ Grilling lean cuts of beef to prepare healthy meals

▶ Creating favorite south-of-the-border beef entrees the healthy way

▶ Bringing burgers back to the table

▶ Preparing healthy pork dishes with a new twist

lthough beef and pork are naturally low glycemic (because they don't contain carbohydrates), they've long been blacklisted from the world of health because of their higher saturated fat contents. The general recommendation in the past few years has been to decrease the amount of beef and pork products you eat, and while that's not a bad idea, for many people, taking away these meats is like taking away their morning coffee!

If you count yourself in this group, don't worry. We're here to show you how to keep beef and pork in your diet and live a low-glycemic and lowfat lifestyle at the same time.

To help you incorporate beef and pork into your diet in a healthy way, follow these tips when planning and preparing your daily meals:

✔ Use leaner cuts of beef and pork (see Chapter 7 for a complete list); some cuts have less fat and fewer calories per serving and can be just as tasty when prepared the right way.

 ✔ Incorporate other ingredients like low-glycemic vegetables and grains (see Chapters 13 and 14 for recipe ideas) into your meals so the amount of beef and pork you eat is less.

 ✔ Balance the higher-fat cuts with lower-fat foods during the day.

We're here to show you that you really can eat beef and pork and maintain a low-glycemic diet. This chapter explores just how to do that with tasty, low-glycemic, lower-fat recipes.

Grilling a Few Healthy Beef Entrees

Good news! Beef can be part of a healthy diet. It is, after all, a great source of protein and iron. You just have to find ways to cut back on the fat content without losing the nutrients. Using lean beef cuts like sirloin and tenderloin is a great way to incorporate beef into your low-glycemic diet. Another great way to go is to find beef products that are completely grass fed so you get even leaner beef cuts. You can find grass-fed beef at your local grocery store.

The risk you take in cooking lean beef, however, is that it may wind up tough and chewy. This section explores some lean cuts of beef and shows you how to add moisture before grilling so you aren't left with a tough cut of meat, but a tasty, juicy entree instead!

When cooking ground beef, you want to cook it completely to a temperature of 160 degrees with no pink in the middle to avoid any risk of e-coli contamination. With steaks, you have a little more leeway and can cook them medium-rare with an internal temperature of 145 degrees or medium at 160 degrees. You can also cook them well-done to 170 degrees, depending on your taste.

Whenever you're grilling, be sure to prepare your grill by cleaning it with a grill brush and spraying with nonstick cooking spray prior to heating it to avoid any dangerous flames.

Grilled Soy-Ginger Sirloin

Prep time: 5 min, plus refrigerating time • **Cook time:** 10 min, plus resting time • **Yield:** 4 servings

Ingredients	*Directions*
4 tablespoons low-sodium soy sauce ¼ cup shallot, minced 1 tablespoon rice wine vinegar 2 tablespoons sesame oil 2 teaspoons light brown sugar 2 teaspoons ground ginger 1 pound top-sirloin steak (about 1-inch thick) Nonstick cooking spray	*1* Combine the soy sauce, shallot, vinegar, sesame oil, brown sugar, and ginger in a shallow dish with a lid. Place the steak in the mixture, cover the dish, and refrigerate it for 2 hours, turning the steak over after 1 hour.
	2 Spray the grill with nonstick cooking spray; then heat it to medium-high. Grill the steak until it reaches the desired doneness, about 5 minutes per side for medium-rare.
	3 Transfer the steak to a cutting board, and let it sit for 3 to 5 minutes. Cut it diagonally into thin slices, and serve.

Per serving: Calories 234 (From Fat 129); Glycemic Load 0 (Low); Fat 14g (Saturated 5g); Cholesterol 74mg; Sodium 203mg; Carbohydrate 1g (Dietary Fiber 0g); Protein 23g.

Tip: If you have leftover sirloin, serve it over a salad of mixed greens the next day!

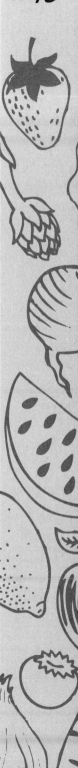

Tenderloin Steaks with Mushroom Sauce

Prep time: 10 min • **Cook time:** About 15 min • **Yield:** 4 servings

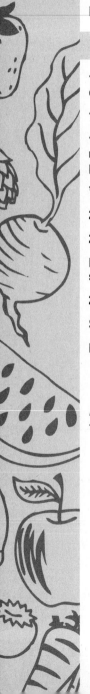

Ingredients	Directions
1 tablespoon extra-virgin olive oil	**1** Heat the oil in a medium skillet over medium heat. Sauté the shallots briefly, until softened. Stir in all the mushrooms, and sauté them until they're tender, about 3 minutes. Pour in the red wine, and simmer for 3 minutes. Stir in the beef broth and tomato paste, and simmer for 6 minutes, or until the sauce has thickened. Remove from the heat.
1 shallot, chopped	
1 pound sliced assorted mushrooms (cremini, portobello, and shiitake)	
½ cup dry red wine	
2 cups beef broth	**2** While the sauce is simmering, pat the steaks dry, and sprinkle each side with the thyme and salt and pepper to taste.
2 tablespoons tomato paste	
Four 5-ounce tenderloin steaks, about ¾-inch thick	**3** Spray the grill with nonstick cooking spray; then heat it to medium-high. Cook the steaks until they reach the desired doneness, about 3 to 5 minutes on each side, depending on thickness, for medium-rare.
2 teaspoons dried thyme	
Salt and pepper to taste	
Nonstick cooking spray	**4** Place the steaks on plates. Top each steak with ¼ of the mushroom sauce.

Per serving: Calories 390 (From Fat 171); Glycemic Load 0 (Low); Fat 19g (Saturated 7g); Cholesterol 118mg; Sodium 482mg; Carbohydrate 5g (Dietary Fiber 1g); Protein 41g.

Marinated Sirloin Steak

Prep time: 5 min, plus refrigerating time • **Cook time:** 6–10 min • **Yield:** 4 servings

Ingredients	*Directions*
2 tablespoons extra-virgin olive oil ¼ cup dry red wine 1 tablespoon Worcestershire sauce 2 tablespoons low-sodium soy sauce 1 tablespoon lemon juice 2 cloves garlic, minced ½ teaspoon dried rosemary ½ teaspoon dried thyme Four 5-ounce sirloin steaks, ¾-inch thick Nonstick cooking spray Salt and pepper to taste	**1** Combine the oil, wine, Worcestershire sauce, soy sauce, lemon juice, garlic, rosemary, and thyme in a 9-x-13-inch pan. Add the steaks, and turn them over to coat them with the marinade. **2** Cover and refrigerate the steaks for 4 to 8 hours, turning them occasionally. **3** Spray the grill with nonstick cooking spray; then heat it to high. Remove the steaks from the refrigerator and discard the marinade. Sprinkle the steaks with salt and pepper to taste, and grill them until they reach the desired doneness, about 3 to 5 minutes on each side for medium-rare. Serve.

Per serving: Calories 199 (From Fat 79); Glycemic Load 0 (Low); Fat 9g (Saturated 3g); Cholesterol 79mg; Sodium 145mg; Carbohydrate 1g (Dietary Fiber 0g); Protein 27g.

Tip: If you like a lot of flavor, marinate your steak for the entire time listed in this recipe; if you like just a hint of flavor, marinate it for 1 to 2 hours instead. Either way, this marinade makes for a very delicious sirloin! Check out this dish in the color section.

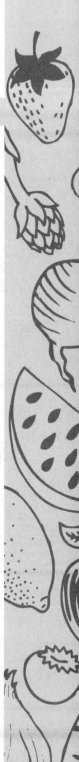

Honey Mustard Beef Skewers

Prep time: 10 min, plus refrigerating time • **Cook time:** 2–3 min, plus resting time • **Yield:** 4 servings

Ingredients	*Directions*
1 pound sirloin steak	*1* Cut the sirloin lengthwise in half, and then cut each half lengthwise in half again. Slice the four strips crosswise to make 1-inch pieces. Thread about 6 to 8 steak pieces onto each skewer by piercing the skewer through the center part of the beef.
1 tablespoon Dijon mustard	
1 tablespoon extra-virgin olive oil	
4 cloves garlic, finely chopped	*2* In a medium bowl, mix together the mustard, oil, garlic, vinegar, soy sauce, honey, thyme, salt, and pepper.
1 tablespoon white-wine vinegar	
1 tablespoon low-sodium soy sauce	*3* Place the skewers in a long baking dish or on a baking sheet, pour half the marinade over them, and turn them to coat all sides of the steak. Cover with plastic wrap and place in the refrigerator for 1 to 2 hours.
1 tablespoon honey	
1 tablespoon finely chopped fresh thyme leaves	
¼ teaspoon salt	*4* Spray the grill with nonstick cooking spray; then heat it to high. Grill the steak skewers until golden brown, slightly charred, and cooked to the desired doneness, about 2 to 3 minutes for medium-rare; turn the skewers over after about 1 minute, brush them with the remaining marinade, and cook for an additional 1 to 2 minutes.
¼ teaspoon black pepper	
Nonstick cooking spray	
	5 Let the skewers sit for 5 minutes after you remove them from the grill. Then place them on plates and serve either hot or at room temperature.

Per serving: Calories 203 (From Fat 85); Glycemic Load 3 (Low); Fat 9g (Saturated 3g); Cholesterol 63mg; Sodium 439mg; Carbohydrate 7g (Dietary Fiber 0g); Protein 22g.

Spicing Up Supper with "Fiesta" Beef

One thing we love about Mexican-inspired entrees is that they're so easy to put together. Plus, you can easily change up the recipes to be spicier by adding some hot peppers, to be tangier by adding some citrus (like lime), or to be more savory by using bolder flavors like cumin.

Following a low-glycemic diet plan is really easy to do with south-of-the-border entrees because they're loaded in low-glycemic ingredients like lean meats, cheese, vegetables, beans, and tortillas. This section explores some new twists on some old favorite recipes — fiesta style!

You'll find many types of ground beef in the grocery store. Go for 90 to 95 percent lean beef to help you lower the saturated fat content and calories.

Beef Tacos

Prep time: 15 min • **Cook time:** 12 min • **Yield:** 8 servings

Ingredients	Directions
1 tablespoon canola oil 1 pound lean ground beef 1 medium onion, chopped 1 jalapeño, seeded and finely chopped 1½ teaspoons ground cumin 2 teaspoons paprika 1 teaspoon salt Eight 8-inch low-carb or whole-wheat flour tortillas ¼ cup lowfat sour cream ½ head iceberg lettuce, shredded ½ cup diced tomatoes ½ cup grated Monterey Jack cheese ¼ cup chopped fresh cilantro (optional) 8 lime wedges	**1** In a large nonstick skillet, heat the oil over medium-high heat. Add the beef, onion, and jalapeño. Cook until the beef is thoroughly browned, about 8 minutes; break up the meat with a spoon as it cooks. **2** Add the cumin, paprika, and salt, and cook until the beef is completely cooked through, about 4 more minutes. **3** Heat the tortillas in the microwave for about 10 seconds. Layer each tortilla with ¼ of the sour cream, lettuce, tomatoes, beef mixture, cheese, and cilantro (if desired); squeeze the lime juice of one wedge on top. Fold each tortilla in half and serve.

Per serving: Calories 267 (From Fat 114); Glycemic Load 16 (Medium); Fat 13g (Saturated 4g); Cholesterol 45mg; Sodium 488mg; Carbohydrate 18g (Dietary Fiber 9g); Protein 21g.

Tip: You can use lowfat cheese to help lower the fat and calories in this meal.

Vary It! While we prefer soft tacos, you can use either soft tortillas or hard shells in this recipe. For hard shells, just layer the meat and toppings from bottom to top before serving.

Mexican Bake

Prep time: 10 min • **Cook time:** 28 min • **Yield:** 6 servings

Ingredients	*Directions*
Nonstick cooking spray **1 teaspoon canola oil**	**1** Preheat the oven to 350 degrees. Spray a 2-quart casserole dish with nonstick cooking spray.
1 small sweet onion, chopped **¾ pound lean ground beef** **Salt and pepper to taste** **1 teaspoon ground cumin** **½ teaspoon chili powder** **½ teaspoon dried oregano**	**2** In a medium skillet, heat the oil over medium-high heat. Add the onion, ground beef, salt, pepper, cumin, chili powder, and oregano. Cook until the beef is browned and cooked through, about 8 minutes, stirring and breaking up the beef with your spoon as it cooks.
One 15-ounce can black beans, drained and rinsed **One 15-ounce can hominy, drained and rinsed** **1 cup plus 1 cup chunky salsa** **One 4-ounce can chopped mild green chile peppers** **2 tablespoons plus 2 tablespoons chopped fresh cilantro**	**3** In a large bowl, combine the beans, hominy, 1 cup of salsa, green chile peppers, and 2 tablespoons of cilantro. Put the bean mixture into the casserole dish. Spoon the ground beef mixture over the bean mixture; then spoon the remaining salsa over the beef. Sprinkle the salsa and beef with the remaining cilantro, and top evenly with the cheese.
1 cup shredded Mexican-blend cheese or mixture of cheddar, Monterey Jack, and colby cheeses	**4** Cover the dish tightly with foil, and bake for 15 minutes. Remove the foil, and bake for 5 more minutes, or until the cheese is melted.

Per serving: Calories 287 (From Fat 115); Glycemic Load 9 (Low); Fat 13g (Saturated 6g); Cholesterol 55mg; Sodium 1,091mg; Carbohydrate 21g (Dietary Fiber 5g); Protein 20g.

Vary It! You can replace the hominy with regular corn. We tend to use hominy because we like the flavor better and it has a lower glycemic load than regular corn.

Tip: You can use spicy or mild salsa to make this recipe fit your tastes.

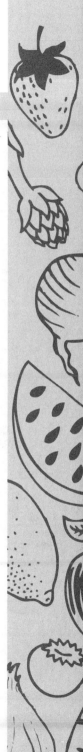

Beef Burritos

Prep time: 15 min • **Cook time:** 28 min • **Yield:** 12 servings

Ingredients	Directions
2 teaspoons canola oil	*1* In a large skillet, heat the oil over medium heat. Cook the ground beef, onion, and garlic until the meat is browned, about 8 minutes; stir the meat often as it cooks to break it up.
¾ pound lean ground beef	
½ cup chopped onion	
1 clove garlic, minced	
½ teaspoon chili powder	*2* Add the chili powder, oregano, cumin, smoked paprika, salt, and pepper; simmer for 10 minutes. Add the black beans and taco sauce. Cover the skillet, turn down the heat to low, and simmer for 10 more minutes.
½ teaspoon dried oregano, crumbled	
1 teaspoon ground cumin	
¼ teaspoon smoked paprika	*3* Heat the tortillas in the microwave for 10 seconds. Spoon about ½ cup of the beef mixture onto each tortilla, and top with about 1 tablespoon of cheese and about 2 tablespoons of tomatoes.
½ teaspoon salt	
¼ teaspoon black pepper	
One 15-ounce can black beans, drained and rinsed	*4* For each burrito, fold over one side of the tortilla, bring the bottom up, and fold over the last side. Serve.
¼ cup red taco sauce	
Twelve 8-inch low-carb or whole-wheat flour tortillas	
1 cup shredded Monterey Jack cheese	
1½ cups diced tomatoes	

Per serving: Calories 215 (From Fat 80); Glycemic Load 18 (Medium); Fat 9g (Saturated 3g); Cholesterol 27mg; Sodium 365mg; Carbohydrate 19g (Dietary Fiber 10g); Protein 17g.

Note: This recipe makes a lot of filling, so it's perfect to have for two nights if you have a smaller family.

Vary It! You can use enchilada sauce in these burritos if you can't find taco sauce. You can also use lowfat cheese to lower the fat and calories.

Beef Enchiladas

Prep time: 25 min • **Cook time:** 32 min • **Yield:** 10 servings

Ingredients	Directions
1 tablespoon canola oil	**1** Preheat the oven to 350 degrees. In a large skillet, heat the oil over medium-high heat. Add the ground beef, shallot, and bell pepper, and cook until the beef is browned, about 8 minutes, stirring often to break up the meat. Drain well.
¾ pound lean ground beef	
1 shallot, chopped	
1 small green bell pepper, seeded and chopped	
1 teaspoon ground cumin	**2** Turn down the heat to medium, and add the cumin, chili powder, oregano, tomato paste, and chicken broth; stir until everything's blended. Cover and simmer until the liquid is absorbed, about 4 minutes.
½ teaspoon chili powder	
½ teaspoon dried oregano	
3 tablespoons tomato paste	**3** Pour ½ cup of the enchilada sauce into the bottom of a 9-x-13-inch glass baking dish. For each tortilla, spread about 3 tablespoons of the meat mixture down the center of the tortilla, add 1 tablespoon of shredded cheese, roll it up, and place it in the baking dish.
⅔ cup chicken broth	
One 12-ounce bottle enchilada sauce	
Ten 8-inch low-carb or whole-wheat flour tortillas	
1¼ cups grated Mexican-blend cheese	**4** Pour the remainder of the enchilada sauce over the filled tortillas. Sprinkle the top of the enchiladas with the remainder of the cheese and the sliced olives.
One 2.25-ounce can sliced black olives, drained	
	5 Bake uncovered in the oven for 20 minutes, or until the cheese is melted and the sauce is well heated. Serve one enchilada per serving.

Per serving: *Calories 245 (From Fat 119); Glycemic Load 14 (Medium); Fat 13g (Saturated 4g); Cholesterol 38mg; Sodium 290mg; Carbohydrate 17g (Dietary Fiber 9g); Protein 16g.*

Vary It! If you like, you can use grated cheddar or Monterey Jack cheese in place of the Mexican blend. You can also substitute lowfat cheese to lower the fat and calories.

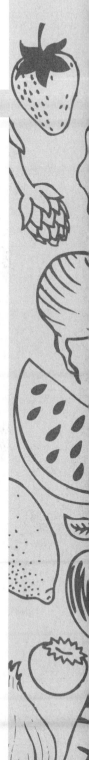

Satisfying Your Burger Craving the Low-Glycemic Way

Who doesn't love a good hamburger? Although a plain old burger with just a little salt and pepper sounds good once in a while, sometimes you may want to punch it up a notch. Burgers are a fun entree to make when you're feeling adventurous because they offer so many ways to experiment with flavor.

In general, burgers are low glycemic, and by using lean beef, you can lower the saturated fat content. (As we note in the previous section, you want to look for ground beef that is 90 to 95 percent lean with only 5 to 10 percent fat content.) The bun raises your glycemic index a bit, but you can keep it under control by using small- to medium-sized, whole-wheat buns. Avoiding the huge-sized buns is the key to keeping your glycemic load down for your meal.

This section offers you a few new ideas when you're in the mood for a little more flavor with your burgers.

Use a meat thermometer to see whether a burger is cooked through, as shown in Figure 16-1. Use an instant-read thermometer to make sure your burger is cooked to 160 degrees.

CHECKING FOR BURGER DONENESS

Figure 16-1:
Checking
a burger to
see whether
it's cooked
through.

I FEEL GREAT! CAN I GO OUT AND PLAY NOW?

160°

INSERT A MEAT THERMOMETER AT A HORIZONTAL ANGLE INTO A HAMBURGER PATTY SO THE THERMOMETER DOESN'T TOUCH THE PAN! WHEN THE THERMOMETER REGISTERS 160°, THE BURGER IS DONE!

Fresh Basil Burgers

Prep time: 10 min • **Cook time:** 8 min • **Yield:** 8 servings

Ingredients	*Directions*
2 pounds lean ground beef **1 tablespoon Worcestershire sauce** **2 tablespoons shallots, minced** **4 ounces shredded Parmesan cheese** **¼ cup chopped fresh basil**	*1* In a large bowl, mix together the ground beef, Worcestershire sauce, shallots, cheese, and basil, and form the mixture into 8 hamburger patties.
Nonstick cooking spray **8 whole-wheat hamburger buns**	*2* Spray the grill with nonstick cooking spray; then heat it to medium-high. Cook the burgers until they're cooked through, about 4 minutes on each side for medium doneness.
8 slices lettuce **8 slices tomato**	*3* Serve each burger on a whole-wheat hamburger bun with 1 slice each of lettuce and tomato.

Per serving: Calories 396 (From Fat 156); Glycemic Load 16 (Medium); Fat 17g (Saturated 8g); Cholesterol 92mg; Sodium 572mg; Carbohydrate 24g (Dietary Fiber 4g); Protein 36g.

Tip: We suppose you could call this recipe an Italian-inspired burger without the marinara sauce — although that may be a delicious topping to add when you're feeling extra adventurous!

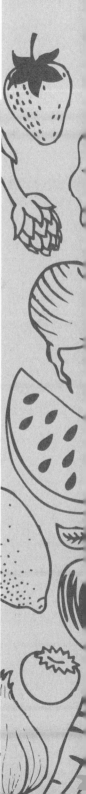

South-of-the-Border Burgers

Prep time: 10 min • **Cook time:** 8 min • **Yield:** 8 servings

Ingredients	*Directions*
2 pounds lean ground beef	*1* In a large bowl, mix together the ground beef, salsa, cumin, chili powder, and salt, and form the mixture into 8 hamburger patties.
½ cup mild salsa	
1 teaspoon ground cumin	
½ teaspoon chili powder	*2* Spray the grill with nonstick cooking spray; then heat it to medium-high. Cook the burgers until they're cooked through, about 4 minutes on each side for medium doneness.
¼ teaspoon salt	
Nonstick cooking spray	
8 whole-wheat hamburger buns	*3* Serve each burger on a whole-wheat bun with 1 slice of cheese and 2 slices of avocado.
8 slices cheddar cheese	
1 ripe avocado, peeled, pitted, and sliced	

Per serving: Calories 478 (From Fat 230); Glycemic Load 16 (Medium); Fat 26g (Saturated 11g); Cholesterol 111mg; Sodium 645mg; Carbohydrate 25g (Dietary Fiber 5g); Protein 37g.

Vary It! This recipe works well with regular beef burgers as well as turkey burgers, so pick a meat and give it a try. You can even try these burgers bunless with a dollop of salsa!

Tip: Use lowfat cheese if you prefer to lower the fat and calories.

Savory Burgers

Prep time: 10 min • **Cook time:** 8 min • **Yield:** 8 servings

Ingredients	*Directions*
2 pounds lean ground beef	*1* In a large bowl, combine the ground beef, red wine, red onion, garlic salt, bread crumbs, parsley, and lemon juice; mix well. Form the mixture into 8 hamburger patties.
¼ **cup dry red wine**	
¼ **cup minced red onion**	
2 teaspoons garlic salt	
¼ **cup fresh Italian bread crumbs**	*2* Spray the grill with nonstick cooking spray; then heat it to medium-high. Cook the burgers until they're cooked through, about 4 minutes on each side for medium doneness.
1 tablespoon minced fresh flat-leaf parsley	
1 tablespoon lemon juice	*3* Serve each burger on a whole-wheat bun with 1 slice each of provolone cheese, tomato, and lettuce.
Nonstick cooking spray	
8 whole-wheat hamburger buns	
8 slices provolone cheese	
8 slices tomato	
8 slices lettuce	

Per serving: Calories 445 (From Fat 187); Glycemic Load 16 (Medium); Fat 21g (Saturated 10g); Cholesterol 100mg; Sodium 830mg; Carbohydrate 27g (Dietary Fiber 4g); Protein 38g.

Tip: You can use lowfat cheese to lower the fat and calories.

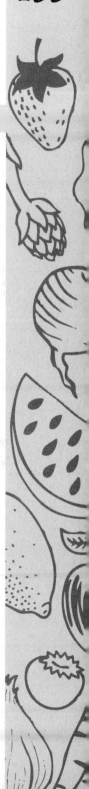

Enjoying New Pork Favorites

Although we aren't sure why, pork has gotten a bad rap as being a high-fat food choice. Yes, ham and pork sausage can be pretty high in fat and calories, but many other cuts of pork are as lean as chicken breasts (see Chapter 15 for some delicious chicken recipes). Pork cutlets, chops, and tenderloins are all healthy, lean cuts that you can add to your weekly menu for a little variety. Let's face it, part of the reason why you may have difficulties making changes to your diet is feeling restricted. This section provides some fresh, new ways to add lowfat and low-glycemic pork entrees to your meal plan. The recipes we include here fall into two general categories:

- **Pork chops and cutlets:** *Pork chops* can vary in size depending on whether they come from the pig's center loin chops or shoulder chops. They tend to be a little bit tougher cut of meat so you don't want to overcook them! *Pork cutlets* are a thin cut of meat, so they cook quickly and take up the flavor of any sauce well.

- **Pork tenderloin:** *Pork tenderloin* is a lean cut of pork that retains a lot of the flavor and moisture of marinades. It's the most tender cut of pork and appears as a long round steak.

To get an accurate read on a tenderloin's temperature, use a meat thermometer (preferably an instant-read variety) and test in the thickest part of the meat. You want to make sure your pork tenderloin is cooked to an internal temperature of 160 degrees to avoid getting infections like trichinosis.

Garlic and Lemon Grilled Pork Chops

Prep time: 5 min, plus refrigerating time • **Cook time:** 5 min, plus resting time • **Yield:** 4 servings

Ingredients	*Directions*
1 tablespoon extra-virgin olive oil	*1* In a small bowl, mix the olive oil, lemon juice, sage, thyme, onion powder, and garlic. Put the pork chops in a large sealable bag, pour in the marinade, and refrigerate the marinating pork for 2 to 3 hours.
3 tablespoons lemon juice	
1 teaspoon finely chopped fresh sage	
½ teaspoon finely chopped fresh thyme	*2* Spray the grill with nonstick cooking spray; then heat it to medium-high. Drain and discard the marinade from the meat and pat the meat dry. Sprinkle the pork chops with salt and pepper to taste.
¼ teaspoon onion powder	
2 cloves garlic, minced	*3* Place the pork chops on the grill, and cook them for 3 minutes on one side. Turn and cook an additional 2 minutes on the other side, or until the internal temperature reads 155 degrees. Pull the pork chops off the grill, and let them sit for 5 more minutes — the internal temperature should rise to 160 degrees.
Four ½-inch-thick boneless pork chops, fat trimmed	
Nonstick cooking spray	
Salt and pepper to taste	

Per serving: *Calories 241 (From Fat 136); Glycemic Load 0 (Low); Fat 15g (Saturated 5g); Cholesterol 71mg; Sodium 195mg; Carbohydrate 2g (Dietary Fiber 0g); Protein 23g.*

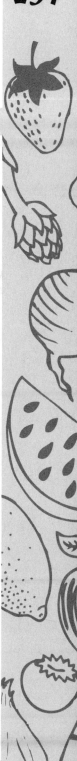

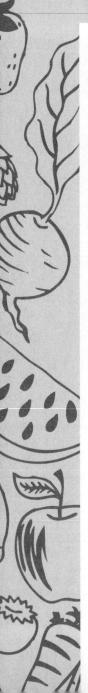

Pork Cutlets with Apricot Sauce

Prep time: 5 min • **Cook time:** 16 min • **Yield:** 6 servings

Ingredients	*Directions*
2 teaspoons plus 1 teaspoon extra-virgin olive oil	*1* In a large nonstick skillet, heat 2 teaspoons of olive oil over medium heat. Season the cutlets with the salt and pepper. When the oil is hot, add the pork and cook until lightly browned, or about 3 minutes per side. Remove the pork from the skillet and set aside.
6 boneless pork loin cutlets, about ¾-inch thick	
¼ teaspoon salt	
Black pepper to taste	
1 small onion, cut in half, thinly sliced	*2* In a medium saucepan, heat the remaining 1 teaspoon of olive oil. Add the onion, and sauté it until tender, about 2 minutes. Add the garlic, and sauté for 1 minute. Then add the apricot preserves and broth, and bring the mixture to a boil. Reduce the heat, and simmer until the liquid is reduced by half, about 2 minutes.
1 clove garlic, minced	
½ cup apricot preserves	
½ cup low-sodium chicken broth	*3* Return the pork cutlets to the skillet you browned them in, sprinkle them with parsley, and heat them through, about 5 minutes. Place the cutlets on a serving platter, and drizzle the apricot sauce evenly over each one.
2 tablespoons chopped fresh flat-leaf parsley	

Per serving: Calories 301 (From Fat 134); Glycemic Load 7 (Low); Fat 15g (Saturated 50g); Cholesterol 70mg; Sodium 168mg; Carbohydrate 18g (Dietary Fiber 1g); Protein 24g.

Curry and Apple Pork Chops

Prep time: 15 min • **Cook time:** About 30 min • **Yield:** 4 servings

Ingredients	*Directions*
Four 1-inch-thick boneless pork chops	*1* Preheat the oven to 400 degrees. Season the pork chops with salt and pepper. In a large skillet, heat the oil on medium-high heat; then add the pork chops and brown on each side, about 3 minutes per side. Spray a 9-x-13-inch baking dish with nonstick cooking spray, and arrange the pork chops inside the dish.
Salt and pepper to taste	
2 teaspoons canola oil	
Nonstick cooking spray	
1 teaspoon butter	*2* In the same skillet, melt the butter; add the onions and apples, cooking and stirring them until they're caramelized, about 4 minutes. Add the applesauce, apple juice, wine, chicken bouillon granules, garlic, curry powder, cumin, and cinnamon, and stir until well heated, about 2 minutes.
1 large sweet onion, diced	
2 large red delicious, gala, or fuji apples, cored and diced	
1½ cups unsweetened applesauce	*3* Pour the mixture over the pork chops, and cover the baking dish with foil. Bake for 15 to 20 minutes, or until the pork chops are cooked through, checking with a thermometer that the internal temperature is 160 degrees.
1 cup apple juice	
½ cup dry white wine	
2 tablespoons chicken bouillon granules	
2 cloves garlic, minced	
2 tablespoons ground curry powder	
1 teaspoon ground cumin	
1 teaspoon ground cinnamon	

Per serving: Calories 406 (From Fat 149); Glycemic Load 4 (Low); Fat 17g (Saturated 5g); Cholesterol 74mg; Sodium 760mg; Carbohydrate 41g (Dietary Fiber 6g); Protein 25g.

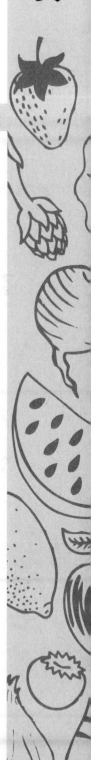

Roasted Pork Tenderloin with Rosemary and Garlic

Prep time: 10 min, plus refrigerating time • **Cook time:** 40–45 min, plus resting time • **Yield:** 4 servings

Ingredients	Directions
2 tablespoons extra-virgin olive oil 1 tablespoon balsamic vinegar ½ cup apple juice 4 large cloves garlic, minced 1 tablespoon chopped fresh rosemary 1 tablespoon Dijon mustard 1 pound pork tenderloin Nonstick cooking spray	**1** In a medium bowl, combine the olive oil, vinegar, apple juice, garlic, rosemary, and mustard, and mix well. Pour ⅓ cup of the mixture in a bowl with a lid, cover, and refrigerate. **2** In a large resealable plastic bag, combine the pork and the remaining marinade. Seal the bag and turn it to coat the pork evenly. Refrigerate the pork overnight, or for 12 hours. **3** Preheat the oven to 350 degrees. Drain and discard the marinade from the pork. Spray a roasting pan with non-stick cooking spray, and place the pork in the pan. Pour the reserved marinade on top of the pork. **4** Bake the pork, uncovered, for 40 to 45 minutes, or until a meat thermometer reads 160 degrees. Let the tenderloin stand for 10 minutes before slicing and serving.

Per serving: Calories 228 (From Fat 109); Glycemic Load 1 (Low); Fat 12g (Saturated 3g); Cholesterol 65mg; Sodium 142mg; Carbohydrate 6g (Dietary Fiber 0g); Protein 23g.

Vary It! If you don't have fresh rosemary on hand, feel free to substitute 2 teaspoons of dried rosemary.

Marinated Grilled Pork Tenderloin

Prep time: 5 min, plus refrigerating time • **Cook time:** 12–15 min, plus resting time • **Yield:** 4 servings

Ingredients	*Directions*
2 tablespoons extra-virgin olive oil	*1* In a medium bowl, combine the olive oil, honey, soy sauce, Worcestershire sauce, wine, garlic, onion powder, cinnamon, cumin, and cayenne pepper, and mix well. Set aside a third of the marinade; cover and refrigerate.
2 tablespoons honey	
¼ cup low-sodium soy sauce	
2 tablespoons Worcestershire sauce	*2* Pour the remainder of the marinade into a large sealable plastic bag and add the tenderloin. Seal the bag and turn to coat the pork evenly. Refrigerate the pork for 8 hours, turning occasionally.
¼ cup dry white wine or cooking sherry	
3 cloves garlic, minced	
½ teaspoon onion powder	*3* Drain and discard the marinade from the pork. Spray the grill with nonstick cooking spray; then heat it to medium-high. Grill the meat, uncovered, over indirect medium-high heat for about 12 to 15 minutes, turning the tenderloin every 3 to 4 minutes and basting with the reserved marinade.
½ teaspoon ground cinnamon	
½ teaspoon ground cumin	
¼ teaspoon cayenne pepper	
1 pound pork tenderloin	*4* Cook the tenderloin until a meat thermometer reads 155 degrees and the juices run clear. Remove the pork from the heat and let it stand for 5 minutes so that the temperature reaches 160 degrees before slicing and serving.
Nonstick cooking spray	

Per serving: Calories 197 (From Fat 76); Glycemic Load 5 (Low); Fat 8g (Saturated 3g); Cholesterol 78mg; Sodium 225mg; Carbohydrate 3g (Dietary Fiber 0g); Protein 25g.

Note: Although you can use many different marinades to create a delicious pork dish, we like this one best because it brings out that smoky and sweet grilled flavor. (You can see this dish in the color section.)

Tip: Check the temperature of the pork periodically after 10 minutes to help avoid overcooking.

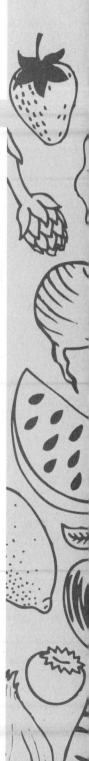

Chapter 17

Sailing the Sea for Some Sensational Seafood Entrees

....

In This Chapter

▶ Creating quick and family-friendly fish entrees

▶ Finding fresh ways to incorporate different fish into your seafood dishes

▶ Cooking up delicious shellfish entrees

....

Seafood is without a doubt one of the healthiest foods you can eat because it's a great source of protein and contains important omega-3 fatty acids that are essential for good health. *Omega-3 fatty acids* are found in fatty fish like salmon and halibut as well as other seafood like sardines and shrimp. These fatty acids offer the following benefits:

✔ Lower triglycerides for heart health

✔ Increase good cholesterol for heart health

✔ Decrease anxiety and depression to improve your mood

✔ Act as an anti-inflammatory

✔ Help decrease your risk of stroke or heart attack by preventing your blood from clotting

Although seafood comes with many benefits, it can contain toxins such as mercury or PCBs (polychlorinated biphenyls), so research recommends eating seafood no more than two to three times a week. Pregnant women and children are especially susceptible to these toxins, so they should limit certain fish such as king mackerel and swordfish. See Chapter 7 for your best low-toxin seafood picks.

Even with all these great benefits, however, seafood is still one of those foods that many people find hard to cook. We've heard countless clients say that they enjoy fish but have no idea how to cook it. Rest easy! What we love about seafood is that you don't have to doctor it up too much to create delicious meals. Simple additions like lemon and seasonings do the trick.

Our goal for this chapter is to show you how easy it is to cook seafood to fit into a low-glycemic diet. For those of you who are already champions at cooking seafood, you'll find some fresh new low-glycemic recipes to add to your recipe box.

If you're looking for something to serve with the seafood recipes in this chapter, turn to Chapters 13 and 14 for some yummy vegetable and pasta sides that go well with almost any meal.

Seafood doesn't take a terribly long time to cook. Fish flakes apart with a fork but is still moist when it's done cooking. Shellfish (such as shrimp) turns opaque in color when it's done. You don't want to overcook seafood, or the taste will suffer.

Quick and Easy Fish Favorites

Maybe you're having one of those nights when you want to cook something healthy but you don't have tons of time to prep. Or you're looking for a no-fuss-no-mess seafood recipe that's kid friendly, too. This section combines lowfat seafood with easy-to-cook (and low-glycemic!) recipes for those nights when you want to serve something healthy, tasty, and super simple.

Grilled Salmon with Maple Glaze

Prep time: 5 min • **Cook time:** 8 min • **Yield:** 4 servings

Ingredients	*Directions*
2 teaspoons low-sodium soy sauce	*1* Combine the soy sauce, maple syrup, and orange juice in a small bowl; set aside.
2 tablespoons pure maple syrup	
2 tablespoons orange juice	*2* Spray a grill tray with nonstick cooking spray, and heat the grill to high heat. Drizzle the salmon fillets evenly with the olive oil, and sprinkle them with salt and pepper to taste. Place the fish on the grill tray, and place the tray on the hot grill.
Nonstick cooking spray	
Four 5-ounce salmon fillets, skinned	
1 tablespoon olive oil	*3* Grill the fillets for 3 minutes on each side. Set aside half the marinade and brush the other half over each side of the salmon with a basting brush; cook it for 1 more minute per side. Serve immediately, drizzling the other half of the marinade mixture over the fish as a glaze.
Salt and pepper to taste	

Per serving: Calories 241 (From Fat 79); Glycemic Load 5 (Low); Fat 9g (Saturated 1g); Cholesterol 81mg; Sodium 351mg; Carbohydrate 8g (Dietary Fiber 0g); Protein 31g.

Tip: The fact that all you have to do is baste the salmon on the grill makes this a great recipe when you're short on time.

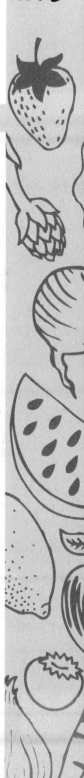

Home-Baked Halibut Fish Sticks

Prep time: 15 min • **Cook time:** 10–12 min • **Yield:** 4 servings

Ingredients	*Directions*
1 pound halibut fillet, skin removed, cut into ½-inch sticks	*1* Preheat the oven to 425 degrees. Place the fish sticks on a plate, and squeeze the lemon juice evenly over the fish. Let the fish sit for 5 minutes.
Juice of 1 lemon	
½ cup lowfat milk	*2* Pour the milk into a shallow bowl. In another shallow bowl, combine the bread crumbs, Parmesan cheese, salt, pepper, garlic powder, and parsley.
⅔ cup plain, dry bread crumbs	
⅓ cup shredded Parmesan cheese	*3* Spray a baking sheet with nonstick cooking spray. Dip the fish sticks into the milk and then into the bread crumb mixture to coat completely. Place the fish sticks on the prepared baking sheet.
½ teaspoon salt	
¼ teaspoon black pepper	
¼ teaspoon garlic powder	*4* Bake the fish for 10 to 12 minutes, or until the fish flakes easily and the outside is browned.
½ teaspoon dried parsley	
Nonstick cooking spray	*5* Transfer the sticks to a serving platter, and serve with the lemon wedges.
1 lemon cut into wedges	

Per serving: Calories 233 (From Fat 48); Glycemic Load 6 (Low); Fat 5g (Saturated 2g); Cholesterol 42mg; Sodium 647mg; Carbohydrate 17g (Dietary Fiber 1g); Protein 29g.

Tip: For a darker crust, turn the oven to the broil setting and cook the fish sticks for an additional 1 minute on each side.

Oven-Fried Fish Sandwiches

Prep time: 10 min • **Cook time:** 15–20 min • **Yield:** 4 servings

Ingredients	*Directions*
1 pound white fish (haddock, cod, or halibut), skin removed, cut into four 4-ounce squares	*1* Preheat the oven to 400 degrees. Place the pieces of fish on a plate, and squeeze the lemon juice evenly over all the pieces; let the fish sit for 5 minutes.
Juice of 1 lemon	
1 egg, lightly beaten	*2* In a shallow bowl, mix together the egg and milk. In another shallow bowl, mix together the bread crumbs, salt, pepper, garlic powder, and parsley.
¼ cup lowfat milk	
⅔ cup plain, dry bread crumbs	
½ teaspoon salt	*3* Spray a baking sheet with nonstick cooking spray. Dip each piece of fish into the egg mixture and then into the bread crumb mixture to coat completely. Place the fish pieces on the prepared baking sheet, and spray them very lightly with the cooking spray.
¼ teaspoon black pepper	
¼ teaspoon garlic powder	
½ teaspoon dried parsley	
Nonstick cooking spray	*4* Bake the fish for 15 to 20 minutes until it's flaky and browned on the top.
4 whole-wheat buns	
4 slices iceberg lettuce	*5* Serve each piece of fish on a whole-wheat bun with 1 slice each of lettuce and tomato and 1 teaspoon of tartar sauce.
4 slices tomato	
4 teaspoons tartar sauce	

Per serving: Calories 338 (From Fat 64); Glycemic Load 16 (Medium); Fat 7g (Saturated 1g); Cholesterol 136mg; Sodium 649mg; Carbohydrate 39g (Dietary Fiber 4g); Protein 30g.

Tip: We like this sandwich with a little tartar sauce, but you can save yourself some calories and fat by omitting that topping.

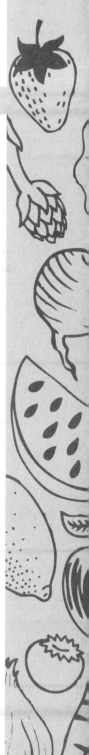

Fabulous Fish Dishes for Your Main Course

Let's face it: There are countless recipes in the world for chicken (see Chapter 15 for some of them), but when it comes to fish, the recipes out there are either too boring or too elaborate. We know it's easy to get stuck in a rut when you're cooking fish, so, in this section, we include a few classic recipes that have stood the test of time as well as some fresh new ones that you're sure to love as much as the old standbys. The recipes we share with you here are just what you need to make eating fish enjoyable and delicious! We use several different kinds of fish in these dishes:

- ✔ **Halibut:** Halibut is a wonderful fish to include in your low-glycemic diet because it's tasty and a good source of omega-3 fatty acids. It's also a larger, thick white fish with the light flavor of a small white fish.

- ✔ **Red snapper:** Red snapper is a popular white fish found in most supermarkets. It has a firm texture and works well with many different flavors. If you're feeling like cooking up some fish but don't know what to get, red snapper is a great pick.

- ✔ **Salmon:** Salmon seems to be the king of fish. It's most people's go-to fish choice and is another great source of omega-3 fatty acids. Salmon has such a great flavor that you don't have to doctor it up too much. A little seasoning goes a long way.

- ✔ **Tilapia:** Tilapia is a small, moist white fish with a wonderful light and somewhat sweet flavor, perfect for a light summer meal. It's another great source of lean protein along with omega-3 fatty acids.

Eating fish two to three times a week is a great way to reach some important health goals; as we note earlier in this chapter, fish is a lean protein source and the best way to incorporate omega-3 fatty acids into your diet.

Halibut with Tomatoes and Green Peppers

Prep time: 10 min • **Cook time:** 20 min • **Yield:** 4 servings

Ingredients	*Directions*
Four 5-ounce halibut fillets, skinned **Juice of 2 lemons** **Salt and pepper to taste** **2 teaspoons butter** **3 Roma tomatoes, sliced thinly** **½ green bell pepper, sliced thinly**	*1* Preheat the oven to 350 degrees. Place a large piece of foil (enough to cover all the fish) in a 9-x-13-inch glass baking dish; arrange the fish on top of the foil. Squeeze the lemon juice evenly on the fish, and let it sit for 5 minutes.
	2 Season the fish with salt and pepper to taste. Place a ½-teaspoon pat of butter on the center of each piece of fish. Place the sliced tomatoes and peppers on top of the fish, and wrap the foil over the top to cover tightly.
	3 Bake until the fish is flaky but still moist, about 20 minutes. Serve.

Per serving: Calories 185 (From Fat 43); Glycemic Load 0 (Low); Fat 5g (Saturated 1g); Cholesterol 52mg; Sodium 231mg; Carbohydrate 5g (Dietary Fiber 1g); Protein 32g.

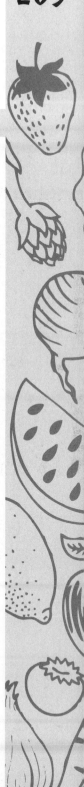

Chipotle Fish Tacos

Prep time: 20 min • **Cook time:** 6 min • **Yield:** 8 servings

Ingredients	Directions
One 1-pound halibut fillet, skinned	**1** Place the fish fillets in a shallow bowl. In a separate small bowl, whisk together ¼ cup of the lime juice and the salt and pepper. Pour the mixture over the fish fillet, and let it sit for 5 to 10 minutes.
¼ cup plus 2 tablespoons lime juice	
Salt and pepper to taste	
Nonstick cooking spray	**2** Spray a grill tray with nonstick cooking spray, and preheat the grill and tray to medium-high heat. Remove the fish from the marinade, and place it on the grill tray. Grill until the fish is cooked through and flaky but still moist, about 3 minutes on each side. Set the fish aside.
½ cup lowfat Greek yogurt	
⅓ cup lowfat sour cream	
1 chipotle pepper in adobo sauce, finely chopped	
¼ cup chopped red onion	**3** In a small bowl, combine the yogurt, sour cream, chipotle pepper, remaining 2 tablespoons of lime juice, red onion, and cilantro.
¼ cup chopped fresh cilantro	
Eight 8-inch low-carb or whole-wheat flour tortillas	**4** Heat the tortillas in the microwave for 10 seconds, and flake the fish with a fork. Spread 1 tablespoon of the chipotle mixture over each tortilla. Top each tortilla with an equal amount of fish, cabbage, and avocado.
1 cup shredded green cabbage	
1 avocado, sliced	

Per serving: Calories 231 (From Fat 75); Glycemic Load 17 (Medium); Fat 8g (Saturated 2g); Cholesterol 22mg; Sodium 264mg; Carbohydrate 20g (Dietary Fiber 10g); Protein 22g.

Red Snapper with Tomatoes and Green Chiles

Prep time: 10 min • **Cook time:** 15–20 min • **Yield:** 4 servings

Ingredients	Directions
Four 4- to 5-ounce red snapper fillets	**1** Preheat the oven to 350 degrees. Place a large sheet of foil (enough to cover all the fish) in a 9-x-13-inch glass baking dish. Arrange the fish on the foil (leaving enough foil to cover it), and squeeze the lime juice over the top of each fillet. Let the fish sit for 5 minutes.
Juice of 1 lime	
Salt and pepper to taste	
2 teaspoons butter	
One 2.25-ounce can diced fire-roasted green chiles	**2** Sprinkle the fish with salt and pepper to taste, and place a ½-teaspoon butter pat on the center of each fish fillet. In a small bowl, mix together the chiles, tomatoes, onion, garlic powder, and cilantro to make the salsa. Spoon the salsa evenly over each fish fillet, and wrap the other end of the foil over the fish tightly.
3 Roma tomatoes, finely diced	
¼ cup chopped sweet onion	
¼ teaspoon garlic powder	
¼ cup chopped fresh cilantro	**3** Bake the fish in the oven until it's flaky but still moist, about 15 to 20 minutes.

Per serving: Calories 145 (From Fat 32); Glycemic Load 0 (Low); Fat 4g (Saturated 2g); Cholesterol 45mg; Sodium 258mg; Carbohydrate 5g (Dietary Fiber 1g); Protein 23g.

Tip: We like to use fire-roasted chiles if we can find them; look for them right where you find the regular canned diced green chiles. If you can't find them, feel free to use the regular diced green chiles instead.

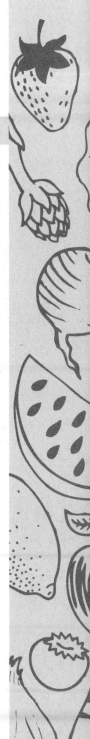

Grilled Salmon with Rosemary-Garlic Butter

Prep time: 10 min • **Cook time:** 8 min • **Yield:** 4 servings

Ingredients	Directions
One 1-pound salmon fillet, skinned	**1** Place the salmon in the middle of a large piece of aluminum foil, leaving enough foil to cover. Squeeze the lemon juice over the fish, and let it sit for 5 minutes.
Juice of 1 lemon	
½ teaspoon salt	**2** Sprinkle the fish with the salt and black pepper. In a small bowl, blend together the butter and garlic. Spread the garlic-butter mixture over the fish, and place the rosemary sprigs on top of the buttered fish. Close the sides of the aluminum foil, and fold up the ends so the fish is completely covered.
¼ teaspoon black pepper	
2 teaspoons butter	
2 cloves garlic, minced	
2 to 3 sprigs fresh rosemary	
	3 Heat the grill to medium-high heat, and grill the fish until it's flaky but still moist, about 8 minutes total. Place the foil-wrapped salmon on a large plate or a small metal tray to transfer. Discard the rosemary sprigs, cut the fish into four 4-ounce portions, and serve.

Per serving: Calories 167 (From Fat 56); Glycemic Load 0 (Low); Fat 6g (Saturated 2g); Cholesterol 70mg; Sodium 374mg; Carbohydrate 2g (Dietary Fiber 0g); Protein 25g.

Teriyaki Salmon Kabobs

Prep time: 15 min, plus refrigerating time • **Cook time:** About 10 min • **Yield:** 4 servings

Ingredients	*Directions*
2 tablespoons sesame oil	*1* In a small bowl, mix together the sesame oil, soy sauce, honey, ginger, garlic powder, and lime juice. Place the salmon cubes in a sealable plastic bag, and pour the sesame marinade over them. Seal the bag, turn it to coat the salmon evenly, and place it in the refrigerator for 30 minutes.
3 tablespoons low-sodium soy sauce	
1 tablespoon honey	
2 teaspoons ground ginger	
¼ teaspoon garlic powder	*2* Thread the salmon cubes evenly on 4 skewers. Then thread the green peppers, red peppers, and pineapple chunks on 4 more skewers. Discard the marinade.
2 tablespoons lime juice	
One 14-ounce salmon fillet, skinned and cubed	
1 green bell pepper, sliced in 1½-inch squares	*3* Spray the grill with nonstick cooking spray; then heat it to medium. Grill the vegetable/fruit skewers for 5 minutes. Turn and cook an additional 5 minutes, or until soft and browned.
1 red bell pepper, sliced in 1½-inch squares	
Twelve to sixteen 1-inch pineapple chunks	*4* Add the salmon skewers midway through the vegetable cooking time and cook for 2 minutes on one side. Turn the salmon skewers, and cook an additional 1 to 2 minutes, or until the salmon is golden on the outside and flaky on the inside.
Nonstick cooking spray	

Per serving: *Calories 184 (From Fat 51); Glycemic Load 6 (Low); Fat 6g (Saturated 1g); Cholesterol 57mg; Sodium 188mg; Carbohydrate 11g (Dietary Fiber 2g); Protein 23g.*

Note: Kabobs may take a little more prep time, but cooking them is a breeze. Plus, you can make extras for leftovers.

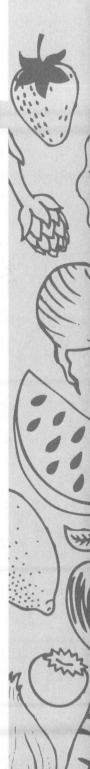

Grilled Salmon with Mango Salsa

Prep time: 15 min • **Cook time:** 8 min • **Yield:** 4 servings

Ingredients	*Directions*
One 1-pound salmon fillet, skinned	*1* Place the fish on a large sheet of aluminum foil on an oblong dish or pan. Squeeze the lemon juice over the salmon, and then let it sit for 5 minutes.
Juice of 1 lemon	
1 ripe mango, peeled, pitted, and diced	*2* In a medium bowl, mix together the mango, red bell pepper, red onion, jalapeño, cilantro, lime juice, and orange juice; add salt and pepper to taste. Set aside.
1 red bell pepper, chopped	
½ medium red onion, finely chopped	
1 jalapeño chile, minced	*3* Rub the salmon with additional salt and pepper to taste, cumin, and chili powder.
¼ cup chopped fresh cilantro	
2 tablespoons fresh lime juice	*4* Spray a grill tray with nonstick cooking spray, and heat the tray on the grill to medium-high heat. Grill the salmon until it's flaky but still moist, about 4 minutes on each side. Top with the mango salsa and serve.
2 tablespoons orange juice	
Salt and pepper to taste	
½ teaspoon cumin	
½ teaspoon chili powder	
Nonstick cooking spray	

Per serving: Calories 198 (From Fat 42); Glycemic Load 4 (Low); Fat 5g (Saturated 1g); Cholesterol 65mg; Sodium 235mg; Carbohydrate 14g (Dietary Fiber 2g); Protein 26g.

Note: Mango salsa is the perfect accompaniment to grilled salmon. This recipe (which you can see in the color section) adds a little kick to the salmon with cumin and chili powder.

Vary It! If you prefer less spice in your meal, simply omit the cumin and chili powder; the salmon is still wonderful with the mango salsa.

Lemon-Baked Tilapia

Prep time: 10 min • **Cook time:** 20 min • **Yield:** 4 servings

Ingredients	*Directions*
Four 5-ounce tilapia fillets, skinned	**1** Preheat the oven to 350 degrees. Place a large sheet of foil (enough to cover all the fish) in a 9-x-13-inch glass baking dish. Arrange the fillets on the foil. Squeeze the lemon juice over the fillets, and let them sit for 5 minutes.
Juice of 1 lemon	
½ teaspoon Old Bay Seasoning	
1 tablespoon butter, softened	**2** Sprinkle the Old Bay Seasoning over the fish evenly. In a small bowl, combine the softened butter with the garlic and parsley. With a knife, gently spread the butter mixture evenly over each fish fillet.
1 clove garlic, minced	
1 teaspoon dried parsley	
1 lemon, sliced into 8 slices, bottom and top thinly removed	**3** Place two lemon slices over each fish fillet, wrap the aluminum foil over the top of the fish tightly, and bake until the fish is flaky yet still moist, about 20 minutes.

Per serving: Calories 178 (From Fat 53); Glycemic Load 0 (Low); Fat 6g (Saturated 3g); Cholesterol 72mg; Sodium 231mg; Carbohydrate 3g (Dietary Fiber 0g); Protein 30g.

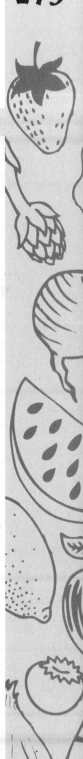

Grilled Tilapia with Parmesan Polenta

Prep time: 10 min　•　**Cook time:** About 30 min　•　**Yield:** 4 servings

Ingredients	Directions

Ingredients

1¼ cups lowfat milk

¼ cup fat-free half-and-half

¾ cup cornmeal

¾ cup water

¼ cup freshly grated Parmesan cheese

¼ teaspoon black pepper

Four 4- to 6-ounce tilapia fillets, skinned

Juice of 1 lemon

Salt and pepper to taste

1 teaspoon canola oil

Directions

1 Preheat the oven to 350 degrees. In a medium saucepan, stir together the milk and half-and-half and simmer over low heat for 2 minutes. Remove the milk mixture from the heat, cover, and let stand for 5 minutes.

2 Gradually stir the cornmeal into the milk mixture, and then return the pan to low heat. Simmer the cornmeal mixture on low, stirring continuously until smooth. Add the water, and stir until creamy, about 20 minutes. Add the Parmesan and pepper. Then remove the mixture from heat, cover with a lid, and set aside (it'll firm up as it sits).

3 Place the tilapia fillets on a plate, and squeeze the lemon juice evenly over them. Let the fish sit for 5 minutes. Then sprinkle the fillets with salt and pepper to taste.

4 Heat the oil in a nonstick skillet over medium-high heat. Add the fish fillets to the skillet, and cook them until they're opaque in the center and flaky, about 4 minutes on each side.

5 Serve each tilapia fillet on top of ½ cup of polenta.

Per serving: Calories 319 (From Fat 63); Glycemic Load 11 (Medium); Fat 7g (Saturated 3g); Cholesterol 72mg; Sodium 354mg; Carbohydrate 27g (Dietary Fiber 2g); Protein 37g.

Note: The cheesy polenta in this recipe is a delicious, sweet addition to the tilapia. Plus, it's a great way to include a low-glycemic grain in your dinner (see Chapter 14 for additional healthy side dish ideas). Add a steamed vegetable, and you have a complete meal.

Sublime Shellfish

Despite health scares about the high cholesterol levels found in shellfish, you can make shrimp, crab, and other similar foods a part of a healthy low-glycemic diet. As a matter of fact, shrimp and crab both contain omega-3 fatty acids that promote heart health, and the cholesterol found in shellfish doesn't contribute to your cholesterol levels as much as saturated fats do.

This section shows you some delicious (and low-glycemic) ways to say yes to shellfish.

The American Heart Association recommends limiting your daily cholesterol intake to fewer than 300 milligrams. If you have heart disease, you need to limit your intake to fewer than 200 milligrams a day. A 3-ounce serving of shrimp contains 166 milligrams of cholesterol, and a 3-ounce serving of crab contains 85 milligrams. As you can see, they both fall under the recommended thresholds, so you don't have to steer clear of shellfish as part of your heart-healthy, low-glycemic diet.

Parmesan Shrimp and Broccoli

Prep time: 10 min • **Cook time:** About 8 min • **Yield:** 4 servings

Ingredients	Directions
1 tablespoon canola oil	*1* In a large skillet or wok, heat the oil over medium heat. Add the garlic and broccoli, and cook for 5 minutes.
2 cloves garlic, minced	
2 cups broccoli florets, cut small	
1 pound medium fresh or thawed frozen deveined shrimp, tails removed	*2* Add the shrimp and sauté for 2 to 3 minutes, or until the shrimp is almost cooked through. Add the wine, lemon juice, and parsley, and cook until the shrimp is pink and cooked through, about 30 seconds.
3 tablespoons dry white wine	
3 teaspoons lemon juice	*3* Sprinkle the Parmesan cheese evenly over the shrimp and broccoli, and serve.
1 teaspoon dried parsley	
2 tablespoons grated Parmesan cheese	

Per serving: Calories 142 (From Fat 48); Glycemic Load 0 (Low); Fat 5g (Saturated 1g); Cholesterol 170mg; Sodium 250mg; Carbohydrate 3g (Dietary Fiber 1g); Protein 20g.

Tip: Use a dry white wine such as a Chardonnay or Pinot Grigio.

Tip: Serve this dish with a half cup of your favorite low-glycemic grain like brown rice or quinoa for a complete meal (flip to Chapter 14 for some yummy grain side dishes).

Spicy Ginger and Lime Shrimp

Prep time: 5 min, plus refrigerating time • **Cook time:** 2–4 min • **Yield:** 4 servings

Ingredients	*Directions*
½ cup fresh lime juice 2 tablespoons sesame oil 1½ tablespoons ground ginger 2 garlic cloves, minced ⅛ teaspoon black pepper ¼ teaspoon cayenne pepper ¼ teaspoon salt	*1* In a large shallow dish with a lid, mix together the lime juice, sesame oil, ginger, garlic, black pepper, cayenne pepper, and salt.
	2 Add the shrimp, put the lid on the dish, and shake it until the shrimp is well coated. Refrigerate the shrimp for 30 to 45 minutes.
1 pound medium fresh or thawed frozen deveined shrimp, tails removed **Nonstick cooking spray** **4 lemon wedges**	*3* Preheat the broiler, and spray a small-rimmed baking sheet with nonstick cooking spray. Put the shrimp on the baking sheet, and broil the shrimp until it's pink and cooked through, about 2 to 4 minutes. Place the shrimp on a plate, and serve with lemon wedges.

Per serving: Calories 107 (From Fat 24); Glycemic Load 0 (Low); Fat 3g (Saturated 1g); Cholesterol 168mg; Sodium 230mg; Carbohydrate 2g (Dietary Fiber 0g); Protein 18g.

Vary It! If you like mild heat, use the recipe as it is, but if you want to crank it up a notch, add a little more cayenne pepper and you'll be on your way!

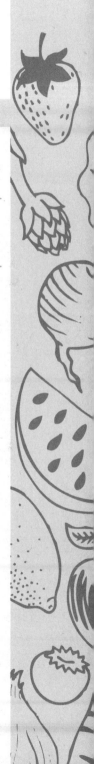

Shrimp and Vegetable Stir-Fry

Prep time: 15 min • **Cook time:** 8 min • **Yield:** 4 servings

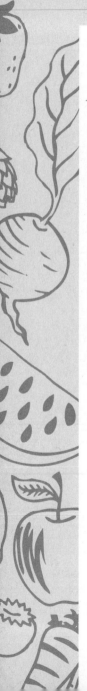

Ingredients	Directions
1 tablespoon canola oil	*1* In a large nonstick skillet, heat the oil over medium-high heat. Add the garlic, red bell pepper, and carrots, and sauté until the vegetables begin to soften, about 4 minutes.
1 teaspoon minced garlic	
1 red bell pepper, thinly sliced	
1 carrot, thinly sliced on the diagonal	*2* Add the shrimp, sugar snap peas, and ginger, and cook until the shrimp is almost cooked through, about 2 minutes.
¾ pound large fresh or thawed frozen deveined shrimp, tails removed	
½ cup sugar snap peas	*3* Add the wine, soy sauce, and red pepper flakes. Continue to cook until the shrimp is completely cooked through and well coated with the liquid ingredients, about 2 more minutes. Serve with a half cup of your favorite low-glycemic grain, such as brown rice or quinoa.
2 teaspoons ground ginger	
2 tablespoons dry white wine	
3 tablespoons low-sodium soy sauce	
¼ teaspoon dried red pepper flakes	

Per serving: Calories 132 (From Fat 39); Glycemic Load 0 (Low); Fat 4g (Saturated 1g); Cholesterol 126mg; Sodium 612mg; Carbohydrate 7g (Dietary Fiber 2g); Protein 15g.

Tip: Use a dry white wine such as a Chardonnay or Pinot Grigio.

Tip: Check out Chapter 14 for some delicious grain side dish recipes.

Grilled Garlic-Lemon Prawns

Prep time: 5 min, plus refrigerating time • **Cook time:** 2–4 min • **Yield:** 4 servings

Ingredients	_Directions_
2 tablespoons canola oil	_1_ In a shallow dish with a lid, combine the oil, mustard, garlic, lemon juice, wine, parsley, salt, and pepper. Add the prawns, place the lid on the dish, and shake it until the prawns are well coated. Marinate the prawns in the refrigerator for 30 minutes.
1 teaspoon Dijon mustard	
3 cloves garlic, minced	
Juice of 1 lemon	
2 tablespoons dry white wine	_2_ Thread the prawns onto skewers, about 5 prawns per skewer.
½ teaspoon dried parsley	
¼ teaspoon salt	_3_ Spray the grill with nonstick cooking spray; then heat it to medium-high. Cook the prawns until they're opaque and cooked through, about 1 to 2 minutes on each side. Serve with your favorite low-glycemic side dish, such as the Cheesy Quinoa with Spinach in Chapter 14.
¼ teaspoon black pepper	
20 fresh or thawed frozen tiger prawns, deveined	
Nonstick cooking spray	

**Per serving:** Calories 129 (From Fat 25); Glycemic Load 0 (Low); Fat 3g (Saturated 0g); Cholesterol 168mg; Sodium 238mg; Carbohydrate 2g (Dietary Fiber 0g); Protein 23g.

**Note:** The great thing about all shellfish is the way their already-amazing flavor mixes with any marinade you add to them. Grilling prawns (a large form of shrimp) is an easy way to have an incredible dinner.

**Tip:** Use a dry white wine such as a Chardonnay or Pinot Grigio.

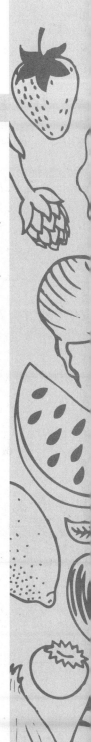

Crab Cakes

Prep time: 15 min • **Cook time:** 12–16 min • **Yield:** 8 servings

Ingredients	*Directions*
½ cup chopped onion	**1** In a large bowl, combine the onion, parsley, garlic, bell pepper, lemon juice, Worcestershire sauce, egg white, yogurt, mayonnaise, black pepper, salt, mustard, and paprika. Add the crabmeat and ¼ cup of the bread crumbs. Lightly toss to coat the crabmeat.
1 teaspoon dried parsley	
2 cloves garlic, minced	
½ cup finely chopped red bell pepper	
1 tablespoon lemon juice	**2** Form 8 patties; coat them with the remaining bread crumbs, pressing the crumbs in place.
½ teaspoon Worcestershire sauce	
1 egg white, lightly beaten	**3** Coat a large skillet with nonstick cooking spray, and heat it over medium-high heat. Add 4 of the crabmeat patties, and cook for 6 to 8 minutes, or until lightly browned on both sides, turning the patties after 3 or 4 minutes. Transfer the patties to a plate, and repeat this step for the remaining patties, wiping away any crumbs left on the skillet. Serve.
1 tablespoon lowfat plain yogurt	
2 tablespoons lowfat mayonnaise	
¼ teaspoon black pepper	
¼ teaspoon salt	
¼ teaspoon dried mustard	
½ teaspoon paprika	
1 pound lump crabmeat, flaked	
¼ cup plus ½ cup plain, dry bread crumbs	
Nonstick cooking spray	

Per serving: Calories 100 (From Fat 49); Glycemic Load 7 (Low); Fat 6g (Saturated 0g); Cholesterol 32mg; Sodium 528mg; Carbohydrate 11g (Dietary Fiber 1g); Protein 10g.

Note: The next time you feel a crab-cake craving coming on, use this recipe to save yourself about one-third of the calories and fat you'd get from a fried crab cake.

Chapter 18

Going Vegetarian with Some Hearty Entrees

In This Chapter

▶ Creating delicious meals out of whole grains and lentils

▶ Cooking vegetarian entrees that are just as filling and tasty as meat meals

*E*ating vegetarian entrees is a great wellness strategy whether you consider yourself a vegetarian or not. Eating more plant-based foods like vegetables, beans, lentils, and whole grains can help decrease your risk of chronic diseases like heart disease, cancer, and diabetes. (For those of you who aren't vegetarians, don't worry. This chapter isn't a lecture on becoming one; it's simply a way to use some vegetarian entrees in your weekly meals to add a little balance and variety to your diet.)

In this chapter, we share some hearty vegetarian entrees that are both delicious and low glycemic. The benefits you get from these entrees are great, and you don't have to become committed to the lifestyle if you don't want to. So what are you waiting for? Give them a try!

Because we really love cheese, many of the recipes you see here use cheese in some way. However, you can easily make any of the recipes in this chapter vegan by omitting the cheese or replacing it with soy cheese.

Making the Most of Grains and Lentils

Using low- to medium-glycemic grains, such as barley, brown rice, polenta, and quinoa, as the main ingredients in your entrees works well when you're trying to create hearty vegetarian meals. You can easily add spices and herbs for flavoring and soy, cheese, and nuts for protein.

Combining lentils with veggies creates not only an amazing flavor but also a low-glycemic, high-fiber, and iron-rich entree. Lentils also add protein to your meal to replace the animal proteins you don't get in vegetarian meals.

The recipes in this section demonstrate how to incorporate delicious meals featuring grains and lentils into your diet without tipping the glycemic index scale too high. The recipes you find here fall into these five categories:

- **Barley:** Pearl barley has a creamy texture and can provide a great low-glycemic base for a hearty vegetarian meal. We use pearl barley rather than regular hulled barley throughout this book for convenience and ease of cooking; other forms of barley can be difficult to find in grocery stores. Because pearl barley is processed, it doesn't have as high a nutritional value as regular barley, but it's still a good source of fiber and B vitamins. If you can find regular hulled barley, feel free to give it a try! A half cup of pearl or hulled barley has a low glycemic load, and up to a cup still has a medium glycemic load. Just don't exceed a cup!

- **Brown rice:** Brown rice cooks very similarly to traditional white rice, but it offers a nuttier flavor, a chewier consistency, and more fiber! Plus, it's low to medium glycemic compared to the high-glycemic white rice varieties.

- **Lentils:** Lentils are a great source of fiber and folate, and they're low glycemic. As an added bonus, they're easy to cook, and you don't have to worry about the long soaking time you need with dry beans.

- **Polenta:** Polenta is a cornmeal mush that has a tasty sweet corn flavor and works well with all sorts of recipes. It's a great base to use for vegetarian meals, and it's easy to make. All you need is a little water, cornmeal, and salt (see the recipe for Basic Polenta in Chapter 14).

- **Quinoa:** Quinoa is a great grain to use in any vegetarian meal. Not only is it low glycemic and high in fiber, but it's also a complete protein providing all the essential amino acids vegetarian meals sometimes lack. Plus, it's easy to cook and super tasty to eat!

Mediterranean Bean and Barley Salad

Prep time: 15 min • **Cook time:** 33–35 min • **Yield:** 6 servings

Ingredients	Directions
1 cup pearl barley	**1** In a large saucepan, bring the barley and broth to a boil over high heat. Reduce the heat to medium-low, cover the pan, and simmer for about 25 minutes.
2½ cups low-sodium vegetable broth	
One 15-ounce can white beans (cannellini or great Northern), rinsed and drained	**2** Stir in the white beans, sun-dried tomatoes, garlic, wine, and balsamic vinegar; simmer until the liquid is absorbed, about 8 to 10 minutes.
¼ cup chopped sun-dried tomatoes, not packed in oil	
2 medium cloves garlic, minced	**3** Fold in the basil, olives, and artichoke hearts until well blended. Divide equally into 6 serving bowls, and sprinkle each serving with 1 tablespoon of feta cheese.
2 tablespoons dry white wine	
1 tablespoon balsamic vinegar	
½ cup chopped fresh basil	
¼ cup sliced kalamata olives	
¼ cup chopped frozen artichoke hearts, thawed	
6 tablespoons crumbled feta cheese	

Per serving: Calories 218 (From Fat 38); Glycemic Load 15 (Medium); Fat 4g (Saturated 2g); Cholesterol 8mg; Sodium 491mg; Carbohydrate 38g (Dietary Fiber 8g); Protein 8g.

Note: Although you may think of pasta as the main ingredient in any satisfying Mediterranean dish, barley can be a great replacement thanks to its hearty texture and flavor.

Tip: A Chardonnay or Pinot Grigio works well in this recipe.

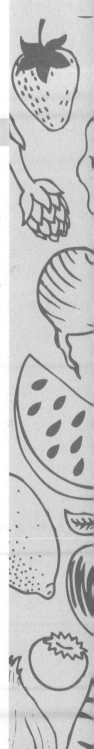

Barley Risotto with Mushrooms and Peas

Prep time: 15 min • **Cook time:** 28–40 min • **Yield:** 6 servings

Ingredients	Directions
6 cups low-sodium vegetable broth	*1* In a medium saucepan, heat the vegetable broth over low heat; let it simmer while you follow Steps 2 and 3.
1 tablespoon butter	
1 teaspoon extra-virgin olive oil	*2* In a large saucepan, combine the butter, oil, and onion over medium-high heat. Sauté the mixture until the onion is soft, about 3 minutes.
1 onion, finely chopped	
2 cloves garlic, minced	*3* Add the garlic and mushrooms to the onion mixture, and continue to sauté for 5 minutes. Stir in the barley, and sauté for 2 minutes, or until the barley is lightly golden. Gradually add the wine, and stir until the barley has absorbed the liquid. Mix in the thyme and bay leaf.
1 cup finely chopped button mushrooms	
½ cup finely chopped crimini mushrooms	
1½ cups pearl barley	
⅔ cup dry white wine	*4* Add 1 cup of the hot vegetable broth to the barley mixture, and stir until the barley has absorbed the liquid. Continue adding broth, 1 cup at a time, and stir until the barley absorbs all the liquid. (Adding all the broth takes about 18 to 30 minutes, or 3 to 5 minutes per cup.)
2 teaspoons chopped fresh thyme	
1 bay leaf	
¾ cup frozen peas, thawed	*5* Remove the mixture from heat, take out the bay leaf, and stir in the peas and Parmesan. Season the risotto with salt and pepper to taste.
⅓ cup grated Parmesan cheese	
Salt and pepper to taste	

Per serving: Calories 282 (From Fat 47); Glycemic Load 5 (Low); Fat 5g (Saturated 2g); Cholesterol 9mg; Sodium 179mg; Carbohydrate 50g (Dietary Fiber 11g); Protein 10g.

Note: You know the barley mixture is finished in Step 4 when the barley grains are tender and the whole dish is a nice, creamy consistency. You may not need all the broth to hit this desired creaminess. On the other hand, you may need more broth than the recipe calls for and may need to add an additional cup, depending on how you like your risotto cooked.

Vary It! For all the vegans out there, you can simply omit the Parmesan cheese in Step 5 and use trans-fat-free margarine in place of butter.

Stuffed Sweet Peppers

Prep time: 25 min • **Cook time:** About 40 min • **Yield:** 6 servings

Ingredients	*Directions*
1½ cups cooked brown rice	**1** Preheat the oven to 350 degrees. In a large bowl, mix together the rice, tomatoes, onion, kidney beans, olives, pine nuts, salt, and black pepper.
3 small Roma tomatoes, chopped	
1 small sweet onion, chopped	**2** Place the peppers in a microwavable dish with about ½ inch of water in the bottom. Microwave the peppers on high for 6 minutes.
⅔ cup canned red kidney beans, rinsed and drained	
One 4.25-ounce can sliced ripe olives	**3** While the peppers are in the microwave, mix together the tomato sauce, water, garlic, oregano, and basil in a small saucepan, and bring to a boil over high heat. Reduce the heat to low, and simmer for 10 minutes.
¼ cup pine nuts	
1 teaspoon salt	
½ teaspoon black pepper	
6 large orange or yellow peppers, cored and seeded with bottoms intact	**4** Spray a 9-x-13-inch baking pan or casserole dish with nonstick cooking spray. In a large bowl, mix together the rice mixture and half of the tomato sauce mixture, and blend well.
One 8-ounce can tomato sauce	
¼ cup water	**5** Place the peppers bottom-side down in the sprayed dish, and stuff them to the top with the rice-tomato mixture. Pour the remaining tomato sauce mixture over the peppers. Sprinkle each pepper with 1 tablespoon of mozzarella cheese, cover loosely with aluminum foil, and bake for 25 minutes. Remove the cover, and bake for an additional 5 minutes.
1 clove garlic, crushed	
1 teaspoon dried oregano	
½ teaspoon dried basil	
Nonstick cooking spray	
6 tablespoons grated mozzarella cheese	

Per serving: Calories 221 (From Fat 63); Glycemic Load 8 (Low); Fat 7g (Saturated 2g); Cholesterol 6mg; Sodium 820mg; Carbohydrate 34g (Dietary Fiber 6g); Protein 9g.

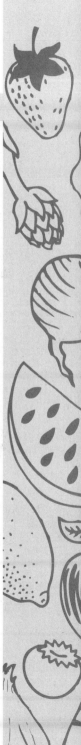

Roasted Vegetables with Lentils

Prep time: 15 min • **Cook time:** About 35 min • **Yield:** 4 servings

Ingredients	Directions
Nonstick cooking spray	**1** Preheat the oven to 400 degrees. Spray a roasting pan with nonstick cooking spray; set aside.
1 eggplant, cut into 1-inch chunks	
1 large zucchini, cut into 1-inch chunks	**2** In a large bowl, mix together the eggplant, zucchini, potatoes, onion, olive oil, and garlic until the vegetables are well coated. Spread the vegetables in the roasting pan, and bake them until they're tender, about 30 minutes; turn the vegetables once during cooking.
2 new potatoes, cut into 1-inch chunks	
1 onion, sliced	
1 tablespoon extra-virgin olive oil	**3** While the veggies are cooking, mix together the lentils, broth, vinegar, wine, tomato sauce, oregano, and parsley in a large pot; bring the mixture to a boil over high heat. Turn the heat down to low, and simmer for 30 minutes, or until the lentils are tender.
1 clove garlic, chopped	
⅔ cup brown lentils, rinsed	
1 cup low-sodium vegetable broth	**4** Stir in the roasted vegetables, season with salt and pepper to taste, and cook over low heat until the flavors are well blended, about 5 minutes.
2 teaspoons balsamic vinegar	
¼ cup dry white wine	**5** Ladle the vegetable-lentil mixture into serving bowls, and sprinkle each serving with 1½ tablespoons of Parmesan cheese.
½ cup tomato sauce	
1 teaspoon dried oregano	
2 tablespoons chopped fresh parsley	
Salt and pepper to taste	
6 tablespoons grated Parmesan cheese	

Per serving: Calories 324 (From Fat 60); Glycemic Load 11 (Medium); Fat 7g (Saturated 2g); Cholesterol 6mg; Sodium 298mg; Carbohydrate 52g (Dietary Fiber 14g); Protein 17g.

Tip: The roasted vegetables topped with tomato sauce make this dish a tasty dinner for any night of the week. Just make sure to give yourself enough time to roast the veggies.

Polenta Lasagna

Prep time: 15 min, plus standing time • **Cook time:** 29–32 min • **Yield:** 8 servings

Ingredients	*Directions*
Nonstick cooking spray	*1* Preheat the oven to 375 degrees. Spray a 9-x-13-inch baking dish with nonstick cooking spray; set aside.
2 teaspoons extra-virgin olive oil	
2 zucchini, cut lengthwise into ¼- to ⅛-inch-thick slices	*2* In a large skillet, heat the oil over medium heat. Add the zucchini, mushrooms, and onions, and salt and pepper to taste; cook until the veggies are softened, about 6 to 8 minutes. Drain any liquid, and set aside.
2 portobello mushrooms, thinly sliced	
½ yellow onion, thinly sliced	*3* Arrange a single layer of polenta in the bottom of the prepared baking dish. Spread the pesto over the polenta. Spread the sautéed vegetables over the pesto, and sprinkle with the basil, thyme, and ½ cup of the mozzarella cheese. Spread 1 cup of the marinara sauce over the cheese and herbs, and arrange the next layer of polenta on top. Top with the remaining sauce.
Salt and pepper to taste	
One 18-ounce package polenta, cut into ¼-inch-thick slices	
¼ cup basil pesto	
2 tablespoons chopped fresh basil	
1 tablespoon chopped fresh thyme	*4* Bake, uncovered, for 20 minutes. Top the polenta with the remaining mozzarella cheese, and turn on the broiler to broil the lasagna until the cheese lightly browns, about 3 to 4 minutes, watching the cheese carefully to make sure it doesn't burn. Let the lasagna sit for 5 to 10 minutes before cutting and serving.
½ cup plus ½ cup shredded mozzarella cheese	
1 cup plus 1 cup marinara sauce	

Per serving: Calories 191 (From Fat 86); Glycemic Load 19 (Medium); Fat 10g (Saturated 4g); Cholesterol 15mg; Sodium 649mg; Carbohydrate 19g (Dietary Fiber 3g); Protein 8g.

Note: Feel free to use the Basic Polenta recipe from Chapter 14 to make your own polenta for this recipe instead of using packaged polenta.

Vary It! You can change the sautéed vegetables to anything you enjoy, like squash or even fresh spinach.

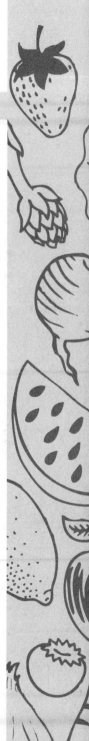

Autumn Vegetable and Polenta Ragout

Prep time: 12 min • **Cook time:** 41–52 min • **Yield:** 6 servings

Ingredients	Directions
1 tablespoon extra-virgin olive oil	**1** Preheat the oven to 400 degrees. In a large bowl, mix together the olive oil and garlic. Add the onion, carrots, squash, and black pepper, and stir to coat the vegetables evenly.
3 cloves garlic, minced	
1 onion, peeled and cut into 1-inch chunks	
2 carrots, peeled, ends trimmed, and cut into 1-inch chunks	**2** Spray a roasting pan with nonstick cooking spray. Put the vegetable mixture in the roasting pan, and bake for 15 minutes. Stir the veggie mixture with a wide spatula; then bake for another 10 to 15 minutes, or until the vegetables are tender enough to be pierced with a fork.
2½ pounds butternut squash, peeled, seeded, and cut into 1-inch chunks	
¼ teaspoon black pepper	**3** Steam the kale in a 6- to 8-quart saucepan with a steamer basket until wilted, about 2 to 3 minutes. Use a slotted spoon to lift the kale out of the pan, and immerse it in a bowl filled with cold water until cool.
Nonstick cooking spray	
1 pound kale, rinsed and leaves torn into bite-size pieces	
1½ cups canned white beans (cannellini or great Northern), rinsed and drained	**4** In the same pan you used in Step 3, combine the white beans, broth, thyme, roasted vegetables, tomatoes with their juices, and olives. Bring the mixture to a boil over high heat. Reduce heat to low, and simmer for 15 to 20 minutes until most of the liquid is absorbed. Add the kale, and cook until it's hot, 1 to 2 minutes. Add salt and pepper to taste.
2 cups low-sodium vegetable broth	
1 teaspoon chopped fresh thyme	
One 28-ounce can diced tomatoes	**5** Place a ½-cup mound of soft polenta on dinner plates or in shallow bowls, and ladle the vegetable mixture over the polenta.
½ cup sliced pitted kalamata olives	
Salt and pepper to taste	
3 cups soft cooked polenta	

Per serving: Calories 325 (From Fat 55); Glycemic Load 13 (Medium); Fat 6g (Saturated 1g); Cholesterol 0mg; Sodium 755mg; Carbohydrate 62g (Dietary Fiber 14g); Protein 10g.

Vary It! If you aren't a fan of kale, feel free to replace it with spinach.

Note: For this recipe, you can use either prepackaged polenta or the Basic Polenta recipe we include in Chapter 14.

Quinoa with White Beans and Tomatoes

Prep time: 10 min • **Cook time:** 30 min • **Yield:** 3 servings

Ingredients	Directions
1 cup quinoa, rinsed and drained	*1* In a medium saucepan, bring the quinoa and broth to a boil over high heat. Reduce the heat to medium-low, cover, and simmer until the quinoa is tender, about 20 to 25 minutes.
2 cups low-sodium vegetable broth	
1 cup white beans (cannellini or great Northern), rinsed and drained	*2* Stir in the white beans, and cook for 5 minutes.
6 cherry tomatoes, chopped	*3* Remove the quinoa-bean mixture from the stove and stir in the tomatoes, green onions, lime juice, cumin, and basil until well blended and heated. Divide into 3 bowls and serve.
2 green onions, chopped	
1 tablespoon lime juice	
1 teaspoon ground cumin	
3 tablespoons chopped fresh basil	

Per serving: Calories 314 (From Fat 38); Glycemic Load 16 (Medium); Fat 4g (Saturated 0g); Cholesterol 0mg; Sodium 70mg; Carbohydrate 57g (Dietary Fiber 8g); Protein 12g.

Tip: Serve this entree with a big side salad like the Cranberry Walnut Salad in Chapter 12 for a complete and balanced meal.

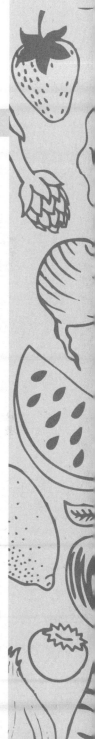

Quinoa with Black Beans and Vegetables

Prep time: 10 min • **Cook time:** 25 min • **Yield:** 4 servings

Ingredients	Directions
2 cups low-sodium vegetable broth	**1** In a large pot, bring the vegetable broth and quinoa to a boil over high heat. Reduce the heat to low, and simmer for 20 minutes, or until the quinoa is tender.
1 cup quinoa, rinsed and drained	
1 cup canned black beans, rinsed and drained	**2** Add the black beans, hominy, bell pepper, green onions, and tomatoes, and cook for an additional 5 minutes. Remove from heat.
½ cup canned hominy, rinsed and drained	
1 red bell pepper, chopped	**3** In a small bowl, mix the lime juice, vinegar, salt, cumin, and cayenne pepper until well blended. Pour the dressing into the quinoa mixture, and stir until the dressing coats the quinoa.
2 green onions, chopped	
6 cherry tomatoes, halved	
¼ cup fresh lime juice, or to taste	**4** Mix in the cheese and cilantro, and serve.
1 teaspoon balsamic vinegar	
1 teaspoon salt	
1 teaspoon ground cumin	
¼ teaspoon cayenne pepper	
½ cup grated queso fresco	
¼ cup chopped fresh cilantro	

Per serving: *Calories 312 (From Fat 55); Glycemic Load 15 (Medium); Fat 6g (Saturated 2g); Cholesterol 10mg; Sodium 191mg; Carbohydrate 51g (Dietary Fiber 9g); Protein 14g.*

Vary It! If you like more spice in your food, throw in a chopped jalapeño or add a little more cayenne pepper.

Tip: If you can't find queso fresco cheese, you can replace the same amount with a shredded Mexican blend or Monterey Jack.

1 Can't Believe It's Not Meat!

Eating vegetarian meals doesn't mean you have to succumb to eating twigs and berries, tasteless tofu, or fake soy products. In fact, you can create healthy, low-glycemic meals that are as hearty and filling as any meat entree.

For those of you who are just venturing into trying some vegetarian meals, you're sure to love this section. You won't know you're missing any meat thanks to the delicious flavors of these entrees, which we've split into the following three categories:

- ✔ **Beans:** Beans are great for vegetarian meals because they're low-glycemic carbohydrates and good sources of protein. Not to mention, they're high in fiber and folate. In this section, you find some of the good, old bean basics like burritos and burgers. Remember, even if you aren't a vegetarian, these meals are great additions to your weekly menu.

- ✔ **Mushrooms:** Mushrooms are a great addition to vegetarian meals because they add a meatlike texture that helps make the meal more satisfying. They're also low in calories and oh-so enjoyable to eat.

- ✔ **Soy products:** Soy is a wonderful source of protein and works great in a vegetarian diet. You can create all kinds of delicious dishes with two different varieties of soy products: tofu and tempeh.

Bean and Cheese Burritos

Prep time: 10 min • **Cook time:** 20 min • **Yield:** 4 servings

Ingredients	Directions
1 tablespoon canola oil	**1** In a small saucepan, heat the oil over medium-high heat. Add the shallot, and cook until it's softened, about 3 minutes. Stir in the pinto beans and jalapeño pepper, and cook for 2 minutes, lightly mashing the mixture against the side of the pan as it cooks.
1 shallot, finely chopped	
One 15.5-ounce can pinto beans, rinsed and drained	
1 jalapeño pepper, seeded and chopped finely	
½ cup low-sodium vegetable broth	**2** Stir the broth into the bean mixture, and bring it to a boil over medium-high heat. Turn the heat down to low, and simmer for about 10 minutes, continuing to mash the mixture until it has thickened. Stir in the corn and tomatoes, and cook until everything is heated through, about 5 minutes. Stir in the lime juice, remove the mixture from heat, and set aside.
1¼ cups canned corn kernels, rinsed and drained	
2 cups diced tomatoes	
Juice of ½ lime	
Four 8-inch low-carb or whole-wheat flour tortillas	**3** Heat the tortillas in the microwave for 10 seconds. Sprinkle 2 tablespoons of the cheese in the center of each tortilla, and spoon about ¼ cup of the bean mixture on top of the cheese. Fold the tortilla burrito-style, and serve with ¼ cup of salsa per serving.
½ cup shredded Monterey Jack cheese	
1 cup salsa	

Per serving: Calories 334 (From Fat 98); Glycemic Load 19 (Medium); Fat 11g (Saturated 3g); Cholesterol 13mg; Sodium 498mg; Carbohydrate 44g (Dietary Fiber 14g); Protein 16g.

Tip: To lower the calorie and fat content of this recipe, you can replace the Monterey Jack cheese with a lowfat cheddar.

Black Bean and Cheese Enchiladas

Prep time: 20 min • **Cook time:** 25–35 min • **Yield:** 5 servings

Ingredients	*Directions*
1 tablespoon canola oil	*1* Preheat the oven to 350 degrees.
1 shallot, chopped	
1 small green bell pepper, seeded and chopped	*2* In a large skillet, heat the oil over medium-high heat. Add the shallot and green bell pepper, and sauté them until they begin to soften, about 4 minutes. Add the cumin, chili powder, and oregano, and stir for about 30 seconds.
1 teaspoon ground cumin	
½ teaspoon chili powder	
½ teaspoon dried oregano	*3* Turn down the heat to medium, and add the tomato paste and broth; stir until everything is well blended and the liquid has been absorbed. Add the black beans, mix well, and remove from heat.
3 tablespoons tomato paste	
¼ cup low-sodium vegetable broth	
One 15-ounce can black beans, rinsed and drained	*4* Pour ½ cup of enchilada sauce in the bottom of a 9-x-13-inch glass baking dish. For each tortilla, spread about 2 tablespoons of the black bean mixture down the center, and top with 1 to 2 tablespoons of shredded cheese. Roll the tortillas, and place them in a row in the bottom of the pan. Repeat until all tortillas are filled.
One 12-ounce bottle red enchilada sauce	
Ten 8-inch low-carb or whole-wheat flour tortillas	
1¼ cups grated Mexican-blend cheese	*5* Pour the remaining enchilada sauce over the top of the enchiladas, and sprinkle them with the remaining cheese. Bake for 20 to 30 minutes until the cheese is melted and everything is warmed through.
5 tablespoons lowfat sour cream	
	6 Serve 2 enchiladas per serving with a small dollop (about 1 tablespoon) of sour cream on top.

Per serving: Calories 436 (From Fat 136); Glycemic Load 19 (Medium); Fat 16g (Saturated 8g); Cholesterol 36mg; Sodium 582mg; Carbohydrate 48g (Dietary Fiber 8g); Protein 18g.

Vary It! If you don't like or can't find a Mexican-blend cheese, you can use grated cheddar or Monterey Jack instead.

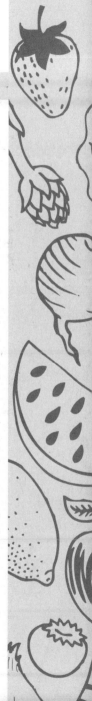

Black Bean Burgers

Prep time: 10 min • **Cook time:** 6–8 min • **Yield:** 4 servings

Ingredients	*Directions*
One 15-ounce can black beans, rinsed and drained ¼ cup plain, dry bread crumbs ¼ cup finely chopped onion	*1* In a medium bowl, mash the beans with a fork. Mix in the bread crumbs, onion, salsa, Worcestershire sauce, cumin, chili powder, oregano, and cilantro.
1 tablespoon salsa 1 tablespoon Worcestershire sauce	*2* Wet your hands with a little bit of water; then shape the bean mixture into four 3- to 4-inch patties.
1 teaspoon ground cumin ½ teaspoon chili powder ¼ teaspoon dried oregano 2 tablespoons chopped fresh cilantro	*3* Spray a large nonstick skillet with nonstick cooking spray, and heat it over medium-high heat. Place the burgers in the pan, and cook them until they're heated through, about 3 to 4 minutes per side.
Nonstick cooking spray 4 slices cheddar cheese 4 small whole-wheat hamburger buns (optional) 4 slices lettuce 4 slices tomato	*4* Place 1 slice of cheese on the top of each burger, and continue to cook the burger until the cheese begins to melt. Serve each burger on a whole-wheat bun (if desired) with 1 slice each of lettuce and tomato.

Per serving: Calories 218 (From Fat 95); Glycemic Load 19 (Medium); Fat 11g (Saturated 6g); Cholesterol 30mg; Sodium 431mg; Carbohydrate 18g (Dietary Fiber 5g); Protein 12g.

Tip: Although this version is pan-fried, you can also grill these burgers in the summer (or any time it's warm outside!).

Tip: Omit the bun for a lower-calorie, lower-glycemic meal. Omitting the bread makes the esti-mated glycemic load 10. You can also replace the cheese with lowfat cheddar to save some cal-ories and fat.

Stuffed Portobello Mushrooms

Prep time: 10 min • **Cook time:** 14 min • **Yield:** 6 servings

Ingredients	*Directions*
1 tablespoon extra-virgin olive oil 1 shallot, minced	*1* In a large skillet, heat the olive oil over medium heat. Add the shallot, and cook until it's softened, about 3 minutes.
2 tablespoons dry white wine 4 cups fresh baby spinach ⅓ cup chopped sun-dried tomatoes, not packed in oil	*2* Add the wine, spinach, and sun-dried tomatoes, and cook, stirring occasionally, until the spinach is just wilting, about 1 minute. Remove from heat, and place the mixture in a small bowl to cool completely.
One 4-ounce container crumbled goat cheese 6 medium portobello mushrooms, stems removed and inside gills scraped out with a spoon	*3* After the spinach mixture is cool, stir in the goat cheese. Place the mushrooms with their openings facing up on a large plate. Fill each mushroom with the spinach-cheese mixture until it's filled slightly over the top.
Nonstick cooking spray Salt and pepper to taste	*4* Spray the grill with nonstick cooking spray; then heat it to medium-high heat. Place the stuffed mushrooms on the grill, and cook them uncovered until the mushrooms are moist and softened, about 10 minutes. Season the mushrooms with salt and pepper to taste, and serve.

Per serving: *Calories 124 (From Fat 73); Glycemic Load 1 (Low); Fat 8g (Saturated 4g); Cholesterol 15mg; Sodium 286mg; Carbohydrate 7g (Dietary Fiber 2g); Protein 6g.*

Note: This recipe is super simple and delicious, and it makes a great presentation for guests. Even your meat-loving friends and family will enjoy these! (Check them out for yourself in the color section.)

Note: Depending on the size of your mushrooms, you may end up with leftover stuffing. You can use it for more mushrooms or blend it into some cooked quinoa for a lovely cheesy quinoa similar to the Cheesy Quinoa with Spinach in Chapter 14.

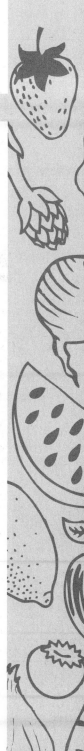

Lemon and Thyme Veggie Tofu Strips over Mixed Greens

Prep time: 15 min, plus standing time • **Cook time:** 8 min • **Yield:** 4 servings

Ingredients	Directions
1 tablespoon extra-virgin olive oil	*1* In a large mixing bowl, combine the olive oil, garlic, chopped thyme, lemon zest, and lemon juice. Toss the soy strips with the garlic-oil mixture, and let sit for 5 to 10 minutes. Remove the strips from the marinade; discard the marinade.
1 clove garlic, minced	
6 sprigs fresh thyme, leaves stripped and chopped	
2 teaspoons lemon zest	
⅓ cup lemon juice	*2* Spray a nonstick skillet with the cooking spray, and heat it over medium-high heat. Add the soy strips, and cook until they're lightly browned, about 4 minutes per side. Remove them from heat and set aside.
12 ounces soy "chicken" strips, sliced into ½-inch strips	
Olive-oil-flavored cooking spray	*3* Toss together the mixed greens, tomatoes, avocado, and salad dressing to coat everything evenly. Place the salad on 4 plates, lay the soy strips over the salad, and serve.
12 cups mixed salad greens	
2 tomatoes, diced	
1 avocado, peeled, cored, and sliced	
4 tablespoons lowfat Italian salad dressing	

Per serving: Calories 309 (From Fat 153); Glycemic Load 1 (Low); Fat 17g (Saturated 2g); Cholesterol 0mg; Sodium 487mg; Carbohydrate 23g (Dietary Fiber 11g); Protein 22g.

Note: Soy products formed into chicken-like strips are found in most supermarkets and are gaining popularity among vegetarians. Instead of just eating the prepared soy products as they are, though, try adding your own seasonings and lemon to transform them into a delicious entree over mixed salad greens.

Tempeh Stir-Fry

Prep time: 15 min • **Cook time:** 10 min • **Yield:** 4 servings

Ingredients	*Directions*
4 ounces soy tempeh, cut into ½-inch pieces	*1* In a medium bowl, stir together the tempeh, soy sauce, sherry, honey, garlic, ginger, and crushed red pepper. Let the tempeh sit while you complete the next step.
2 tablespoons low-sodium soy sauce	
1 tablespoon cooking sherry	*2* In a small saucepan with a steamer basket, steam the broccoli until it's crisp but tender enough to pierce with a fork, about 3 minutes. Set aside.
1 teaspoon honey	
3 cloves garlic, minced	
1 teaspoon ground ginger	*3* Strain the marinade from the tempeh into a small bowl; set aside the tempeh. Whisk the water and cornstarch into the strained marinade.
⅛ teaspoon crushed red pepper	
2 cups broccoli florets, cut into ½-inch pieces	*4* In a large nonstick skillet, heat the oil over high heat. Add the marinated tempeh and bell pepper, and sauté for 4 minutes.
2 tablespoons water	
1 teaspoon cornstarch	*5* Add the broccoli and marinade mixture, and sauté until the broccoli is heated through and the sauce thickens, about 3 minutes. Serve the tempeh over ½ cup brown rice per serving.
2 teaspoons canola oil	
1 red bell pepper, seeded and thinly sliced	
2 cups cooked brown rice	

Per serving: Calories 225 (From Fat 60); Glycemic Load 14 (Medium); Fat 7g (Saturated 1g); Cholesterol 0mg; Sodium 271mg; Carbohydrate 33g (Dietary Fiber 4g); Protein 10g.

Note: Tempeh originated in Indonesia and is the result of fermenting soybeans into a cakelike form. The trick to cooking with tempeh is marinating it well before you cook it. Doing so gives your meal a basic flavor; from there, you can add any other ingredients you love to complete the meal.

Note: If you can't find tempeh in your local grocery store, you can find it at most health food grocery chains and/or Asian markets.

Tip: If you don't have cooking sherry on hand, you can substitute dry white wine.

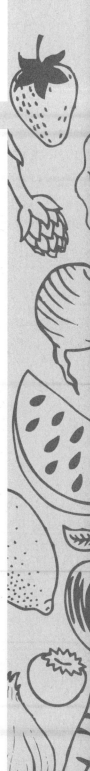

Chapter 19

Satisfying Your Sweet Tooth the Low-Glycemic Way

As dietitians, we can't emphasize enough the importance of creating diet changes that really work in your lifestyle. In other words, moderation is the key to success. We know a few of you can follow a super-strict eating plan for the long haul and be very happy doing so, but research shows that most people end up focusing too much on food and actually sabotage their efforts by being too rigid. Instead of following the all-or-nothing mentality, try adopting a more balanced approach; trust us, doing so will help you get the long-term results you're looking for.

If desserts are an important part of your life, don't panic. We're firm believers that you can conquer your sweet tooth with some dessert options that aren't overloaded in fat, calories, and sugar and some that even incorporate ingredients that are healthy for you. The recipes we include in this chapter are delicious enough to satisfy your sweetest craving, but they also provide the right balance of low fat, low calorie, and low glycemic. Read on to find some great dessert options you can fit into your regular lifestyle; that way, you can save the high-fat/sugar/calorie desserts for special occasions.

One word of caution, especially if you're a brittle diabetic: These recipes are considered low glycemic because they call for low-glycemic ingredients; however, you still need to monitor your blood sugar, pay attention to your total carbohydrate intake, and make sure you're eating the recommended portion sizes so you don't overdo it.

Rediscovering Old Dessert Favorites

The first step to cooking low-glycemic desserts is looking at your old favorites to see which recipes already fit into your low-glycemic lifestyle. You may be surprised to find that some of your recipes work perfectly as they are or that you can make minimal changes to make others fit, too.

To create a healthier version of an old dessert favorite, try making one or more of the following changes:

✔ Decrease the amount of sugar called for by one-fourth.

✔ Decrease the amount of added fats, like butter or oil, called for by one-fourth.

✔ Take advantage of foods that have already undergone clinical testing to show they have low-glycemic loads, like pudding, ice cream, fruits, and peanut butter. (See Chapter 4 for more details on glycemic load; go to www.nutritiondata.self.com to find out the glycemic load of the food you want to eat.)

In this section, we share a few old-favorite dessert recipes that need just a little tweaking to give them a low- to medium-glycemic load.

Custard with Caramel Sauce

Prep time: 10 min • **Cook time:** 30–35 min • **Yield:** 4 servings

Ingredients	*Directions*
1½ tablespoons sugar	*1* Preheat the oven to 325 degrees. In a medium saucepan, heat 3 to 4 cups of water on high to boil.
⅛ teaspoon salt	
½ teaspoon ground cinnamon	*2* In a medium bowl, beat together the sugar, salt, cinnamon, milk, eggs, and vanilla until well mixed.
2 cups evaporated skim milk	
2 eggs	*3* Place 4 ungreased 5-ounce ramekins or custard cups in a 9-inch square pan. Pour the custard mixture into the custard cups, dividing it evenly. Pour the boiling water from Step 1 into the pan around the custard cups to a depth of 1 inch.
½ teaspoon vanilla	
4 tablespoons caramel sauce	
	4 Bake for 30 to 35 minutes, or until a toothpick inserted into the center of one of the cups comes out clean.
	5 Loosen the edges of the custard away from each cup with a knife. Place a dessert plate upside down on top of each custard cup. Quickly turn each plate and custard cup over to release the custard onto the plate. Drizzle 1 tablespoon of caramel sauce on each serving of custard.

Per serving: Calories 209 (From Fat 25); Glycemic Load 18 (Medium); Fat 3g (Saturated 1g); Cholesterol 112mg; Sodium 323mg; Carbohydrate 33g (Dietary Fiber 0g); Protein 13g.

Tip: Simply omit the caramel sauce for fewer calories and a lower glycemic load.

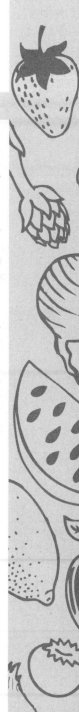

Peanut Butter Cookies

Prep time: 15 min • **Cook time:** 27–30 min • **Yield:** 36 servings

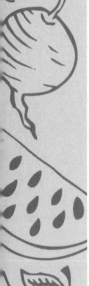

Ingredients	*Directions*
¾ **cup all-purpose flour** 1¼ **cups oat flour** ½ **teaspoon baking soda**	**1** Preheat the oven to 375 degrees. In a small bowl, combine the all-purpose flour, oat flour, and baking soda; set aside.
½ **cup trans-fat-free margarine** ½ **cup sugar** 2 **tablespoons brown sugar** ¾ **cup chunky natural peanut butter, no sugar added**	**2** In a separate bowl, use an electric mixer on low to medium speed to lightly beat the margarine until soft. Add the sugar, brown sugar, and peanut butter. Beat the mixture on low to medium speed until smooth, scraping the bowl's edges as necessary. (Note that the nuts from the chunky peanut butter will make the mixture a little lumpy.)
2 **egg whites** 1½ **teaspoons vanilla**	**3** Add the egg whites and vanilla, and mix well. Add the flour mixture, and beat everything together slowly.
	4 For each cookie, drop 1 tablespoonful of cookie dough onto an ungreased cookie sheet lined with parchment paper. Lightly press down on each cookie with the back of a fork to leave fork lines.
	5 Bake for 9 to 10 minutes, or until the edges turn golden brown.
	6 Place the cookies on wax paper to cool, and bake 2 more batches to use the rest of your dough.

Per serving: Calories 93 (From Fat 48); Glycemic Load 4 (Low); Fat 5g (Saturated 1g); Cholesterol 0mg; Sodium 68mg; Carbohydrate 9g (Dietary Fiber 1g); Protein 2g.

Note: The great thing about peanut butter cookies is that their main ingredient — peanut butter — is naturally low glycemic. Just make sure to buy natural peanut butter with no added sugar — you know, the kind you mix and store in the refrigerator. Other peanut butters contain more sugar and will increase the glycemic load of this recipe.

Note: You can store the cookies in an airtight container for up to a week.

Tip: Every oven is different, so watch your first batch closely to figure out exactly how long you need to bake each batch. It may be less than 9 minutes.

Pumpkin Soufflé

Prep time: 15 min • **Cook time:** 30–45 min • **Yield:** 6 servings

Ingredients	*Directions*
3 egg whites	*1* Preheat the oven to 350 degrees. In a medium bowl, beat the egg whites with a whisk until stiff; set aside.
3 cups canned pumpkin	
¼ cup sugar	*2* In a large bowl, use an electric mixer to blend the pumpkin, sugar, cinnamon, nutmeg, cloves, vanilla, egg yolk, and milk.
2 teaspoons ground cinnamon	
1 teaspoon ground nutmeg	
¼ teaspoon ground cloves	*3* With a large rubber spatula, fold ⅓ of the egg whites into the pumpkin mixture just to blend them. Continue to fold in the egg whites ⅓ at a time until all the egg whites are in the mixture. (Don't overmix, or else the soufflé will fall flat instead of being fluffy.)
½ teaspoon vanilla	
1 egg yolk	
½ cup lowfat milk	
3 teaspoons butter	*4* Grease six 5-inch ramekins or custard cups with ½ teaspoon of butter (or just enough to grease each ramekin). Pour the pumpkin soufflé mix into the ramekins, leaving about ½ inch at the top of each one.
6 tablespoons reduced-fat whipped topping	
	5 Place the cups on a baking pan or a cookie sheet, and bake them for 30 to 45 minutes, or until the tops are dry and browning. Make sure you don't open the oven door while the soufflés are cooking, or else they won't rise properly. Use the oven light to check on them.
	6 Top each cup with 1 tablespoon of whipped topping, and serve immediately.

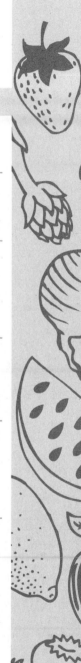

Per serving: Calories 131 (From Fat 37); Glycemic Load 10 (Low); Fat 4g (Saturated 2g); Cholesterol 41mg; Sodium 45mg; Carbohydrate 20g (Dietary Fiber 6g); Protein 5g.

Note: Pumpkin soufflé is a nice change from pumpkin pie, and it works well in a low-glycemic diet. Most soufflé recipes already use low amounts of sugar, and pumpkin itself is a low- to medium-glycemic food, depending on how much you use.

Freshening Things Up with Some Sweet and Fruity Desserts

Fruit is a tasty treat by itself, but you can also use it to add powerful vitamins, minerals, and antioxidants to sweet desserts you can feel good about eating and sharing with your family. How sweet is that!

This section is dedicated to combining healthy ingredients with smaller amounts of sugar and fat to make sweet and fruity desserts that are low glycemic and high in nutrients.

Strawberry Mousse with Chocolate Shavings

Prep time: 10 min • **Yield:** 8 servings

Ingredients	*Directions*
One 10-ounce package frozen unsweetened strawberries, thawed **¼ cup powdered sugar** **One 3.5-ounce package instant vanilla pudding mix** **One 8-ounce package frozen reduced-fat whipped topping, thawed** **8 tablespoons grated dark chocolate**	*1* Put the strawberries and any juices from thawing in a blender, and blend until smooth. Add the sugar and vanilla pudding mix, and whip until thick. Pour the mixture into a large bowl, and fold in the whipped topping until well blended and thick. *2* Divide the strawberry mousse evenly into glass sundae dishes or small water glasses (about ¾ cup of mousse per dish), and sprinkle 1 tablespoon of grated dark chocolate on top of each serving.

Per serving: Calories 162 (From Fat 46); Glycemic Load 10 (Low); Fat 5g (Saturated 4g); Cholesterol 0mg; Sodium 179mg; Carbohydrate 27g (Dietary Fiber 1g); Protein 1g.

Note: This recipe is the perfect solution when you're looking for a quick and easy dessert that's full of flavor but light on calories and sugar. It's also a great way to get in a serving of fruit with frozen strawberries! You can check out this dish in the color section.

Note: You can store the mousse covered in an airtight container in the refrigerator for up to 3 to 4 days.

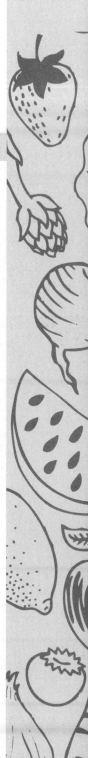

Baked Peaches with Vanilla Frozen Yogurt

Prep time: 5 min • **Cook time:** 13–15 min • **Yield:** 6 servings

Ingredients	Directions
Nonstick cooking spray	**1** Preheat the oven to 400 degrees. Spray a 9-x-9-inch baking dish with nonstick cooking spray, and place the peaches in the dish, sliced sides up.
3 fresh freestone peaches, peeled, sliced in half, and pits removed	
2 tablespoons brown sugar	**2** In a small bowl, mix together the brown sugar and cinnamon until well blended. Sprinkle about 1 teaspoon of the sugar mixture over each peach slice.
½ teaspoon ground cinnamon	
2 cups vanilla frozen yogurt	**3** Bake the peaches in the oven for about 13 to 15 minutes, or until they're tender.
	4 Top each peach with a small scoop of frozen yogurt, about ⅓ cup per serving.

Per serving: Calories 107 (From Fat 8); Glycemic Load 14 (Medium); Fat 1g (Saturated 0g); Cholesterol 3mg; Sodium 41mg; Carbohydrate 22g (Dietary Fiber 1g); Protein 3g.

Tip: Because the baking process makes the fruit naturally sweeter, you don't have to add much to create a delicious, sweet-tooth-satisfying dish. You can serve these peaches with vanilla frozen yogurt (like we do in this recipe) or with 1 tablespoon of reduced-fat whipped topping.

Blueberry Crisp

Prep time: 10 min • **Cook time:** 35 min • **Yield:** 6 servings

Ingredients	Directions
2½ cups fresh blueberries	*1* Preheat the oven to 350 degrees. Rinse the blueberries and drain them, allowing a good amount of water to cling to the berries.
½ teaspoon ground cinnamon	
1 tablespoon plus 2 tablespoons packed light brown sugar	*2* Place the berries in a 9-x-9-inch glass pie dish, and sprinkle them with the cinnamon and 1 tablespoon of brown sugar; stir to blend. Let the berries stand until the sugar dissolves and coats the berries, about 3 minutes.
½ cup quick-cooking oats	
¼ cup oat flour	
¼ teaspoon salt	*3* In a medium bowl, combine the oats, flour, salt, and remaining 2 tablespoons of brown sugar; stir to blend. Add the oil, and rub it in with your fingertips or a fork until moist clumps form. Stir in the almonds, and mix until well blended.
¼ cup canola oil	
¼ cup sliced almonds	
1⅓ cups lowfat vanilla frozen yogurt (optional)	*4* Sprinkle the oat mixture evenly over the blueberries, and bake the crisp until the berries are bubbling and the topping is golden, about 35 minutes. Serve warm with ¼ cup of frozen yogurt per serving.

Per serving: Calories 205 (From Fat 111); Glycemic Load 18 (Medium); Fat 12g (Saturated 1g); Cholesterol 0mg; Sodium 103mg; Carbohydrate 23g (Dietary Fiber 3g); Protein 3g.

Note: Simply omit the frozen yogurt to decrease the calories and glycemic load.

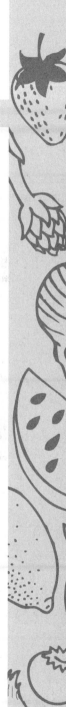

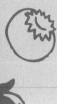

Cream Cheese Pie with Fresh Berries

Prep time: 10 min, plus refrigerating time • **Cook time:** 5–10 min • **Yield:** 8 servings

Ingredients	Directions
Nonstick cooking spray	**1** Preheat the oven to 400 degrees. Spray a 9-x-9-inch glass or metal pie dish with nonstick cooking spray, and set aside.
1½ cups lowfat granola	
¼ cup trans-fat-free margarine	
8 ounces lowfat cream cheese, room temperature	**2** Coarsely grind the granola in a blender or food processor; then transfer the mixture to a medium bowl. Cream in the margarine with a spoon until it makes a batter with the granola.
⅓ cup plus 1 tablespoon powdered sugar	
1 teaspoon vanilla extract	**3** Press the granola mixture into the bottom of the pie pan, and bake until the crust mixture is set and beginning to brown, about 5 to 10 minutes; don't exceed 10 minutes. Place the pie pan on a metal rack, and cool completely.
½ teaspoon almond extract	
½ cup frozen reduced-fat whipped topping, thawed	
1 cup mixed fresh blackberries and raspberries	**4** In a large bowl, combine the cream cheese, ⅓ cup of sugar, vanilla extract, and almond extract. Use a hand mixer to blend the mixture until it's very smooth and thick, occasionally scraping the sides of the bowl. Add the whipped topping, and continue mixing until well blended.
	5 Spread the cream cheese filling over the prepared crust. Refrigerate the pie until the filling is firm, about 2 hours.
	6 Rinse the berries, and drain them, allowing some water to cling to the berries. Arrange the mixed berries over the top of the pie, and sprinkle with 1 tablespoon of powdered sugar; serve immediately.

Per serving: Calories 245 (From Fat 125); Glycemic Load 15 (Medium); Fat 14g (Saturated 7g); Cholesterol 22mg; Sodium 192mg; Carbohydrate 25g (Dietary Fiber 2g); Protein 5g.

Vary It! You can change the berries to whatever you like — perhaps using strawberries or even huckleberries if you live in the Pacific Northwest. Check out this dessert in the color section.

Don't Forget the Chocolate!

Don't worry; we wouldn't dream of writing a dessert chapter without chocolate! You might say we're fans. Many traditional chocolate desserts contain loads of calories, sugars, and fats — which is unfortunate because chocolate itself is actually healthy.

Recent studies show that cocoa and dark chocolate with a high cocoa content contain many heart-healthy antioxidants, including a group of compounds called *flavonoids*. These compounds have been shown to help increase good cholesterol, and decrease risk of stroke, and they may even help prevent certain cancers. Unfortunately, milk chocolate and white chocolate don't offer these same health benefits, so, to get all the chocolaty benefits, stick with cocoa in the kitchen.

Lucky for those of you who, like us, need a chocolate fix from time to time, chocolate-style desserts don't have to be laden with calories and fat. This section offers you some delightful chocolate recipes that are low glycemic as well as low fat and low calorie. The next time you feel a craving coming on, turn to this chapter instead of opening an extra-large chocolate bar!

Chocolate Peanut Butter Ice Dream

Prep time: 10 min, plus freezing time • **Yield:** 10 servings

Ingredients	Directions
Two 3.5-ounce packages instant vanilla pudding mix	*1* Using 3¼ cups of milk or the amount of milk listed in the package directions (whichever is larger), prepare the pudding mixes. Stir in the peanut butter and chocolate chips. Spread the mixture evenly in a 9-x-13-x-2-inch nonstick pan; cover and freeze for 4 hours.
3¼ cups skim milk	
½ cup creamy natural peanut butter, no sugar added	
1 cup semisweet chocolate chips	*2* When you're ready to serve your dessert, pull the ice dream out of the freezer, and let it sit for 5 to 10 minutes, or until it's soft enough to scoop.
	3 Use an ice cream scoop to scoop out about ⅔ cup for each serving; store any extra dessert in the freezer.

Per serving: Calories 298 (From Fat 114); Glycemic Load 19 (Medium); Fat 13g (Saturated 5g); Cholesterol 3mg; Sodium 333mg; Carbohydrate 39g (Dietary Fiber 1g); Protein 8g.

Vary It! You can play around with the flavors in this dessert by adding chocolate with coffee for a mocha flavor or adding fruit in place of the chocolate and peanut butter. The sky's the limit!

Easy Chocolate Mousse

Prep time: 5 min • **Yield:** 8 servings

Ingredients	Directions
One 3.5-ounce package instant chocolate pudding mix	**1** In a medium bowl, mix together the pudding mix, milk, coffee, and whipped topping with a hand mixer until thick.
1¼ cups lowfat milk	
¼ cup brewed coffee, cooled	**2** Divide the mousse evenly into eight glass sundae dishes or small water glasses (about ¾ cup each).
One 8-ounce package frozen reduced-fat whipped topping, thawed	

Per serving: Calories 123 (From Fat 34); Glycemic Load 4 (Low); Fat 4g (Saturated 4g); Cholesterol 2mg; Sodium 197mg; Carbohydrate 19g (Dietary Fiber 0g); Protein 2g.

Tip: Decadent chocolate mousse is a wonderful dessert, but if you don't have the time or equipment (namely, a double boiler) to create the real thing, give this quickie version a try. It's great for an easy, tasty dessert and still satisfies your chocolate fix. We love serving this mousse with sliced strawberries.

Note: You can store the mousse covered in an airtight container in the refrigerator for 3 to 4 days.

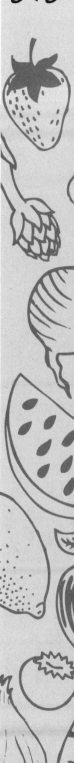

Old-School Chocolate No-Bake Cookies

Prep time: 10 min, plus cooling time • **Cook time:** 2 min • **Yield:** 12 servings

Ingredients	*Directions*
⅓ cup trans-fat-free margarine or butter ¾ cup sugar ½ cup lowfat milk 4 tablespoons cocoa	**1** In a medium saucepan, mix together the margarine (or butter), sugar, milk, and cocoa over medium-high heat. Bring the mixture to a rolling boil. Keep the mixture boiling for 1 minute; then remove the pan from heat.
½ cup chunky natural peanut butter, no sugar added 3 to 3½ cups dry quick-cooking oats	**2** Stir in the peanut butter, oats, and vanilla. For each cookie, drop 1 tablespoonful of cookie dough on wax paper.
2 teaspoons vanilla	**3** Let the cookies cool until set, about 30 minutes.

Per serving: *Calories 242 (From Fat 108); Glycemic Load 18 (Medium); Fat 12g (Saturated 3g); Cholesterol 0mg; Sodium 99mg; Carbohydrate 30g (Dietary Fiber 3g); Protein 6g.*

Note: You can store the cookies in the refrigerator in an airtight container for 4 to 6 days.

Tip: Use 3 cups of oats for very gooey cookies and 3½ cups for less gooey cookies.

Part V
The Part of Tens

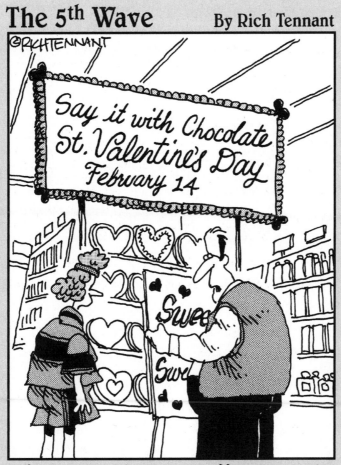

"Of course you're better off eating grains and vegetables, but for St. Valentine's Day, we've never been very successful with 'Say it with Legumes.'"

In this part . . .

Taking a holistic approach to wellness will help you stay your healthiest, so in this part, we provide ten healthy lifestyle choices that complement a low-glycemic diet and help you create a complete health plan. We also explore ten tips for sticking to your low-glycemic lifestyle during special occasions, such as parties and holidays, so you can bake your cake and eat it, too!

Chapter 20

Ten Healthy Choices to Complement a Low-Glycemic Diet

In This Chapter

▶ Realizing that one health strategy doesn't work without a few others

▶ Discovering ways to improve your health with small daily changes

*A*s we discuss throughout this book, a low-glycemic diet isn't a stand-alone solution for your overall health and weight-loss goals; it's part of a much bigger picture. To be successful with your health goals, you need to take a more holistic approach and consider your physical, emotional, and psychological health. For example, if your goal is weight loss, don't expect to see many results if you don't pay attention to your physical activity and stress levels in addition to your diet. Or if you want to decrease your cholesterol, you can't focus solely on diet and exercise because stress and sleep may also play a role. Like many other aspects of life, health questions rarely have just one solution.

This chapter covers our top-ten lifestyle choices, in addition to maintaining a low-glycemic diet, that provide a holistic approach for meeting your health goals.

Enjoy Some Exercise

Regular exercise is an important part of your overall health. We know you've probably heard this message before, but it's certainly worth repeating. Although you may think of exercise as being important first and foremost for weight management, it's also crucial for your body's overall well-being; it's essential to your body's ability to work at its best capacity. The benefits of regular exercise include

✔ Increased energy

✔ Improved mood

✔ A lower risk of chronic diseases like heart disease and diabetes

✔ Better bone health

✔ Reduced stress

When you're first starting an exercise routine (or simply changing an existing one), try to include both cardiovascular exercise to get your heart rate up and strength training to build your muscles and optimize your metabolism. Some people love the gym and others don't, so before you get started, think of the types of physical activities you enjoy. Maybe just walking is the thing for you, or perhaps swimming is more your style. Whatever you do, try to incorporate 20 to 30 minutes of exercise into your routine each day.

Always check with your doctor before starting an exercise program to make sure it's appropriate for your unique situation.

Sleep Blissfully

Sleep is one of those things that people are getting less and less of, yet it's still an important part of your overall health. You may be surprised to find out just how much a lack of sleep can put you at risk of certain health issues.

According to the National Sleep Foundation, chronic lack of sleep is linked to high blood pressure, heart disease, stroke, depression, and diabetes. Research published in the *Annals of Internal Medicine* also found a connection between lack of sleep and weight gain.

Getting seven to eight hours of sleep a night is an important health strategy to put into place, so, in addition to eating right, make sure you're getting the right sleep, too. If you have sleeping problems, contact your healthcare provider to get more information on steps you can take to get back on track.

Get Your Omega-3 Fatty Acids

Research in recent years has shown just how important omega-3 fatty acids are for your health. In fact, studies show that these fatty acids act as an anti-inflammatory, which is a major health benefit because inflammation in the body is at the root of many diseases, including heart disease, cancer, and Alzheimer's. Omega-3 fatty acids can also lower *triglycerides* (a form of fat in your blood that is associated with a risk of coronary artery disease when levels are elevated) and reduce the risk of heart attacks, abnormal heart rhythms, and strokes. Essentially, what these studies show is that eating omega-3s regularly is a wonderful gift to your heart. As an added bonus, these fatty acids have been proven to be helpful with depression and anxiety.

 Good sources of omega-3 fatty acids include fatty fish like salmon and plant foods like walnuts, flaxseeds, and canola oil. Your best bet is to have two servings of fish each week. If you don't enjoy fish, ask your healthcare provider about using a fish-oil supplement.

Make Sure You Get Your Vitamin D

New research shows that more and more people are deficient in vitamin D. Lack of vitamin D is associated with bone disease, heart disease, and diabetes. Although you can find some vitamin D in food, it's limited and primarily found in fortified foods like milk.

So what can you do to get more vitamin D? Get more sun! Your body synthesizes vitamin D by being exposed to the sun. According to the National Institute of Health, approximately 5 to 30 minutes at least twice a week of sun exposure without sunscreen between 10 a.m. and 3 p.m. to the face, arms, legs, or back is sufficient to produce vitamin D. Those of you who don't go outside often or who live in cloudy areas with little sunlight, like Seattle, Washington, may be at a greater risk of vitamin-D deficiency. You may also be at greater risk if you have darker skin because the higher amount of melanin in your skin reduces your body's ability to produce vitamin D from sun exposure.

Make sure to get some sun each week, and if you're concerned about your risk factors for vitamin-D deficiency, ask your healthcare provider to test your vitamin D levels with a blood test.

Reduce Your Stress

Stress is one of those things that can damage your body without your really knowing it. In today's day and age, people have become accustomed to feeling stressed on a regular basis, and they do little to combat the physical damage it causes.

If you don't consciously work on ways to reduce your stress levels, you may be at a higher risk for many health problems, like ulcers, migraines, high blood pressure, stroke, heart attack, and lowered immune system, just to name a few. So don't try to lower your blood pressure through diet without also doing something to reduce your stress. Trust us, you won't get very far.

To decrease your stress, try to incorporate deep breathing, meditation, exercise, yoga, massage, guided imagery, or journaling into your daily routine. Also try to pay attention to your responses to situations. Do you catastrophize situations? Procrastinate? By addressing your responses to life's situations, you can help reduce or even eliminate unnecessary stressors. Find one or a few activities you can do to calm your mind each day and/or change the way you respond to life situations, and you'll be on your way to a less-stressful life and a healthier you!

Slow Down

Most people today live very fast-paced lifestyles, and, although jam-packed schedules result in high productivity, they also lead to high stress levels, lack of sleep, and poor eating habits.

Give yourself a small amount of time each day to do something slow! Read a few pages of a book before bed, or just take some time over breakfast to read the newspaper. These quiet, slow moments can reduce stress and help you recharge. You may find they help you sleep better at night, too!

Enjoy Family Meals Together

Eating meals together as a family is an important bonding time for parents and kids alike, but research suggests it may benefit your health, too. When you eat meals as a family, you focus more on the types of foods you're eating, and meal planning begins to take on more importance.

Numerous studies show that families who eat together tend to eat better, take in more nutrients, and consume more fruits and vegetables than families who don't eat together. Research has also found that kids tend to do better in school and have less risk of getting involved with drugs and alcohol when their families share meals together.

Work on making family meals happen in your home. Even if you don't have children, try to sit down for dinner with your partner or spouse. Single? Get together with some friends a few nights a week for a sit-down dinner.

Be Mindful While You Eat

You've heard of being mindful of what you eat, but how about being mindful *while* you eat? One of the biggest obstacles to weight management is eating until you're emotionally or psychologically satisfied, as opposed to physically fulfilled. Have you ever felt super full, but you still went for that last bite of brownie because it simply tasted too good to pass up? If so, you know exactly what we're talking about here.

Although it's easy to ignore your body's fullness cues, doing so regularly can result in unwanted weight gain. If you're someone who eats fast and/or for emotional reasons, you may already be in this cycle of overeating. Being mindful while you eat is a wonderful step to help you break the cycle.

To be mindful while you eat, you need to slow down and truly pay attention to what you're eating. By taking the time to notice the textures, tastes, and smells in your food, you can become satisfied with an average serving size of that food and not feel compelled to continue eating. Try to take at least 20 minutes at mealtime to really enjoy your food.

Find Humor in Your Day

Laughter is the best medicine, right? Although you may think laughter's a strange lifestyle choice to include in this list, research supports the theory that laughter can be helpful for your health. In fact, preliminary research shows that laughter can improve blood flow, increase your immune response, and even improve blood sugar levels in diabetics. Yes, more research is needed in the study of laughter's relationship to good health, but finding a few more reasons to laugh every day certainly won't hurt you!

Look for ways to add a little humor to your day. Maybe you hang up a funny day-to-day calendar at your desk, or you watch a funny television show in the evening. Do whatever works for you, and try to have at least one good belly laugh a day.

Keep a Journal to Track Everything

Keeping a journal is a great way to monitor not only your food intake but also your activity and stress levels. You don't have to keep a long-term journal if you don't want to, but, as you begin to make lifestyle changes, you need to be able to see the progress you're making and also what challenges you're facing. Journaling sets you up for success!

You will meet challenges and obstacles along the way, so you need to expect them as a normal part of your lifestyle-changing process and work on finding solutions. Journaling can help you point out your trouble areas and inspire you to ask the right questions to find the best solutions for your particular situation. For example, during your first week of journaling, you may find that by 8 p.m. every day, you break down in front of the television and graze on unhealthy snacks for the rest of the evening. Seeing that not-so-good habit on paper can guide you in asking yourself important habit-changing questions like "Am I really hungry?" and "What are some other ways I can enjoy a treat in the evening?"

Chapter 21

Ten Tips for Sticking to a Low-Glycemic Diet during Special Occasions

*I*f you've ever had to make diet changes for a health condition or for weight loss, you know how easy it is to slip into old habits during parties, holidays, and vacations. In this book, we talk a lot about balance, which is sometimes easier said than done. You don't want to deny yourself to the point that you're miserable, but you also don't want to go overboard and sabotage all your hard work.

This chapter features ten tips to help you find that elusive balance so you can enjoy yourself during these special events and still continue to meet all your health goals with a low-glycemic diet.

Make Time for Some Fun Movement

To counteract any straying from a low-glycemic diet you do during a party, holiday, vacation, or other special occasion, make sure to add extra exercise to your schedule. Adding some movement may be as simple as going for a walk or taking the stairs rather than the elevator. If you can make your exercise fun and enjoyable, you have a better chance of actually doing it.

If you're on a destination vacation, go for a swim in the ocean or hotel pool, take a hike on a nature trail, or just go for a nice stroll along a beautiful beach. If you're celebrating a special occasion at home, ask one of your friends to go for a walk to catch up, or go on a bike ride with your kids shortly before or after the occasion.

Watch Out for Alcohol

Whether you're having some margaritas at a pool party or hot buttered rum at a holiday gathering, alcoholic drinks add more calories to your diet than you may think. They may even increase your glycemic load a bit as well. To help you stay on track but still have fun, space out your drinks every few hours, and don't go overboard; one to two drinks per party is a good rule of thumb. Don't forget to drink plenty of water as well to help you stay hydrated.

Mixed-fruit drinks like margaritas can be especially troublesome because of their high sugar contents and high number of calories. Enjoy one and then move on to something less sugary.

Beware the Bread Basket

The bread basket is a sneaky, sneaky thing. Picture this: You're sitting unsuspectingly in a nice restaurant when the server casually brings a basket full of yummy little slices of bread. It's so easy to begin eating those tasty little treats when you're engaged in conversation. Before you know it the basket is empty, and you haven't a clue how many slices you ate.

The truth behind the bread basket is that it's full of high-glycemic, high-calorie filler foods that you don't really need. If you love bread, have a slice (yes, we mean *one*), but keep in mind that you're probably having another type of carbohydrate with your meal.

If you're a big bread fan, choose an entree that has only a meat and a low-glycemic vegetable; then use the bread as your starch. If you don't care too much, feel free to omit the bread altogether.

Go Big for One Meal, but Eat Light the Rest of the Day

When you know you're going to have one big meal during a particular day, eat light for the other meals. That way, you don't go overboard in your total glycemic load or calorie intake for the day. For example, imagine that you're going out for your anniversary dinner. Of course you want to indulge and eat something rich and wonderful. Doing so is perfectly fine as long as you try to eat more simply throughout the rest of the day by having something like oatmeal at breakfast and soup and salad for lunch.

Make sure you still eat small meals throughout the day. Skipping meals entirely in preparation for a big meal can negatively affect your metabolism.

This eat-big-for-one-meal-but-light-for-the-rest-of-the-day method should never feel like a punishment. For many people who have participated in a lot of weight-loss diets, tips like this may make them feel like they have to restrict in order to enjoy, but that's not true. We want you to enjoy all your meals, small and big. So your smaller meal can still be something you love — just make it something on the lighter side!

Fill Up on Low-Glycemic Choices at Parties

You know how parties are — you walk into the room and scope out the foods that have been prepared. You may find some dips and other appetizers or full entrees, depending on the type of party you're attending. What should you do now? No, the answer is not to load up a plate with everything in sight!

The best thing to do is find the low-glycemic items in the mix. Load up on those foods, and then pick one or two of your favorite high-glycemic foods and have just a small amount of them. For example, if you're at a barbeque with an array of potato salad, macaroni salad, and tossed green salad, fill your plate with the greens and get smaller portions of the macaroni and potatoes, or, better yet, have only one of the starchy sides to go with your healthy greens.

If you go to a party and can't find any low-glycemic foods, don't feel like you have to starve yourself. Instead, add some small portions of the high-glycemic foods to your plate. Doing so helps you control your overall blood sugar levels for that meal and for the day.

Take a Low-Glycemic Dish to Your Next Pitch-In Party

Potlucks are always fun, but they can turn out to be endless buffets of high-glycemic foods. One great way to ensure you have some of your favorite low-glycemic foods available is to make your pitch-in dish a low-glycemic one. Depending on the party, you may find some good pitch-in ideas in this cookbook. If you need to bring an appetizer, for example, pick a great dip like the Smoked Salmon Dip or the Mango Chutney and Brie Bake from Chapter 10. Need a salad? Take the Cranberry Walnut Salad or the Summer Melon Salad with Lime Dressing from Chapter 12.

The best part about low-glycemic recipes is that they use regular foods, so you don't have to worry about bringing something that other potluck-goers won't like. You don't even have to mention the fact that your dish is low glycemic, especially to those people who don't want "health food" at the gathering. They'll never even know your dish is good for them.

Enjoy a Holiday of Splurges, and Get Back on Track the Next Day

Imagine this scene: It's Thanksgiving Day, the whole family is gathered together, and the house smells like roasted turkey, stuffing, and sugared yams. Let's face it — no one wants to skimp on a day like that, and, we certainly don't want to ask you to. Thanksgiving and similar holidays are one-day deals, so feel free to eat what you want and not worry about it (unless, of course, you're a brittle diabetic and eating whatever you want may increase your risk of major health issues). Just be sure to get back to your low-glycemic lifestyle the day after the holiday.

If you're using a low-glycemic diet for better health or weight management, one day of indulging won't blow it for you. Just focus on getting back on track the next day.

Bake and Give Away Treats during the Holidays

Are you one of those people who really enjoys baking cookies and other goodies during the holidays? If so, don't put an end to this lovely tradition just because you're trying to maintain a low-glycemic diet. However, if you have trouble fighting off the temptation to eat all those tasty treats that sit on your countertops during the holidays, try spreading your holiday cheer through your baked treats.

Set aside a small amount of goodies for yourself and your immediate family; then give the rest away as holiday gifts to other family members and friends. That way, you can continue your baking tradition, have a few treats, but not be tempted by tons of high-glycemic foods for weeks. You can also keep your baked treats in the freezer, and take out a small amount whenever you want them. That way, you don't feel the urge to eat up all the goodies before they spoil.

Avoid the All-or-Nothing Approach during the Holidays

So you're in the middle of the big holiday season and you've just made a secret pact with yourself that starting on January 1st you're going to start paying attention to your diet choices again, but until then you're going to ignore them. Don't feel bad, you're not the only one struggling with this all-or-nothing approach to weight-loss diets.

Instead of letting your holiday-hungry mind lead you to eating every high-calorie, high-fat food in sight, challenge yourself to find a way to eat some holiday treats and maintain your low-glycemic diet at the same time. Keeping a journal with your long-term goals handy is a great way to help you get through those challenging times. You can also enlist a support buddy (friend, spouse, dietitian, or life coach) to help keep you on the right track.

You Can (Almost) Have It All on Vacation

Vacations don't mean a complete vacation from your healthy eating habits. But you also don't have to give up indulging on vacation. Just try to be conscious about your food choices, especially if your vacation lasts for a week or more. For example, avoid eating a high-glycemic breakfast every day, and, instead, eat healthier options like oatmeal with fruit or a poached egg with toast on some days and indulge on the others. You also may choose to have a light breakfast and lunch on the day you're planning a great evening out. However you try to mix your high-glycemic foods with your low-glycemic ones, just try to find that balance each day so you don't end up overeating high-glycemic foods on an everyday basis.

Part VI
Appendixes

The 5th Wave   By Rich Tennant

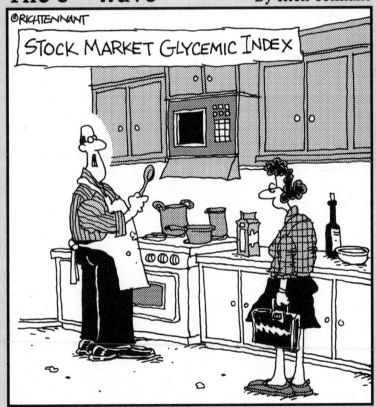

"The Glycemic Index rose 2 points today in active eating, but indicators predict a reversal of this trend due to rising blood sugar."

In this part . . .

The appendixes in this part contain a lot of useful information for implementing a low-glycemic diet. In Appendix A, you find a detailed food list (divided into food groups) showing you the glycemic load of popular foods and beverages; use this appendix to determine which foods to use in moderation and to search for low-glycemic foods to incorporate into your meals.

In case you prefer using the metric system while cooking, Appendix B provides simple conversion tables to make switching from ounces to grams (and more!) a snap.

Appendix A

The Glycemic Load and Common Foods: An At-a-Glance Guide

• •

Consider this appendix your quick-reference guide to the glycemic information for foods used in this book's recipes as well as some other common foods. The easy-to-digest information is presented in tables, with each table listing specific foods, their portion sizes, and their glycemic loads for those portion sizes. (Remember that a glycemic load of 10 or less is considered low, a glycemic load of 11 to 19 is considered medium, and a glycemic load of 20 or more is considered high.) Use this appendix to look up your favorite foods to see where they fall, as well as to help you select low-glycemic foods when planning your meals.

If you want to eat more of an item than the suggested portion size we include here, just know that doing so will likely increase that food's glycemic load a bit. If that food already has a medium-level glycemic load, you may be bumping its glycemic load up to the high range. In this situation, consider sticking to the portion size listed (and if you're still hungry, choose a lower-glycemic food to fill you up).

A good rule of thumb is to keep your total daily glycemic load under 100. If you choose mostly low- and medium-glycemic foods, you shouldn't have a problem doing so.

Bakery Treats

Who doesn't enjoy a donut, muffin, or cupcake every now and then? If you're looking for the healthiest and lowest-calorie options, choose baked goods made with whole grains and fruit. Sweet treats are just that — occasional treats that aren't meant to be an everyday part of your diet. So even though the items in Table A-1 are medium- to high-glycemic, indulging in them once in a while is perfectly okay.

Table A-1	Bakery Treats	
Food Type	*Portion Size*	*Glycemic Load*
Angel food cake	2-ounce slice	Medium
Apple muffin	1 small muffin	Medium
Blueberry muffin	1 small muffin	Medium
Cake with frosting	4-ounce slice	High
Donut	1 donut	Medium

Beverages

What's the healthiest low-glycemic beverage? If you answered water, you're right. Plain, unflavored water quenches your thirst without adding anything, including calories, and it's exactly what your body craves. Make plain water your primary beverage, and enjoy other beverages, such as the ones listed in Table A-2, in small amounts once in a while.

Table A-2	Beverages	
Food Type	*Portion Size*	*Glycemic Load*
Apple juice	1 cup	Medium
Beer	12 fluid ounces	Low
Coffee	1 cup	Low
Cranberry juice cocktail	1 cup	High
Gatorade	1 cup	Medium
Hot chocolate (from powder mixed with water)	1 cup	Medium
Lemonade	1 cup	Medium
Orange juice	1 cup	Medium
Red wine, dry	5 fluid ounces	Low
Rice milk	1 cup	High
Soymilk	1 cup	Low
Tea	1 cup	Low
Tomato juice	1 cup	Low
White wine, dry	5 fluid ounces	Low

Breads and Snacks

Whenever you purchase breads and snacks, look for the phrase *100% whole grain* on the package advertising or the word *whole* listed first in the ingredients. That way, you can be confident that you're purchasing the most wholesome, low-glycemic breads and snack products available. Make even better choices by searching out companies that specialize in producing low-glycemic foods, such as Natural Ovens (www.naturalovens.com). You can also use Table A-3 as a guide.

Table A-3	Breads and Snacks	
Food Type	*Portion Size*	*Glycemic Load*
100% whole-wheat bread	1 ounce	Medium
Air-popped popcorn	3 cups	Low
Baguette	1 ounce	Medium
Corn tortilla	1 small tortilla	Low
Gluten-free bread	1 ounce	Medium
Hamburger bun	1 large bun	Medium
Healthy Choice Hearty 100% Whole-Grain Bread	1 ounce	Low
Healthy Choice Hearty 7-Grain Bread	1 ounce	Low
Hot dog bun	1 bun	Medium
Natural Ovens 100% Whole-Grain Bread	1 ounce	Low
Natural Ovens Hunger Filler Bread	1 ounce	Low
Natural Ovens Multi-Grain Bread	1 ounce	Medium
Pita bread	½ of a 6-inch-diameter pita	Medium
Pretzels	½ cup of small pretzels	Medium
Pumpernickel bread	1 ounce	Low
Rice cakes	2 cakes	Medium

(continued)

Table A-3 *(continued)*

Food Type	Portion Size	Glycemic Load
Rye bread (whole grain or regular)	1 ounce	Low
Ryvita Rye Crispbread	2 slices	Low
Saltine crackers	3 crackers	Medium
White bagel	3 ounces	High
White Wonder bread	1 ounce	Medium

Breakfast Foods

Tread carefully when it comes to choosing breakfast foods so that you incorporate low-glycemic foods as often as possible. Low-glycemic foods fill you up with fewer calories and help you stay satisfied longer than their high-glycemic counterparts, so, if you want to avoid a midmorning energy crash, skip the donuts and choose low-glycemic breakfast foods instead. Check out Table A-4 for guidance on what foods to add to your daily menu.

Table A-4   Breakfast Foods

Food Type	Portion Size	Glycemic Load
Cheerios	1 cup	Medium
Instant oatmeal, unflavored	1 cup	Medium
Kellogg's All-Bran	½ cup	Low
Kellogg's Corn Flakes	1 cup	High
Kellogg's Raisin Bran	½ cup	Medium
Kellogg's Special K	1 cup	Medium
Oatmeal from steel-cut oats	¾ cup	Low
Old-fashioned oats	¾ cup	Medium
Pancake	One 4-inch pancake	Low
Post Grape-Nuts or Grape-Nuts Flakes	⅓ cup	Medium
Waffle	One 4-inch waffle	Low

Dairy Products

Fat-free milk and yogurt are excellent sources of calcium and vitamin D, and they have a low glycemic load. Other dairy products, like the ones listed in Table A-5, are also good choices when you're craving something dairy but don't want to overdo it with calories and fat.

Table A-5	Dairy Products	
Food Type	*Portion Size*	*Glycemic Load*
Chocolate milk	1 cup	Low
Evaporated skim milk	1 cup	Medium
Frozen yogurt	1 cup	Medium
Ice cream (including lowfat and sugar-free varieties)	1 cup	Low
Lowfat instant pudding	½ cup	Low
Milk (skim, 1%, 2%, or whole)	1 cup	Low
Plain yogurt (or any no-sugar-added yogurt)	1 cup	Low

Fruits

Fruit sometimes (and undeservingly!) gets a bad rap because it's a sweet, natural source of carbohydrates. Don't let that stereotype come between you and your daily fruit servings because fruits are quite good for you. They provide fiber, vitamins, minerals, and phytochemicals to promote overall health. The glycemic index and glycemic load can help you make sound decisions about the healthiest types of fruits to enjoy. Refer to Table A-6 and choose fresh fruit as often as possible to take advantage of its lower glycemic load compared to snacks like potato chips and candy bars.

Table A-6	Fruits	
Food Type	**Portion Size**	**Glycemic Load**
Apples	1 medium apple	Low
Bananas	1 medium ripe banana	Medium
Blackberries	½ cup	Low
Blueberries	½ cup	Low
Cantaloupe	¾ cup	Low
Dried cranberries	¼ cup	Medium
Grapefruit	½ medium grapefruit	Low
Grapes (green or red)	¾ cup	Low
Honeydew	¾ cup	Low
Oranges	1 medium orange	Low
Peaches (canned in heavy syrup)	½ cup	Medium
Peaches (canned in juice)	½ cup	Low
Peaches (fresh)	1 large peach	Low
Pears (canned in juice)	½ cup	Low
Pears (fresh)	1 medium pear	Low
Pineapple (fresh)	½ cup	Low
Plums (fresh)	2 medium plums	Low
Raspberries	½ cup	Low
Strawberries	½ cup	Low
Watermelon	1 large slice	Medium

Grains

Choose your grains carefully by searching out whole-grain food products that incorporate the lower-glycemic grains, such as bulgur, buckwheat, quinoa, and wild rice. Replace higher-glycemic grains with lower-glycemic choices whenever possible; Table A-7 lists some of your options.

Table A-7	Grains	
Food Type	*Portion Size*	*Glycemic Load*
Amaranth	1 ounce	High
Buckwheat	½ cup	Low
Bulgur	½ cup	Low
Cheese tortellini	6½ ounces	Low
Couscous	½ cup	Medium
Fettuccini	1½ cups	Medium
Grits	1 cup	Medium
Instant white rice	1 cup	High
Meat-filled ravioli	6½ ounces	Medium
Pearl barley	1 cup	Medium
Polenta	¾ cup	Medium
Quinoa	½ cup	Low
Spaghetti	1½ cups	Medium
Split pea/soya shells	1½ cups	Low
Uncle Ben's Converted White Rice	½ cup	Low
Uncle Ben's Whole-Grain Brown Rice	⅓ cup	Low
Vermicelli	1½ cups	Medium
Whole-wheat spaghetti	1½ cups	Medium
Wild rice	½ cup	Low

Legumes

Legumes, sometimes known as dried beans and peas, are an excellent low-glycemic source of protein and fiber. As an added bonus, they don't contain any saturated fat or cholesterol. Experiment with adding legumes to your favorite grain recipes, such as quinoa or rice pilaf. Consider replacing meat in burritos or tacos with black or pinto beans. Or just enjoy a hearty split pea or lentil soup rather than a stew based on beef or chicken. However you choose to add legumes to your diet, check out Table A-8 for the glycemic loads of the most common ones.

Table A-8	Legumes	
Food Type	**Portion Size**	**Glycemic Load**
Baked beans	½ cup	Low
Black bean dip	½ cup	Low
Black beans	½ cup	Low
Black-eyed peas	½ cup	Low
Cannellini beans	½ cup	Low
Garbanzo beans	½ cup	Low
Hummus	1½ tablespoons	Low
Kidney beans	½ cup	Low
Lentils	½ cup	Low
Lima beans	½ cup	Low
Northern white beans	½ cup	Low
Pinto beans	½ cup	Low
Refried beans	½ cup	Low
Soy beans	1 cup	Low
Split peas	½ cup	Low

Meat Products

Meat, including chicken, seafood, beef, and pork, contains no carbohydrates. Only carbohydrate-containing foods are part of the glycemic index, so we can't provide glycemic data for meat. However, we can tell you that when you add cracker-crumb coating to chicken, dredge fish in flour, or mix dry oatmeal or crushed crackers into hamburger for meatloaf or meatballs, you're incorporating carbohydrates into your meat. The amount usually isn't enough to increase the glycemic load too much, but it's always good to note when you've added some carbohydrate to your meats so you can eat a smaller amount of starches in your side dishes.

Don't forget carbohydrate-containing meat substitutes like soy products. They contain protein and fat but also have some carbohydrates to consider. The good news is that most soy products have a low glycemic load. Products made from vegetable grains vary; you can check out www.nutritiondata.com to check products that aren't listed here.

Table A-9 shows you some meat substitutions that do contain some carbohydrates.

Table A-9	Meat Substitute Products	
Food Type	*Portion Size*	*Glycemic Load*
Tofu	½ cup	Low
Veggie burger	1 patty	Low

Sweeteners and Candy

The glycemic index is just one method of choosing healthy foods. When it comes to sweeteners, the key truly is the amount you consume, which is why Table A-10 can come in really handy. The glycemic load is based on the amount of a particular food you eat, or the amount of that food within an entire meal. For example, if you make a meal out of sugar or other sweeteners, the glycemic load will be high. To help you tame your sweet tooth quite naturally, use small amounts of sugar only when absolutely necessary.

Table A-10	Sweeteners and Candy	
Food Type	*Portion Size*	*Glycemic Load*
Agave syrup	1 tablespoon	Low
Brown sugar	1 teaspoon	Low
Dark chocolate	1 ounce	Low
Grape jelly	1 tablespoon	Low
Honey	1 tablespoon	Low
Jelly beans	6 pieces	Medium
Maple syrup	1 tablespoon	Low
Milk chocolate	1 ounce	Low
Peanut M&M's	1 small packet (1.74 ounces)	Medium
Snickers bar	2 ounces	Medium
White granulated sugar	1 teaspoon	Low

Vegetables

Your mother was right: You really should eat more vegetables. The vast majority of vegetables provide plenty of vitamins and minerals along with a good dose of fiber and very few calories. As you can see in Table A-11, most vegetables even have a low-glycemic load. If you struggle with including more vegetables in your diet, try to get creative. For example, prepare omelets with leftover cooked vegetables or whip up vegetable-based soups for lunch. Making veggies a part of every meal is really easier than you may think (see Parts III and IV for some stellar recipe ideas).

Table A-11	Vegetables	
Food Type	*Portion Size*	*Glycemic Load*
Asparagus	½ cup	Low
Avocado	¼ of 1 large avocado	Low
Baked potato	5 ounces	High
Bell peppers (green, orange, red, and yellow)	3 ounces	Low
Black olives	5 olives	Low
Broccoli	1 cup	Low
Canned pumpkin	3 ounces	Low
Carrots	1 medium carrot	Low
Cauliflower	¾ cup	Low
Celery	2 stalks	Low
Cherry tomatoes	5 tomatoes	Low
Enchilada sauce	¼ cup	Low
Green cabbage	1 cup	Low
Green chiles	1 chile	Low
Green onions	2 onions	Low
Instant mashed potatoes	½ cup	Medium
Italian canned tomatoes	½ cup	Low
Lettuce	1 cup	Low
New potatoes	4 small potatoes	Medium
Onions	½ medium onion	Low
Portobello mushrooms	½ cup	Low
Red-skinned potatoes, boiled or mashed	5 ounces	Medium

Food Type	Portion Size	Glycemic Load
Roasted red peppers (from a jar)	¼ cup	Low
Salsa	2 tablespoons	Low
Shiitake mushrooms	3 small mushrooms	Low
Snow peas	1 cup	Low
Spaghetti sauce	½ cup	Low
Spinach	1 cup	Low
Sun-dried tomatoes	1 cup	Low
Sweet corn	½ cup	Medium
Sweet pickle relish	1 tablespoon	Low
Tomatoes	1 tomato	Low
Zucchini	½ cup	Low

Metric Conversion Guide

● ●

*N**ote:* The recipes in this book weren't developed or tested using metric measurements. There may be some variation in quality when converting to metric units.

Common Abbreviations

Abbreviation(s)	What It Stands For
cm	Centimeter
C., c.	Cup
G, g	Gram
kg	Kilogram
L, l	Liter
lb.	Pound
mL, ml	Milliliter
oz.	Ounce
pt.	Pint
t., tsp.	Teaspoon
T., Tb., Tbsp.	Tablespoon

Volume

U.S. Units	Canadian Metric	Australian Metric
¼ teaspoon	1 milliliter	1 milliliter
½ teaspoon	2 milliliters	2 milliliters
1 teaspoon	5 milliliters	5 milliliters
1 tablespoon	15 milliliters	20 milliliters
¼ cup	50 milliliters	60 milliliters
⅓ cup	75 milliliters	80 milliliters

(continued)

Volume *(continued)*

U.S. Units	Canadian Metric	Australian Metric
½ cup	125 milliliters	125 milliliters
⅔ cup	150 milliliters	170 milliliters
¾ cup	175 milliliters	190 milliliters
1 cup	250 milliliters	250 milliliters
1 quart	1 liter	1 liter
1½ quarts	1.5 liters	1.5 liters
2 quarts	2 liters	2 liters
2½ quarts	2.5 liters	2.5 liters
3 quarts	3 liters	3 liters
4 quarts (1 gallon)	4 liters	4 liters

Weight

U.S. Units	Canadian Metric	Australian Metric
1 ounce	30 grams	30 grams
2 ounces	55 grams	60 grams
3 ounces	85 grams	90 grams
4 ounces (¼ pound)	115 grams	125 grams
8 ounces (½ pound)	225 grams	225 grams
16 ounces (1 pound)	455 grams	500 grams (½ kilogram)

Length

Inches	Centimeters
0.5	1.5
1	2.5
2	5.0
3	7.5
4	10.0
5	12.5
6	15.0
7	17.5

Inches	Centimeters
8	20.5
9	23.0
10	25.5
11	28.0
12	30.5

Temperature (Degrees)

Fahrenheit	Celsius
32	0
212	100
250	120
275	140
300	150
325	160
350	180
375	190
400	200
425	220
450	230
475	240
500	260

Index

Apple & Macs

iPad For Dummies
978-0-470-58027-1

iPhone For Dummies,
4th Edition
978-0-470-87870-5

MacBook For Dummies, 3rd
Edition
978-0-470-76918-8

Mac OS X Snow Leopard For
Dummies
978-0-470-43543-4

Business

Bookkeeping For Dummies
978-0-7645-9848-7

Job Interviews
For Dummies,
3rd Edition
978-0-470-17748-8

Resumes For Dummies,
5th Edition
978-0-470-08037-5

Starting an
Online Business
For Dummies,
6th Edition
978-0-470-60210-2

Stock Investing
For Dummies,
3rd Edition
978-0-470-40114-9

Successful
Time Management
For Dummies
978-0-470-29034-7

Computer Hardware

BlackBerry
For Dummies,
4th Edition
978-0-470-60700-8

Computers For Seniors
For Dummies,
2nd Edition
978-0-470-53483-0

PCs For Dummies,
Windows
7 Edition
978-0-470-46542-4

Laptops For Dummies,
4th Edition
978-0-470-57829-2

Cooking & Entertaining

Cooking Basics
For Dummies,
3rd Edition
978-0-7645-7206-7

Wine For Dummies,
4th Edition
978-0-470-04579-4

Diet & Nutrition

Dieting For Dummies,
2nd Edition
978-0-7645-4149-0

Nutrition For Dummies,
4th Edition
978-0-471-79868-2

Weight Training
For Dummies,
3rd Edition
978-0-471-76845-6

Digital Photography

Digital SLR Cameras &
Photography For Dummies,
3rd Edition
978-0-470-46606-3

Photoshop Elements 8
For Dummies
978-0-470-52967-6

Gardening

Gardening Basics
For Dummies
978-0-470-03749-2

Organic Gardening
For Dummies,
2nd Edition
978-0-470-43067-5

Green/Sustainable

Raising Chickens
For Dummies
978-0-470-46544-8

Green Cleaning
For Dummies
978-0-470-39106-8

Health

Diabetes For Dummies,
3rd Edition
978-0-470-27086-8

Food Allergies
For Dummies
978-0-470-09584-3

Living Gluten-Free
For Dummies,
2nd Edition
978-0-470-58589-4

Hobbies/General

Chess For Dummies,
2nd Edition
978-0-7645-8404-6

Drawing
Cartoons & Comics
For Dummies
978-0-470-42683-8

Knitting For Dummies,
2nd Edition
978-0-470-28747-7

Organizing
For Dummies
978-0-7645-5300-4

Su Doku For Dummies
978-0-470-01892-7

Home Improvement

Home Maintenance
For Dummies,
2nd Edition
978-0-470-43063-7

Home Theater
For Dummies,
3rd Edition
978-0-470-41189-6

Living the
Country Lifestyle
All-in-One
For Dummies
978-0-470-43061-3

Solar Power Your Home
For Dummies,
2nd Edition
978-0-470-59678-4

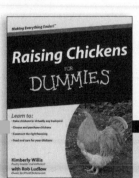

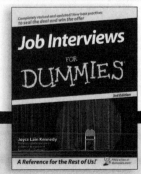

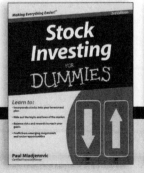

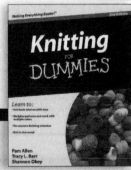

Internet

Blogging For Dummies,
3rd Edition
978-0-470-61996-4

eBay For Dummies,
6th Edition
978-0-470-49741-8

Facebook For Dummies,
3rd Edition
978-0-470-87804-0

Web Marketing
For Dummies,
2nd Edition
978-0-470-37181-7

WordPress
For Dummies,
3rd Edition
978-0-470-59274-8

Language & Foreign Language

French For Dummies
978-0-7645-5193-2

Italian Phrases
For Dummies
978-0-7645-7203-6

Spanish For Dummies,
2nd Edition
978-0-470-87855-2

Spanish
For Dummies,
Audio Set
978-0-470-09585-0

Math & Science

Algebra I
For Dummies,
2nd Edition
978-0-470-55964-2

Biology For Dummies,
2nd Edition
978-0-470-59875-7

Calculus For Dummies
978-0-7645-2498-1

Chemistry For Dummies
978-0-7645-5430-8

Microsoft Office

Excel 2010 For Dummies
978-0-470-48953-6

Office 2010 All-in-One
For Dummies
978-0-470-49748-7

Office 2010 For Dummies,
Book + DVD Bundle
978-0-470-62698-6

Word 2010 For Dummies
978-0-470-48772-3

Music

Guitar For Dummies,
2nd Edition
978-0-7645-9904-0

iPod & iTunes For
Dummies, 8th Edition
978-0-470-87871-2

Piano Exercises
For Dummies
978-0-470-38765-8

Parenting & Education

Parenting For Dummies,
2nd Edition
978-0-7645-5418-6

Type 1 Diabetes
For Dummies
978-0-470-17811-9

Pets

Cats For Dummies,
2nd Edition
978-0-7645-5275-5

Dog Training For Dummies,
3rd Edition
978-0-470-60029-0

Puppies For Dummies,
2nd Edition
978-0-470-03717-1

Religion & Inspiration

The Bible For Dummies
978-0-7645-5296-0

Catholicism For Dummies
978-0-7645-5391-2

Women in the Bible
For Dummies
978-0-7645-8475-6

Self-Help & Relationship

Anger Management
For Dummies
978-0-470-03715-7

Overcoming Anxiety
For Dummies,
2nd Edition
978-0-470-57441-6

Sports

Baseball
For Dummies,
3rd Edition
978-0-7645-7537-2

Basketball
For Dummies,
2nd Edition
978-0-7645-5248-9

Golf For Dummies,
3rd Edition
978-0-471-76871-5

Web Development

Web Design
All-in-One
For Dummies
978-0-470-41796-6

Web Sites
Do-It-Yourself
For Dummies,
2nd Edition
978-0-470-56520-9

Windows 7

Windows 7
For Dummies
978-0-470-49743-2

Windows 7
For Dummies,
Book + DVD Bundle
978-0-470-52398-8

Windows 7 All-in-One
For Dummies
978-0-470-48763-1

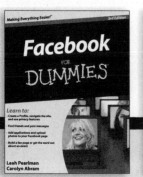
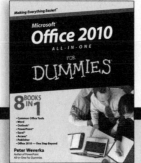
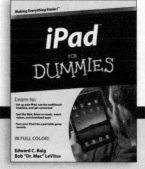
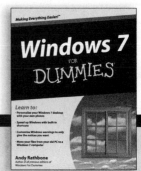

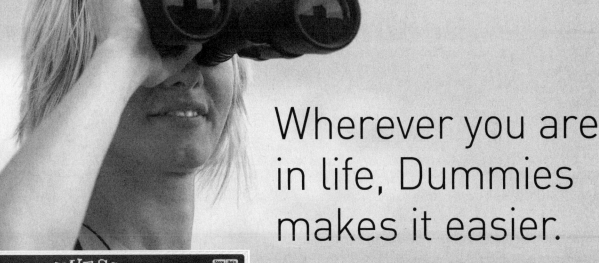

Wherever you are in life, Dummies makes it easier.

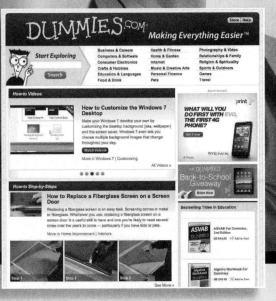

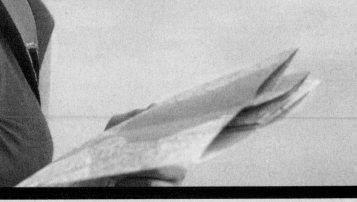

From fashion to Facebook®,
wine to Windows®, and everything in between,
Dummies makes it easier.

Visit us at Dummies.com

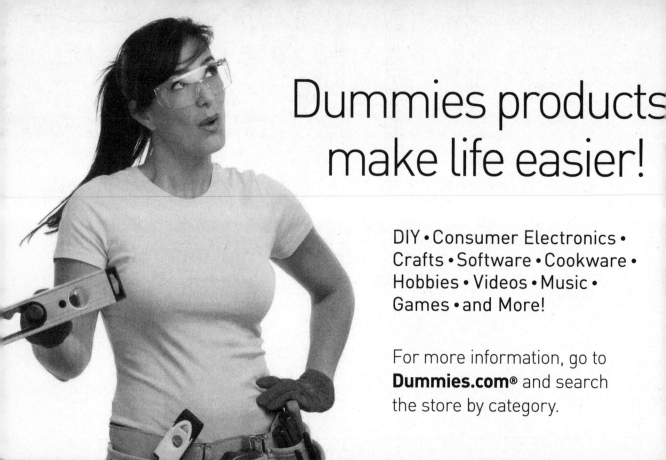
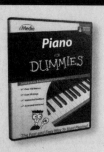
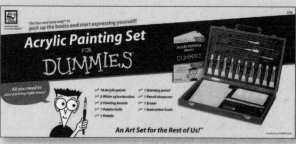
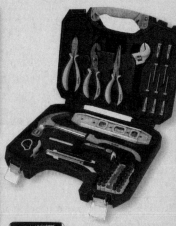
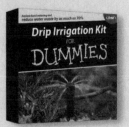
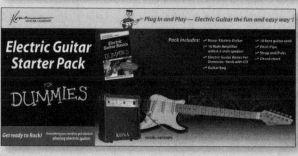
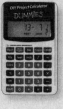
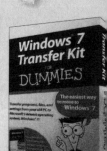
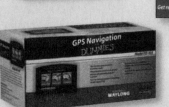
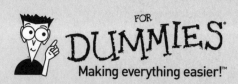